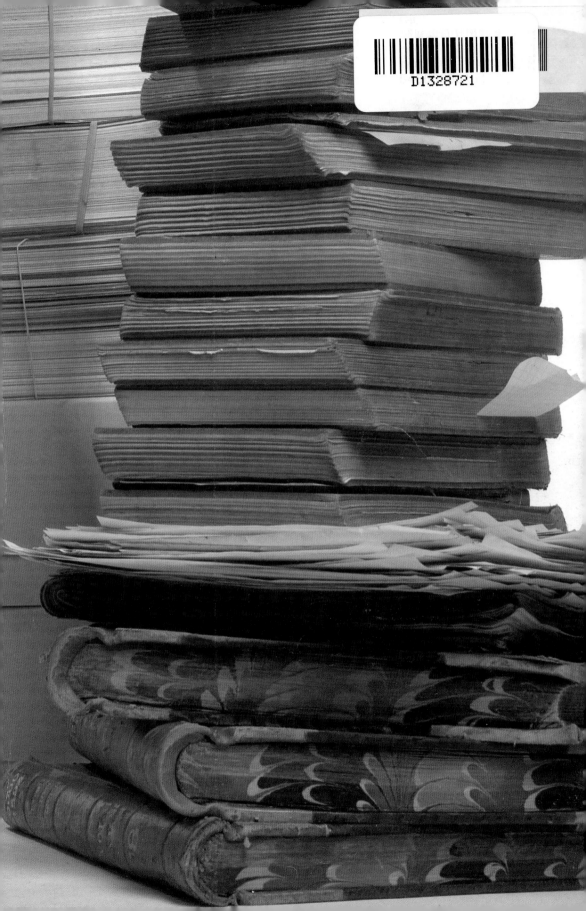

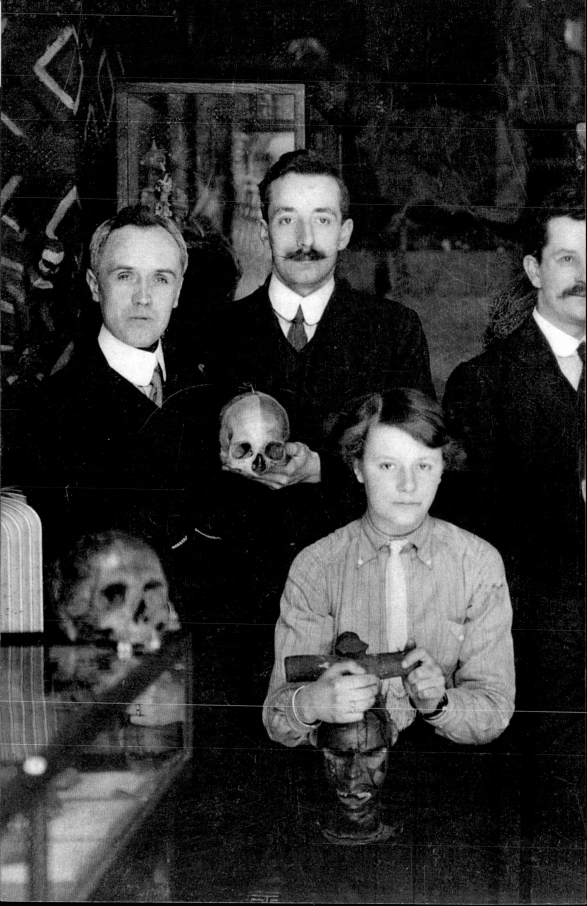

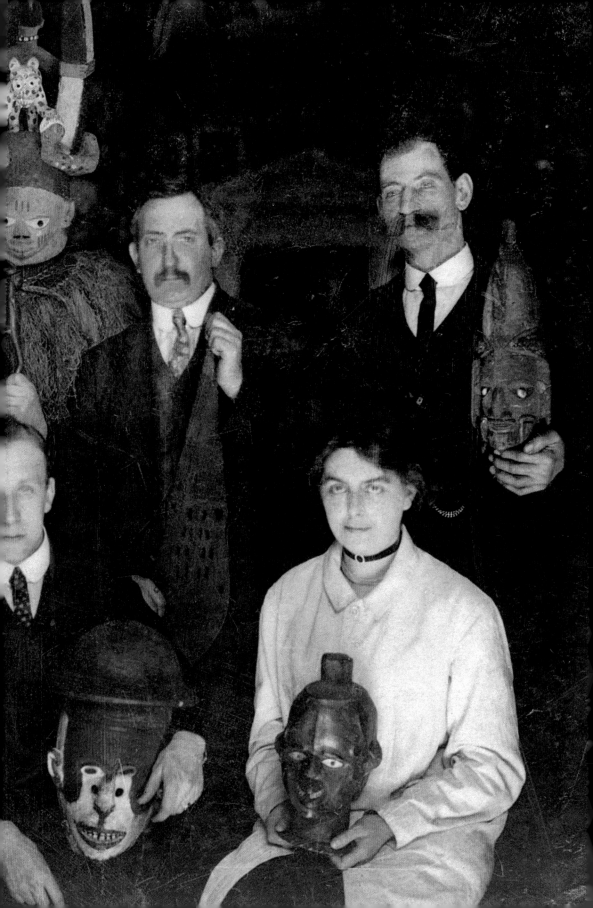

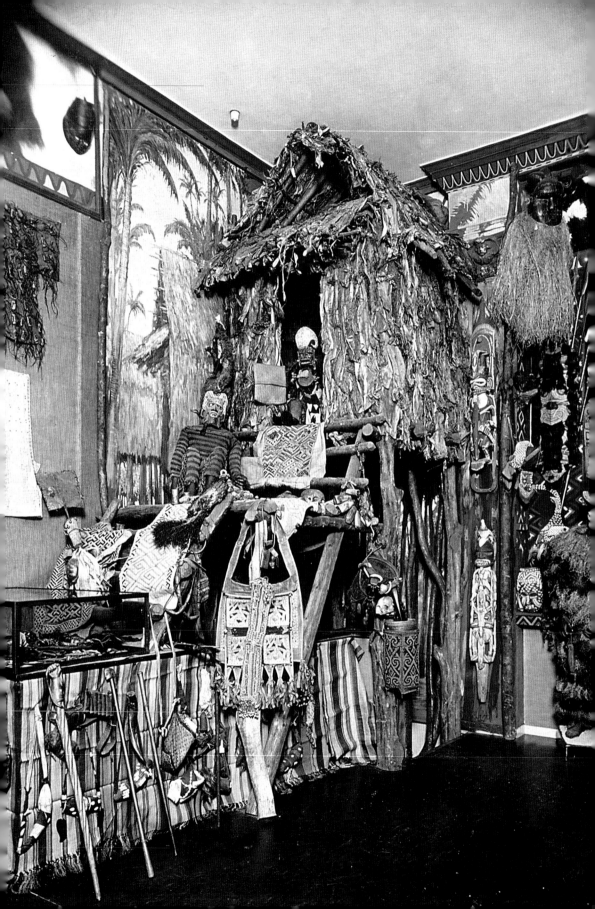

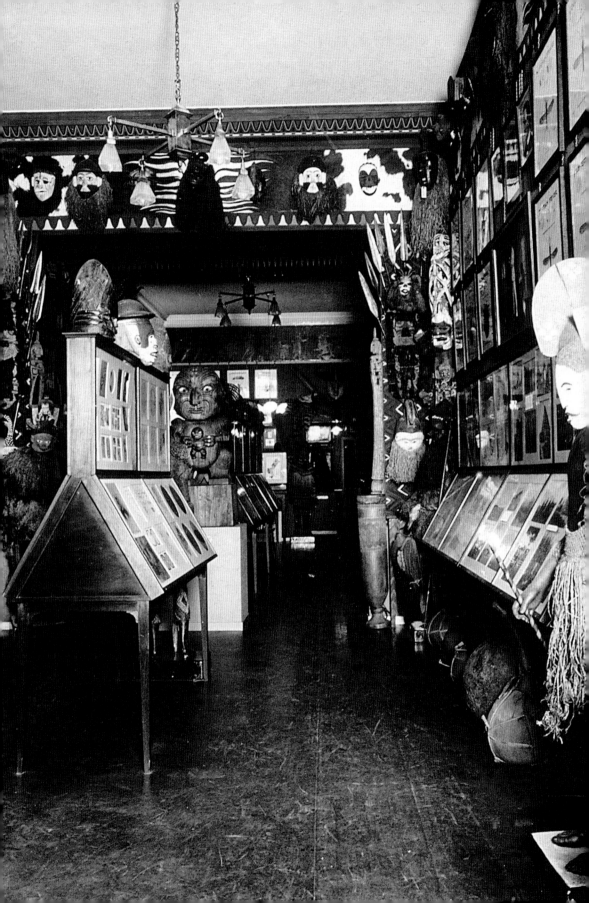

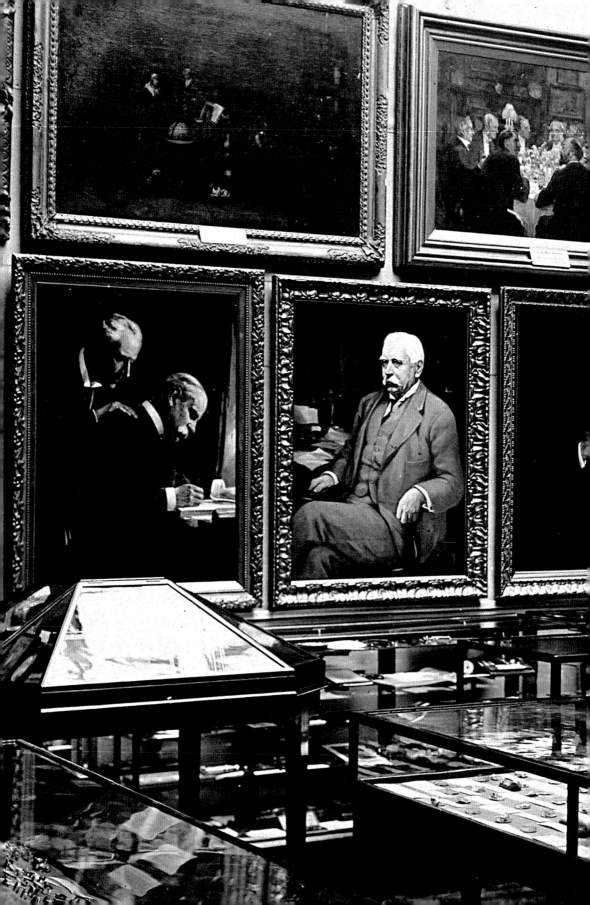

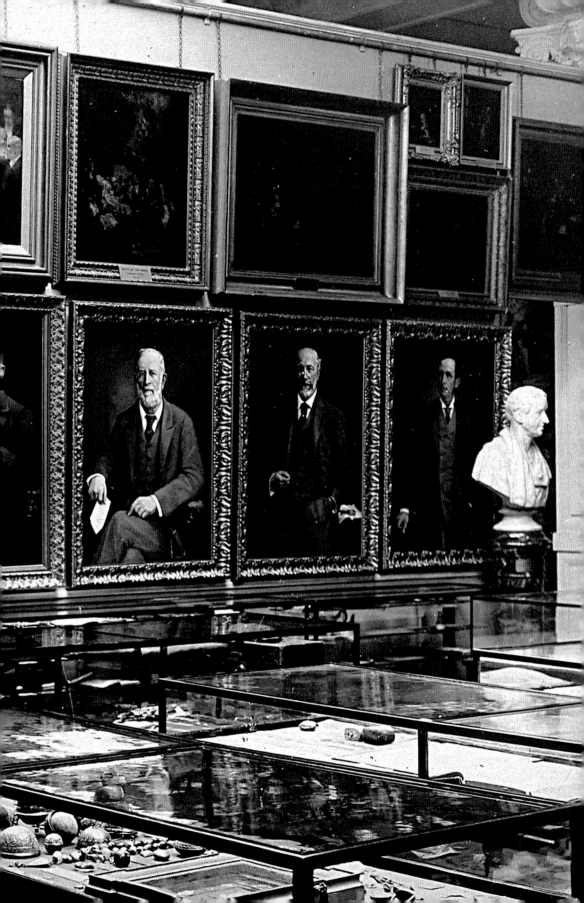

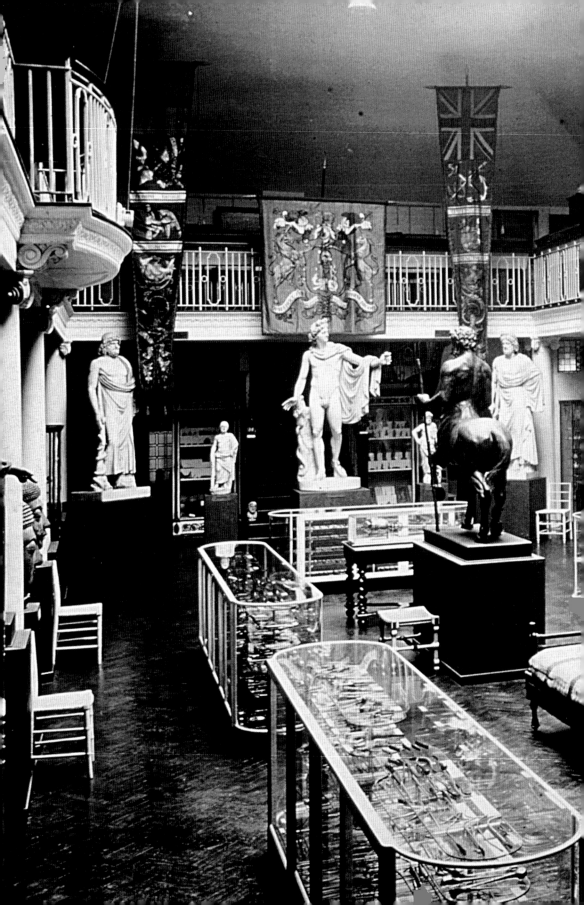

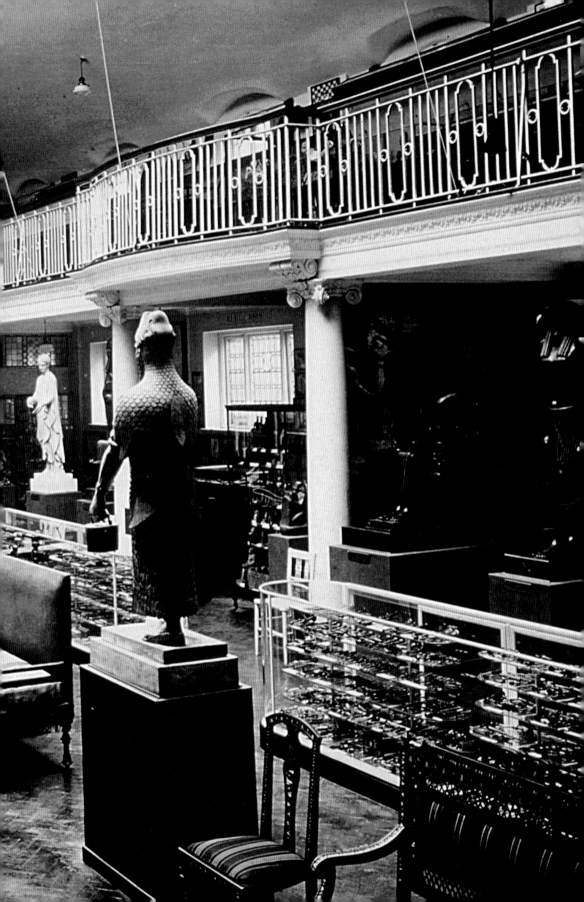

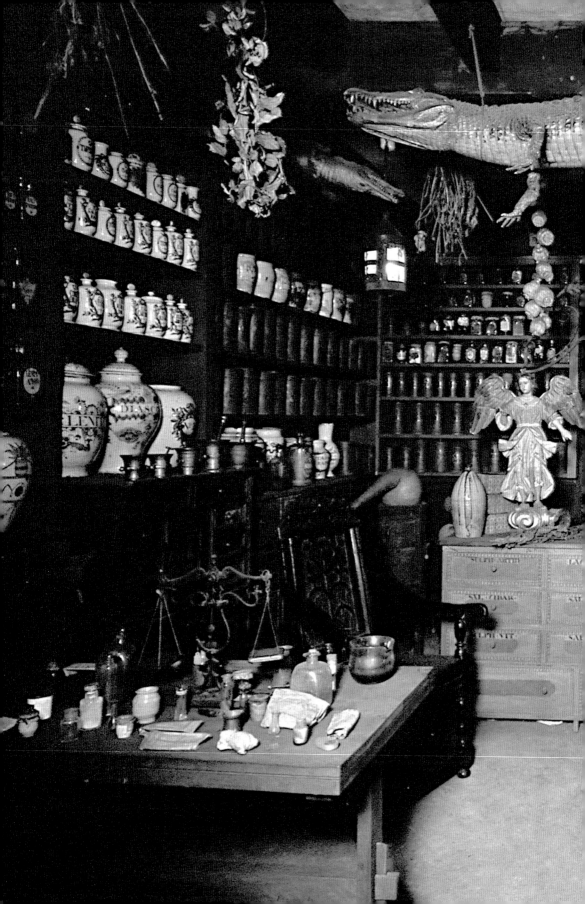

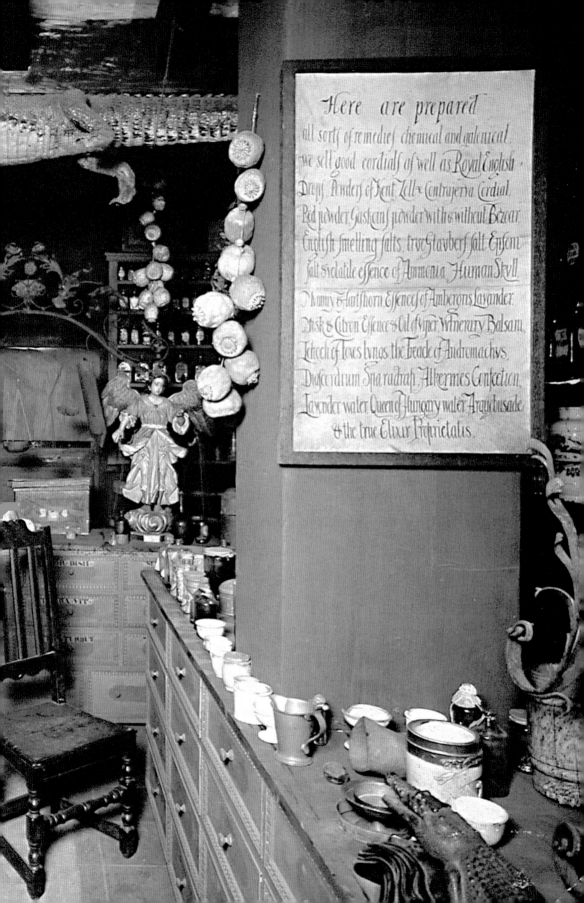

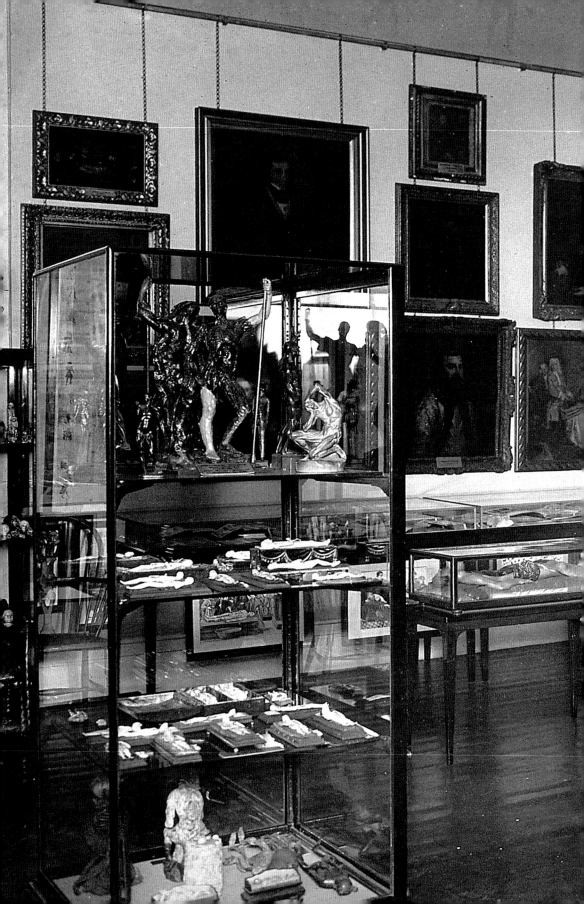

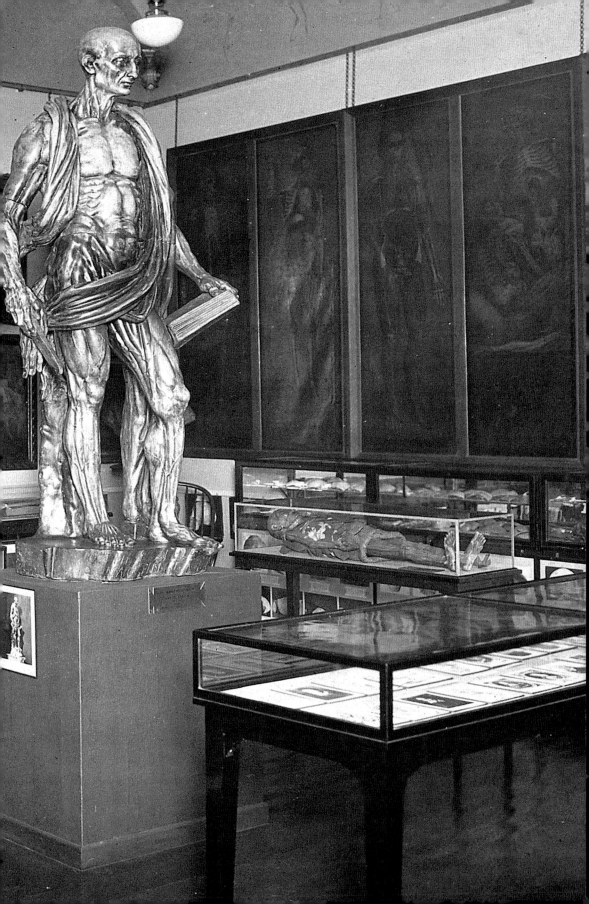

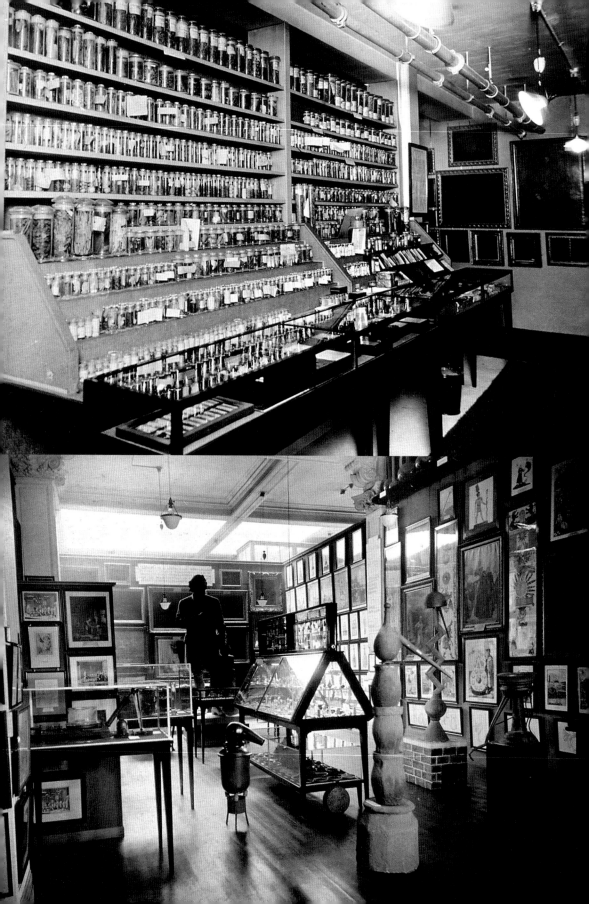

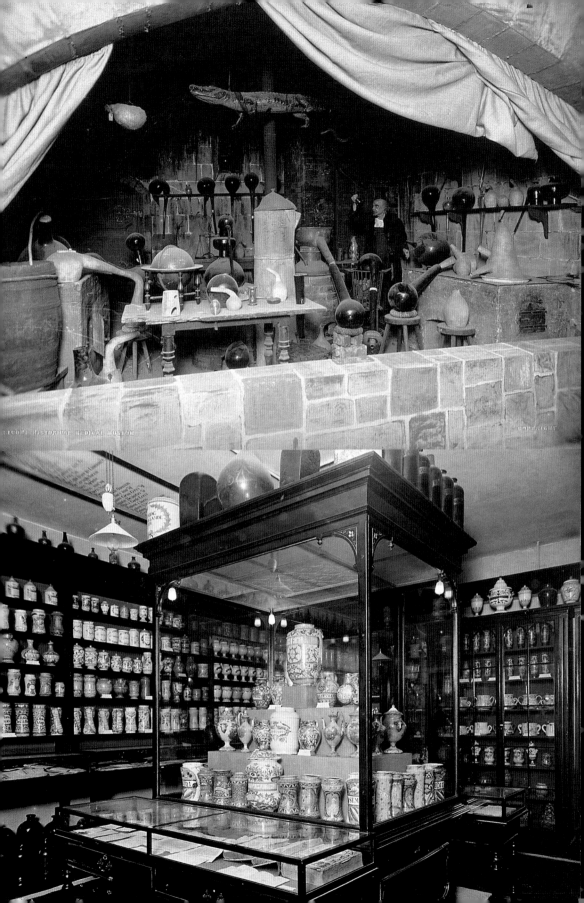

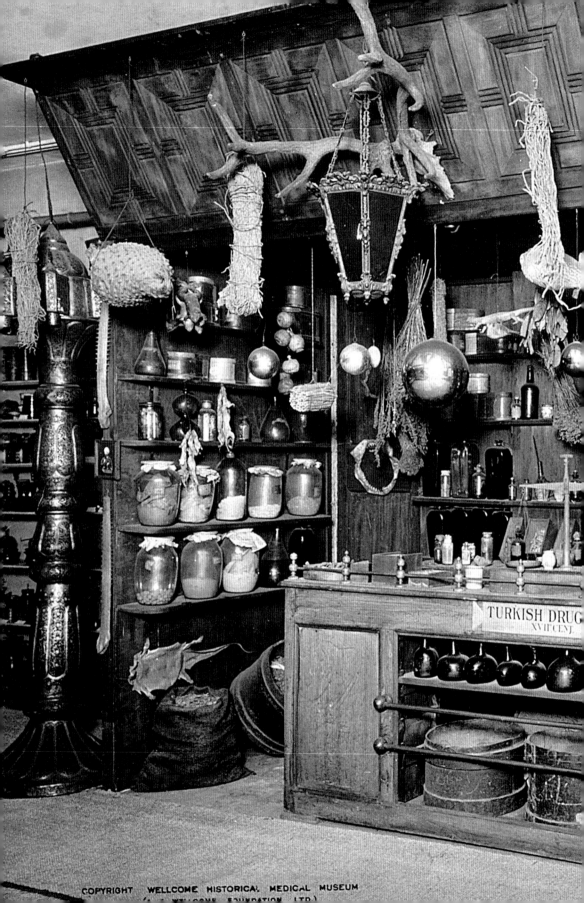

TURKISH DRUG
XVII CENT.

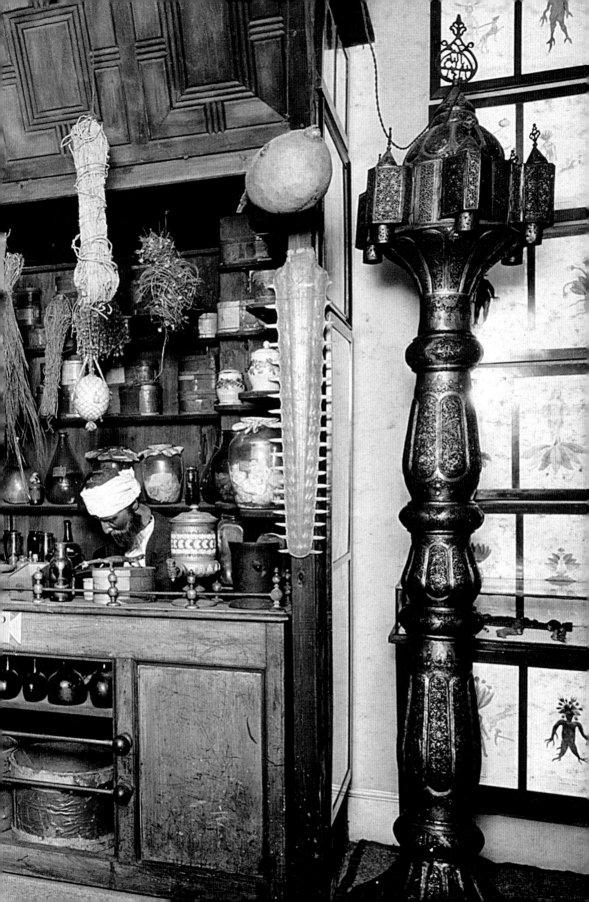

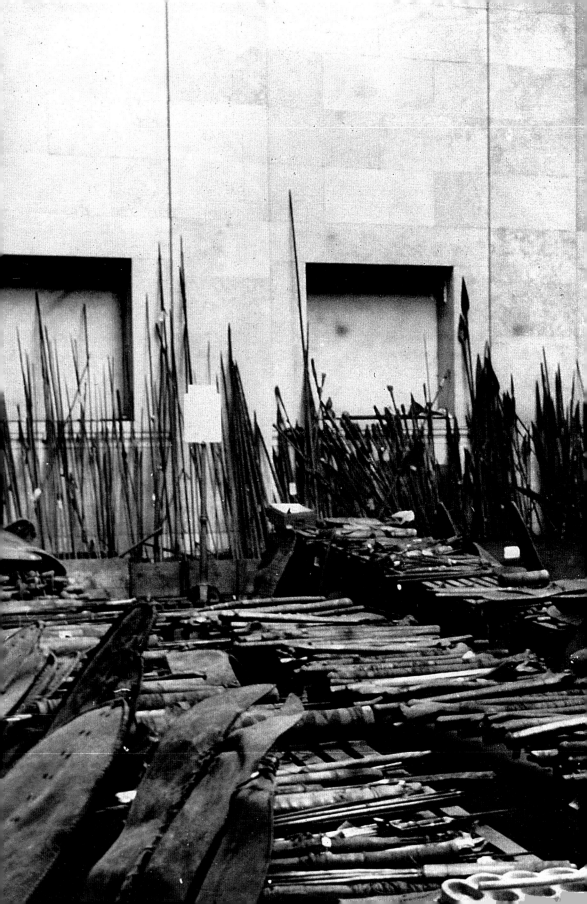

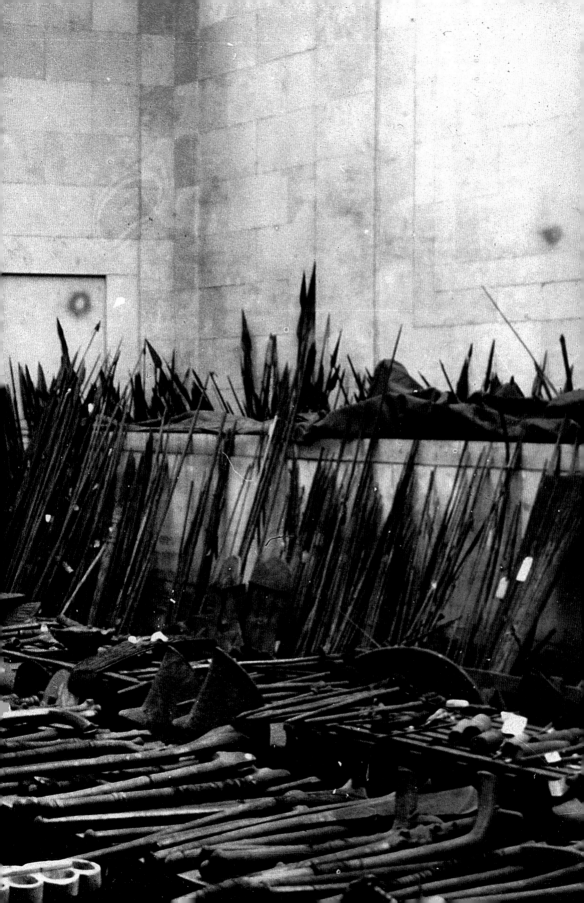

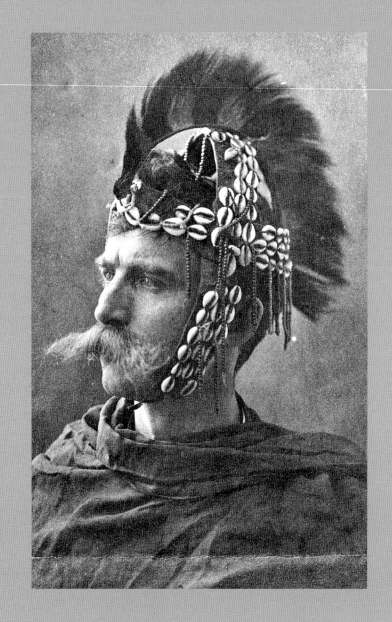

MEDICINE MAN

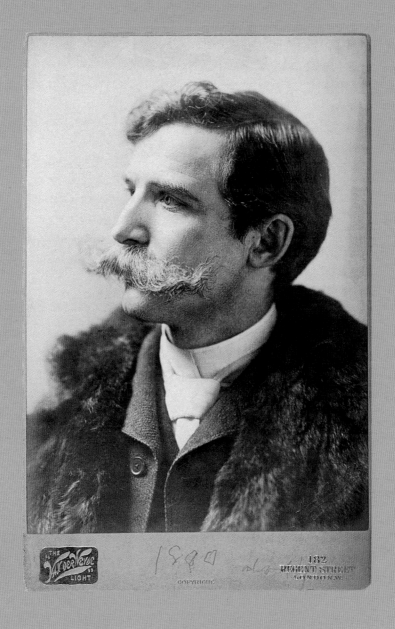

The Forgotten Museum of Henry Wellcome

EDITED BY KEN ARNOLD AND DANIELLE OLSEN

THE BRITISH MUSEUM PRESS

The Wellcome Trust is an independent research-funding charity, established under the will of Sir Henry Wellcome in 1936.

Its mission is to foster and promote research with the aim of improving human and animal health. Its work covers four areas:

Knowledge – improving our understanding of human and animal biology in health and disease, and of the past and present role of medicine in society;

Resources – providing exceptional researchers with the infrastructure and career support they need to fulfil their potential;

Translation – ensuring maximum health benefits are gained from biomedical research;

Public engagement – raising awareness of the medical, ethical, social and cultural implications of biomedical science.

Copyright © The Wellcome Trust 2003

First published in 2003 by The British Museum Press
A division of The British Museum Company Ltd
46 Bloomsbury Street, London WC1B 3QQ

A catalogue record for this book
is available from the British Library

ISBN 0 7141 2794 9

Photography by Chris Carter and Kate Darwin
(unless otherwise stated)

Designed by Harry Green

Typeset in Photina and Akzidenz-Grotesk
Printed in Italy by L.E.G.O. Spa.

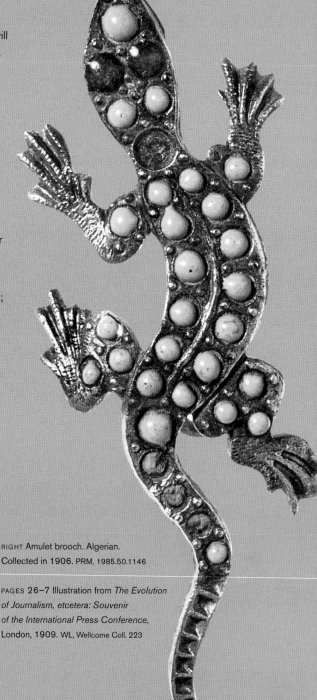

RIGHT Amulet brooch. Algerian.
Collected in 1906. PRM, 1985.50.1146

PAGES 26–7 Illustration from *The Evolution of Journalism, etcetera: Souvenir of the International Press Conference*, London, 1909. WL, Wellcome Coll. 223

Contents

Acknowledgements

First and foremost we wish to thank Christine Bradley who has
worked long and hard to bring this book to life. She has been an
inspiration to work with and it is hard to imagine what the book
would have been without her.

Warm and particular thanks are also due to the contributors
Frances Knight, Chris Gosden, Ghislaine Lawrence, John Mack,
John Pickstone and Ruth Richardson; to Chris Carter, Clive Coward
and Kate Darwin in the Wellcome Trust's Medical Photographic
Library; to Nigel Allan, Richard Aspin, William Schupbach and
John Symons in the Wellcome Library; and to Geoff Bunn,
Stewart Emmens, Alice Nicholls and David Thomas at the Science
Museum; all of whom have been exceptionally generous with their
time, advise and support.

It has also been a real pleasure to work with Ruth Greenberg,
with the team at the British Museum Press – Laura Brockbank,
Teresa Francis, Alasdair MacLeod, Penelope Vogler, Emma Way –
and with designer Harry Green.

In addition we would like to thank Linda Arter, Sarah Ayre, Sue Barnes,
Marla Berns, Robin Boast, Eleanor Boddington, Jackie Britton,
Tim Boon, Caroline Bradley, Sonya Brown, Ben Burt, Ian Carroll,
Herma Chang, Michael Clark, Don Cole, Rachel Collins,
Annie Coombes, John Cooper, Jeremy Coote, Georgina Craufurd,
Alison Deeprose, Catherine Draycott, Cecilia Eklind-Burke,
Amanda Engineer, Heather Ercilla, Diana Fane, Paulette Fontanez,

Stuart Fricker, Philomena Gibbons, Sir Roger Gibbs, Emily Glass,
Claire Griffiths, Miriam Gutierrez-Perez, Lesley Hall, Jim Hammel,
Jane Henderson, Jo Hill, Judith Hill, Christopher Hilton, Jane Hogg,
Isobel Hunter, Sarah Kennington, Hugh Kilmister, Bridget Kinally,
Jonathan King, Helen Kingsley, Chantal Knowles, Fran Krystock,
Marius Kwint, Miriam de Lacy, Emily Lewis, Kristen Lippincott,
Elizabeth Lowe, Peter Mandler, Dan Maslen, Jag Matharu,
Clare Matterson, Graham Matthews, Nick Merriman, Michelle Minto,
Craig Morris, Angela Murphy, Gillie Newman, Helen Nicholl,
Julia Nicholson, Mike O'Hanlon, Venita Paul, David Pearson,
James Putnam, Stephen Quirk, Polly Roberts, Bruce Robertson,
Nathan Schlanger, Julia Sheppard, Nikki Sibley, Laurence Smaje,
Chris Spring, Alan Stevens, Farida Sunada and Phillip Taylor.

PHOTOGRAPHIC ACKNOWLEDGEMENTS

BM   British Museum, London.
         Photos © The Trustees of The British Museum

FMCH UCLA Fowler Museum of Cultural History,
         Los Angeles. Photos: Don Cole

NMS   National Museums of Scotland.
         Photos © The Trustees of the National Museums of Scotland

PRM   Pitt Rivers Museum, University of Oxford

SM   Science Museum, London. Photos: Chris Carter
         and Kate Darwin, Wellcome Library, London

SSPL   Science & Society Picture Library

WL   Wellcome Library, London

UWS   University of Wales, Swansea. Photos © Graham P. Matthews

'Man's earliest chronicle
was his footprint; it told
of his coming, his going,
and of his doings.' HENRY S. WELLCOME

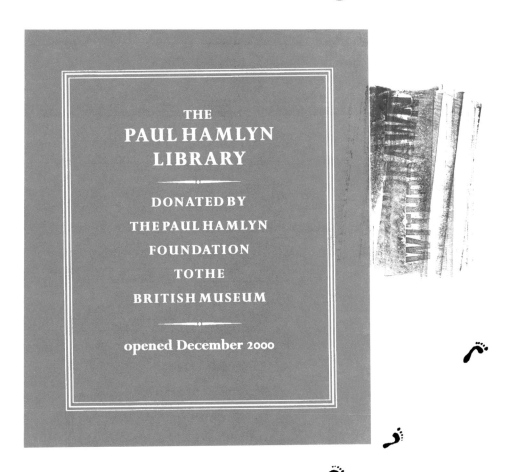

THE
**PAUL HAMLYN
LIBRARY**

❖

**DONATED BY
THE PAUL HAMLYN
FOUNDATION
TO THE
BRITISH MUSEUM**

❖

opened December 2000

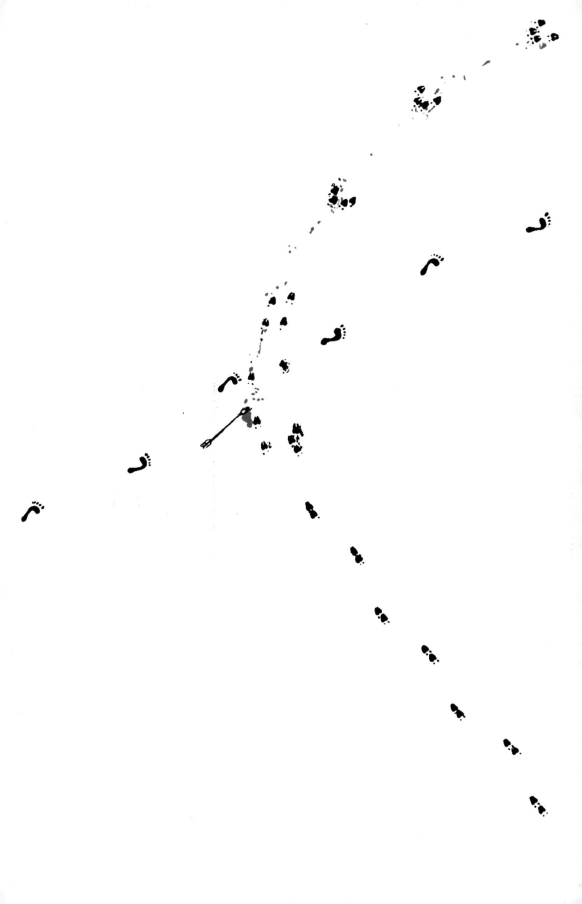

Introduction

Ken Arnold and Danielle Olsen

Henry Solomon Wellcome was a man of many interests, with impressive achievements in a variety of fields. As well as being a collector he was an entrepreneur and international businessman, patron of medical and scientific research, pioneer of tropical medicine and aerial photography, archaeologist and philanthropist (with a particular interest in Sudan and American Indians), close friend of the explorer Henry Stanley, and a father. He was a compulsive networker and had impressive and wide-ranging connections: Andrew Balfour, May French Sheldon, Lord Kitchener, Joseph Chamberlain, Roger Casement, Oscar Wilde, Lady Randolph Churchill and W.M. Flinders Petrie, to name but a few.[1] He had an insatiable curiosity about 'the great past'[2] and led a multi-faceted and unusual life.

Wellcome was born on a pioneer farm in the American Midwest in 1853. His parents, Solomon and Mary, were deeply religious, his father a minister of the Second Adventist Church (fig. 1). When Henry was eight, following the failure of their potato crop, they moved to Garden City, Minnesota, where his uncle, Jacob Wellcome, lived. Jacob was a doctor and, as he owned his own drugstore, was able to provide employment for Solomon. It was in this drugstore that Henry gained his first experience of business and, at the age of sixteen, launched the first Wellcome product on the market – invisible ink (fig. 2).

Wellcome later trained as a pharmacist in Chicago and Philadelphia (fig. 3) and found work with pharmaceutical firms in New York. Whilst working for McKesson & Robbins, he travelled to Ecuador in search of the increasingly rare Cinchona trees, whose bark was the prime source of pure quinine (fig. 4). This was the first of his journeys outside the United States and his subsequent account, published in both American and British *Pharmaceutical Journals*, brought him considerable attention. But it was in 1880 that his real break came when he joined a fellow student, Silas

Mainville Burroughs (1846–95) (fig. 5), in London, to set up the pharmaceutical firm Burroughs Wellcome & Co.

Compressed tablets, with their accurately measured and easily administered doses, had only recently been invented in America and the company set out to market these in Europe. Since there were no big manufacturing chemists in Great Britain, the firm soon became a manufacturing as well as a marketing business (figs 6 and 7). In

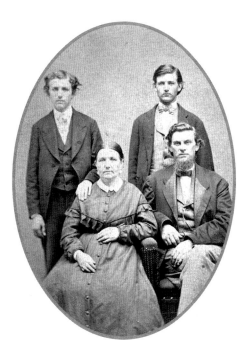

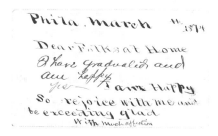

1 Henry Wellcome (standing, left) with his brother, George, and their parents, 1869.

2 TOP RIGHT The first product prepared and sold by Henry Wellcome, 1869.

3 BOTTOM RIGHT Postcard from Henry Wellcome to his parents telling them of his graduation at the Philadelphia College of Pharmacy, March 1874.

1884, to deal with the problem of imitations of their products, Wellcome coined one of the most famous trade names in business history, 'Tabloid'. 'Tabloid' medicine chests, packed with the company's wares, were given away to influential people including King Edward VII and President Theodore Roosevelt, and, carried by explorers of the day, made their way to the North and South Poles and to Mount Everest (fig. 8).

Burroughs Wellcome & Co was a huge success and in 1895, when Burroughs died suddenly, Wellcome became its sole owner. It was around this time that Wellcome began to develop his collecting interests. He had been buying books and objects since his student days but

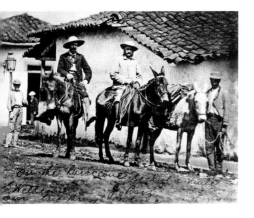

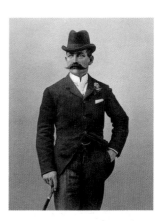

4 LEFT Henry Wellcome
(left) with J. Baiz, his guide
and interpreter, during his
journey through Central
America in 1879.

5 RIGHT Silas Mainville
Burroughs.

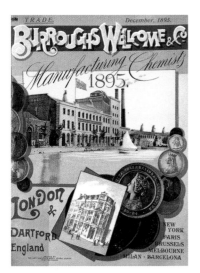

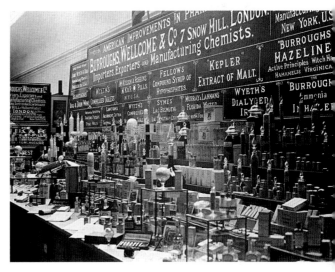

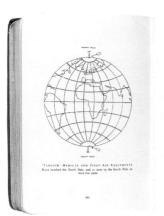

6 ABOVE LEFT A Burroughs Wellcome
& Co. Price list, 1895.

7 ABOVE Burroughs Wellcome
products on display at the International
Medical and Sanitary Exhibition,
London, 1881.

8 LEFT 'Tabloid' products described in
*The Evolution of Journalism, etcetera:
Souvenir of the International Press
Conference*, London, 1909.
WL, Wellcome Coll. 223

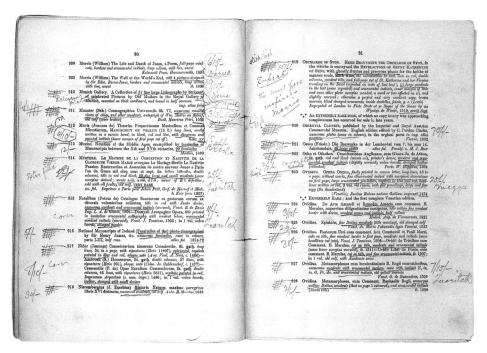

9 Sotheby, Wilkinson & Hodge, Catalogue of a portion of the collection of manuscripts, early printed books, etc. of the late William Morris, 5–10 December 1898. Pages 90 and 91, annotated by Henry Wellcome.

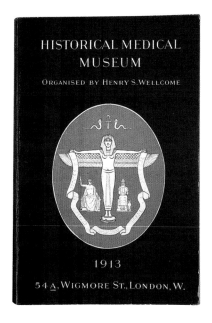

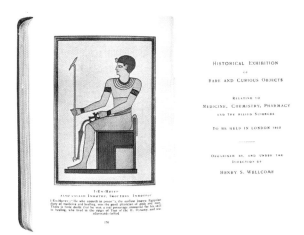

10 LEFT Handbook of the Historical Medical Museum, organised by Sir Henry Wellcome for the XVIIth International Congress of Medicine, London, 1913. WL, BA.AS.43

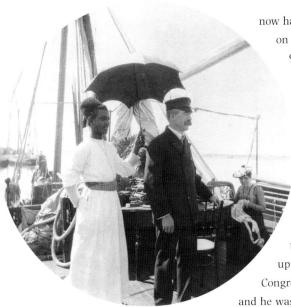

12 Henry Wellcome on the Nile, during his visit to the Sudan, 1900–1901.

now had the means to acquire many more and to do so on an institutional rather than a personal basis (fig. 9). The beginning of a museum can be dated to about 1903 when he took up the idea of holding a Historical Medical Exhibition to celebrate his firm's twenty-fifth year of trading in 1904. He published a short leaflet appealing for historical items and setting out ideas for the content of a museum (fig. 11). In fact, the museum did not open until 1913. 'Wellcome was more interested in the journey than the arrival, and he might have gone on indefinitely collecting for the Museum . . . and letting his acquisitions pile up in store, but fortunately the 17th International Congress of Medicine was being held in London in 1913 and he was persuaded to open the Museum for the conference and to keep it open afterwards' (fig. 10).[3]

It was in 1900 that Wellcome first visited Sudan, not long after Kitchener's defeat of the Khalifa and the establishment of Western rule (fig. 12). The country was in a state of devastation after years of war and Wellcome was appalled by the health conditions that he found there. Determined to do something to improve matters, he set about establishing a tropical research laboratory at Khartoum, including a floating laboratory on the Nile (fig. 13).[4] This did excellent

13 The Wellcome floating laboratory on the Nile, with its tug, the Culex, c. 1907.

11 LEFT Henry Wellcome set out his ideas for the content of his museum in a number of publications including *The Evolution of Journalism, etcetera: Souvenir of the International Press Conference*, London, 1909. WL, Wellcome Coll. 223

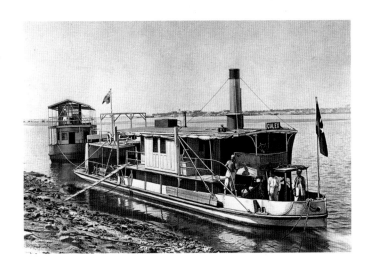

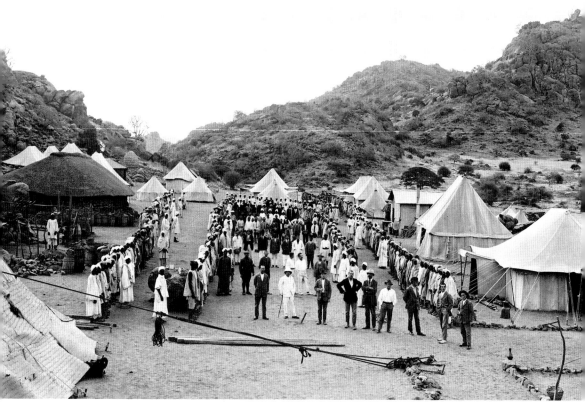

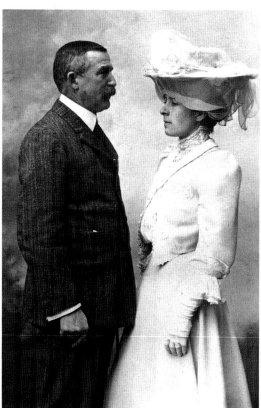

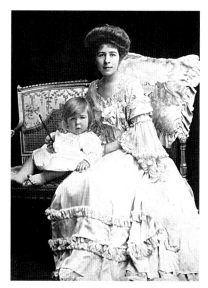

14 TOP Henry Wellcome (centre) at his Jebel Moya camp.

15 LEFT Henry and Syrie Wellcome.

16 ABOVE Syrie and Mounteney Wellcome.

work towards the control of malaria. He later conceived the idea of combining archaeology and philanthropy and, as Chris Gosden describes later in this volume, ended up employing some 4,000 people on his digs in Jebel Moya (fig. 14) and Abu Geili.

Another key chapter in Wellcome's life is that of his marriage to and subsequent divorce from Syrie Barnardo, daughter of the philan-

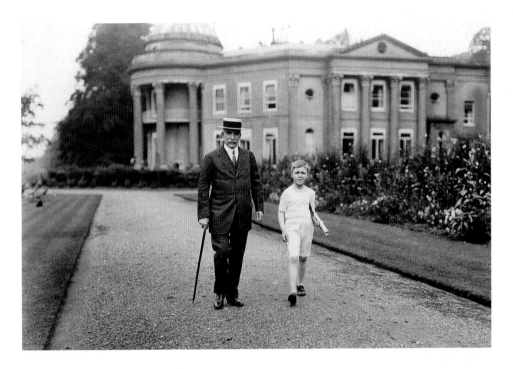

17 Henry and Mounteney Wellcome. Holiday sports at The Mansion, Sundridge Park, Kent, 1913.

thropist Thomas Barnardo (fig. 15). They were married in 1901 when she was twenty-one years old and Wellcome in his late forties; their son Mounteney was born in 1903 (fig. 16). It was an unhappy marriage and they separated in 1910, with Syrie keeping Mounteney. Syrie then had a relationship with William Somerset Maugham – a major scandal at the time. Wellcome filed for divorce in 1916 and was awarded custody of his son. This left Mounteney in a tug of war between his estranged parents: 'Each employed medical and educational experts to support their views on how he should be brought up. While Wellcome favoured a strict regime of exercise, fresh air and instruction, Syrie advocated a governess, afternoon naps and smothering affection' (fig. 17).[5]

18 Photograph taken by Wellcome whilst on tour in 1908. John Ferreira, his courier and interpreter, is seated inside.

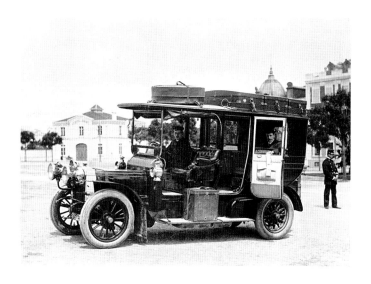

19 Italian, Tunisian and Algerian amulets collected by Walter Leo Hildburgh's father under his instruction. Collected before 1919. PRM, from left to right: 1985.50.1197, 1985.50.685, 1985.50.961, 1985.50.959, 1985.50.15, 1985.50.1028, 1985.50.992, 1985.50.1294, 1985.50.1146, 1985.50.93, 1985.50.639

Since Wellcome destroyed all Syrie's correspondence with him, we have little evidence of their early relationship. But one of the contributory factors to their break-up may well have been her dislike of the amount of time he devoted to his collecting activities (fig. 18):

'I think it only fair to point out to Hal that . . . ever since our marriage, the greater part or our time has been spent, as he well knows, in places I *detested*, collecting curios . . . sacrificing myself in a way I hated, both to please him and gather curios.'[6]

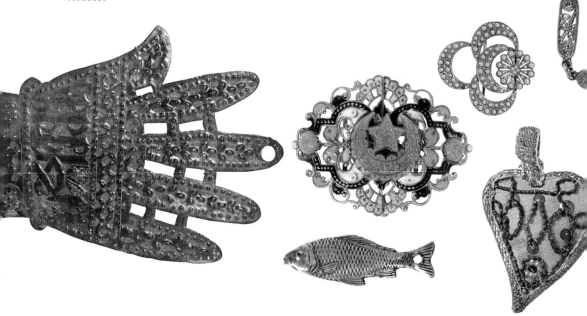

Despite Syrie's misgivings, Wellcome's passion for collecting and for science continued to flourish, taking him all over the world and earning him the respect of many. In 1932 he was knighted and elected a Fellow of the Royal Society, and made an Honorary Fellow of the Royal College of Surgeons - a rare distinction for someone without a medical degree. Wellcome died in 1936 but his commitment to research, whether in the medical sciences or their history, lives on in the Wellcome Trust, an independent charity established under his will.

The scale of the collection

Wellcome built up was one of the world's largest museum collections 'for the purpose of demonstrating by means of objects . . . the actuality of every notable step in the evolution and progress from the first germ of life up to the fully developed man of today'.[7] A grand ambition, this museum was to be a place of scientific research – with objects for data – that would increase our understanding of human history. Central to this endeavour was a study of 'the continuous perils and ravages of disease encountered in the battle of life' and,

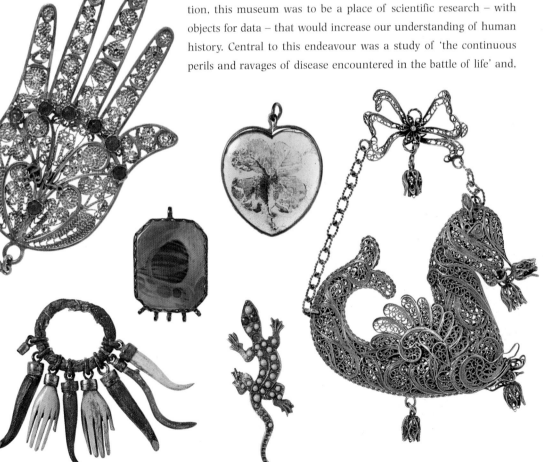

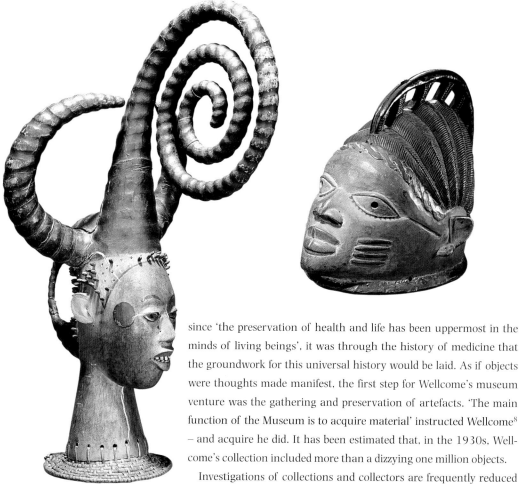

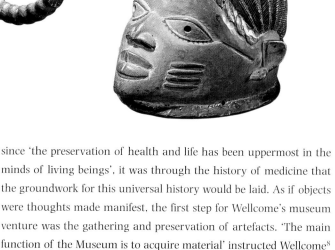

20 Nigerian, Sri Lankan and British Columbian masks.
From left to right: FMCH X65-9043, FMCH X65-4742, SM A62943, FMCH X65-8235, FMCH X65-4273

since 'the preservation of health and life has been uppermost in the minds of living beings', it was through the history of medicine that the groundwork for this universal history would be laid. As if objects were thoughts made manifest, the first step for Wellcome's museum venture was the gathering and preservation of artefacts. 'The main function of the Museum is to acquire material' instructed Wellcome[8] – and acquire he did. It has been estimated that, in the 1930s, Wellcome's collection included more than a dizzying one million objects.

Investigations of collections and collectors are frequently reduced to a matter of lists and numbers, to paper-based exercises that can only gesture at the altogether more powerful experience of wandering through vast storerooms of real stuff. This can so easily become very dull fare indeed. But in Wellcome's case, the length of these lists and the magnitude of the numbers are in themselves an important part of the story. They include thousands of spears, spectacles and amulets (fig. 19); hundreds of votive offerings, pictures and masks (fig. 20); dozens of snuffboxes, anatomical manikins and medicine chests (fig. 21). The sheer scale of the exercise of describing all these things and of placing them into some sort of manageable order was a crucial element of Wellcome's own endeavour, and has also been at the heart of its diaspora since his death.

In fact, this collection was never manageable. Wellcome himself – though he gloriously tried – failed to pull it together during his own lifetime. For over sixty years after his death, heirs to his material culture

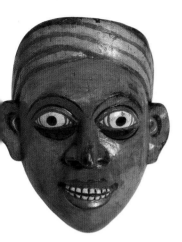

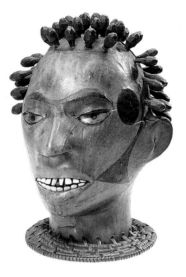

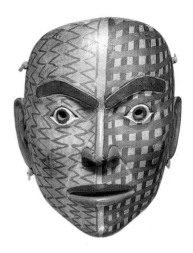

21 BELOW Genoese
medicine chest, c. 1565.
Made for Vincenzo
Giustiniani, the last
Genoese governor of
the island of Chios in the
eastern Aegean Sea. It is
over a metre long with its
drawers extended.
SM, A641515

'fortune' – initially the Trustees of the charity set up in his name, and
then the administrators of the museums to which the collection was
distributed – carried on nobly failing to grasp the magnitude of this
vision. In the Wellcome Library, for example, the task of cataloguing
every picture, photograph and print in the iconographic collection
started in 1993 and still proceeds. The legacy of this hugely diverse
collection is today scattered in numerous institutions across the globe,
from Australia to Zimbabwe, each of which faces – whether acted upon
or not – a similar task of surveying, analysing and organising piles of
objects. Appreciated today in isolated 'bits and pieces', the grand
overview of this fundamental human instinct of 'preserving life and
health' provided by his amassed collection has largely been obscured by
its curatorial and intellectual dispersal.

The exhibition

For reasons practical and memorial, the year 2003 presented
itself as an ideal one in which to mount an exhibition based on the
Wellcome collection, marking Henry Wellcome's 150th birthday. He
happened to be born in the year in which the British Museum
celebrated its centenary. The concurrence of these
anniversaries made the chosen location of this exhibition at the British Museum seem particularly
appropriate. The timely celebration of one man's

personal collection, the scale of which rivalled national museums across Europe and America, within the mother of all those institutions – whose first collections were based primarily on the material legacy of another medical man, Hans Sloane – set up a whole series of intriguing and delightful resonances.

This book, and the exhibition it accompanies, have given us the opportunity to explore some of the many institutions which now accommodate the Wellcome collection; to scan lists of objects and rummage in storerooms, reacquaint ourselves with the better known pieces and discover those lurking in the shadows. We have dipped into the sea of archives which surrounds the collection and met the gate-keepers of various museums who now care for it. Yet still we have only scratched the surface of this vast and generous resource – the remnants of an epic and visionary project – and made the beginnings of an acquaintance with its remarkable founder.

The original intention

Wellcome had grand ambitions for his collection:

> 'In organising this Museum, my purpose has not been simply to bring together a lot of "curios" for amusement. This collection is intended to be useful to students and useful to all those engaged in research. I have found that the study of the roots and foundations of things greatly assists research, and facilitates discovery and invention.'[9]

As Ghislaine Lawrence points out in the first of this volume's essays, Wellcome was not interested in the strange or the beautiful unless it served a 'scientific' purpose in the piecing together of history. He was optimistic about what science could achieve and was less concerned with directly ameliorating the condition of mankind through the provision of education, improved living conditions, or rational amusement. 'It was through science that most benefit would accrue and it was with scientific ventures that he chose to associate his name'.[10] Like the very first medical museums of the Renaissance, Wellcome hoped to create an active place of research. His museum was meant to facilitate the scientific study of the history of mankind and he regarded the systematic arrangement and study of artefacts as furthering knowledge just as much as the work carried out in his physiological and chemical laboratories. Wellcome hoped eventually to create a 'Museum of Man', of which medicine would only be a part; a museum which would 'connect the links in the chain of human experience which stretch back from the present time into the prehistoric period of the early ages'.

With the belief that certain indigenous populations were dying out, and that their material culture was crucial to the 'search for origins', time was of the essence. Retrospectively, Wellcome's rush to acquire ethnographic (which, in the end, constituted more than half of his collection) and other objects might seem rash or deluded. And yet might it not be comparable with today's ecological scramble to collect and preserve the natural world – with the *raison d'être* of the Kew Gardens Seed Bank or Human Genome Projects – or with our continued attempts to document the estimated millions of insects that are yet to be identified? Whilst these grand enterprises are backed by institutions, the Wellcome collection was driven by the passion, determination and purse of one remarkable man. Perhaps, because it had been such a personal ambition, it was inevitable that his vision of a Museum of Man was to die with him. The hundreds and thousands of objects Wellcome collected were never the subject of intensive scientific research and now, scattered around the world in various institutions and disciplinary boxes, it is hard to grasp what, as a whole, they might have revealed.

The history of the medical museum

Henry Wellcome's establishment of a medico-historical museum came at a very particular juncture in a long-standing intermingling of the worlds of medicine and museums. Our own efforts – both with regard to this book and the exhibition it accompanies – inevitably form part of their most recent entanglement. As if to make a circle of the history, we have consciously drawn part of our inspiration for our cultural approach to medicine from strands of similar thinking evident in the very first European Renaissance museums, which were founded on a philosophy of wonder and curiosity.

The cradle for many of these first European museums was in fact provided by the apartments and work places of medical men; many of the curators of these museums came from the healing professions

(physicians, apothecaries and surgeons); and much of their *raison
d'être* was medical. The very earliest examples of 'cabinets of curiosities' in Renaissance Italy were formed in an attempt to manage the
empirical explosion of materials – the sheer flood of new things –
uncovered in travel to unfamiliar countries, in voyages to completely
unknown lands and in the excavation of ancient buildings. Many of
the objects that were found and collected were understood in terms of
medical 'principles' that were held to correspond to a particular
function and part of the body.

These early curators did not just idly admire their collections and
leave them on the shelves to gather dust. They instead engaged with
the objects using all their senses – things were weighed and measured,
tasted, scratched and sniffed, and even set fire to. These museums,
then, were more like studies in which nature was not just gathered
but also experienced and experimented upon, so that museums
became privileged sites of experimental knowledge. They provided the
model for 'theatres of experiments' more generally – places in which,
for example, to test theories about fossils, to explore the magic of lode-
stones, and above all to forge a reform of *materia medica* in order to
make new reliable medicines. In all these projects, experiments
allowed early curators to marshal their objects into facts that served a
particular purpose. It is this Renaissance spirit of experimentation
and application of wonder that seems to have surfaced again in
Wellcome's medical museum, and that has inspired us to draw on and
present his collection in an experimental fashion. As a response to his
material culture legacy, then, *Medicine Man* is offered more as a
Renaissance essay than a definitive modern monograph.

This natural alliance between curiosities and cures also surfaced, as
already mentioned, in the life and work of Hans Sloane (1660–1753),
whose collection formed an uncanny precedent for Wellcome's own.
Trained as a doctor, Sloane's collecting instincts sprang from a curiosity with the material world that was instilled in medical practitioners
eager to balance the natural harm of some substances with the
curative properties of others. Later in the eighteenth century, the
dominant British medical figures of the Hunter brothers both formed
museums: John creating what he saw as an unwritten 'book' embody-
ing his new approach to 'the Animal Oeconomy'; William being more
concerned to establish a teaching museum of anatomy.

The cement that has held together the fields of museums and medicine has throughout its history had a strong didactic ingredient. During the eighteenth century any number of cabinets consisting entirely of samples of *materia medica* were formed and used as the core teaching material for courses of medical instruction, often given publicly for a small fee. And during the nineteenth century the role of museums became more and more exclusively focused on this educational function, with a simultaneous reduction in the use of medical museums for research purposes. Thus their place at the cutting edge of certain scientific disciplines gradually gave way to a secondary one of educating 'tomorrow's scientists'. By the end of the nineteenth century, most of the royal and learned medical societies in Europe and America had gathered collections expressly for the purpose of teaching, more than a few surviving surprisingly intact to this day. Wellcome's museum-making efforts also continued this tradition.

Wellcome seems to have drawn on this 500-year history and then added to it in his own grand fashion. The scale of his ambitions at the beginning of the twentieth century probably accounts for the survival of so much of his museum, whereas many earlier collections have come down to us only in the form of individual relics and published descriptions. Of course, while physically surviving to a remarkable extent, in another fashion Wellcome's museum as an idea and as a vision of material culture has almost disappeared. Indeed, in some meaningful way, one of the world's greatest collections has all but been lost. Scattered as ghostly fragments that have settled in hundreds of institutions, where, except in two or three large repositories, barely a few scholarly keepers with good memories can recall their origins, the Wellcome Museum has all but been forgotten – a phantom of the museum world.

This book

In the following chapters you will find six different perspectives on this forgotten museum. Ghislaine Lawrence, who first wrote about the collection sixteen years ago, reacquaints herself with its history and purpose. Frances Knight, who has more recently embarked on its study, uses the holdings of the Wellcome Library to introduce us to those who did the collecting and to some of the stories that lie behind

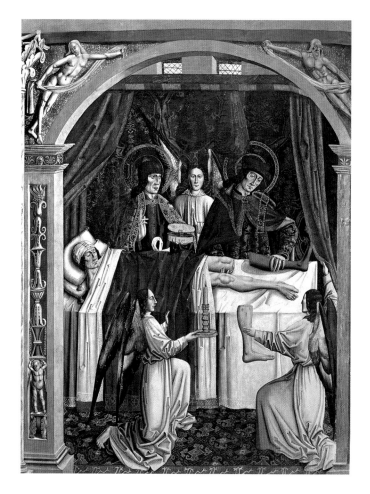

22 Oil painting of Saints
Cosmas and Damian
performing a miraculous feat
of surgery: amputating the
ulcerated leg of a Christian
and transplanting in its place
the undiseased leg of a dead
Moor. Attributed to Alonso de
Sedano, Burgos. *c.* 1495.
WL, 46009i

their acquisitions. Chris Gosden focuses on Wellcome's archaeological interests and discusses what we might learn from objects and their relationships with people. John Mack considers Wellcome's vision of the links between medicine and anthropology. John Pickstone, bringing the histories of medicine, science and technology to the fore, provides us with a tool-box for thinking about the various processes involved in knowledge-making and the role that objects might play therein. Finally, Ruth Richardson invites us into one of the many storerooms which house the collection and evokes its human remains – both literal and metaphorical – echoes of the many lives that have gone before.

Interspersed between these different voices are six visual essays which explore broad themes. For example in the first – 'The beginning of life' – we have clustered a variety of objects to cast a net around the medical context for understanding and dealing with the beginnings of human life. Based on the themes of our exhibition and gesturing towards the adage of knowledge through contrast and comparison, these selections take deliberately diffuse topics around which to bring objects snatched from across history and around the globe. The energy created – sometimes in the form of friction and sometimes harmony – bears witness to our current enchantment with all that lies between and across disciplines.

In these visual essays we have tried to choose things that might delight the eye or challenge the mind. Consequently our cornucopia has the serious rubbing shoulders with the frivolous, the beautiful sharing space with the ugly, and little-known objects spotlighted just as prominently as others more talked about. In a fashion that has inspired much recent work in museums, we too have been motivated by the desires and instincts of collectors and curators from an altogether earlier era of museum history, borrowing something from the spirit of *Wunderkammern*, or 'cabinets of wonder'. In exploring the collection, we were by turns interested in and drawn to the beautiful, the weird, the important and the unusual (figs 22–5), and have selected objects which not only help us to tell medical stories but also which simply stopped us in our tracks. Things with an innate value drawn from a track record of outliving their makers and previous owners – destined no doubt to survive us, too – which either speak volumes about past experiences, or though mute are just wonderful

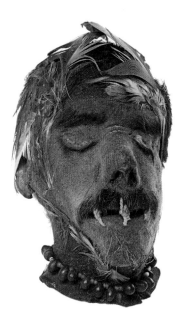

23 A Shuar shrunken head (tsantsa). Ecuador, late nineteenth/early twentieth century. SM, A102935

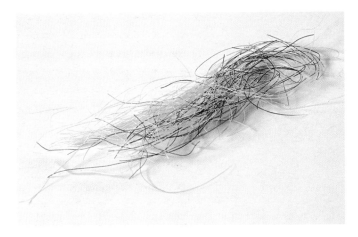

24 A lock of hair said to be from King George III (1760–1820). SM, A1315

and intriguing to behold. Side-stepping the more recent motivation behind museum collections that seeks rational coverage of a history or theme through order and system, what we were particularly drawn to in Wellcome's collection was that which can also be found in Sir John Soane's Museum in Lincoln's Inn Fields in London and the Pitt Rivers Museum in Oxford – the individual, the provocative and the strange.

In working on this book and exhibition we have encountered but a fraction of the Wellcome collection. Out of more than a million objects, fewer than a thousand are depicted here; that is, less than 0.1 per cent of the whole. And so the objects you encounter as you leaf through these pages are not representative of Wellcome's aims. Rather, they reveal a fraction of the things that we have had the pleasure of meeting on our imaginative and intellectual journeys through his collection, and that we have the space to share; a mere glimpse of his epic endeavour. We hope these will give you a flavour of the richness of objects involved and a sense of what it might be like to open drawer after drawer, leaf through print after print, of this wonderful collection.

The objects in Wellcome's collection are nothing if not irrefutable testaments to the fact that medicine and health are as old and as broad as humanity itself. Experienced and understood in dauntingly diverse fashions, they have been driving forces – scientific, cultural, religious, social and personal – for all people, throughout time. In a necessarily impressionistic way then, the objects shown here enable us to contemplate and perhaps reassess how we came to be where we are, as well as illuminate the different ways that different people at different times have understood and dealt with common universal themes – our corporeal existence, the source of its wellbeing, and its relationship to our inner identities, our souls.

If anything, working on this project – with these objects and with our history-of-medicine tinted spectacles – has been a striking reminder of the precariousness and frailty of our lives. Time really is short – so enjoy!

25 Box of appliances designed by George Thomson to be used with his 'Mechanical Substitute for the Arms and Foot Writing Machine'. This apparatus was 'intended for the use of men who have lost both arms'.
SM, A602321

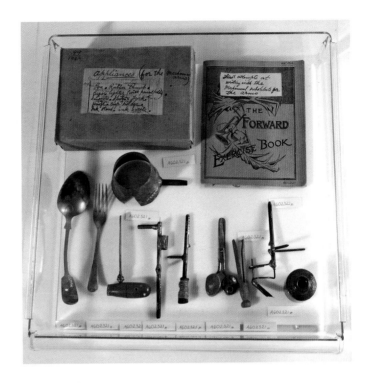

NOTES

1 Engineer, A. 2000. 'Illustrations from the Wellcome Library: Wellcome and "The Great Past"' in *Medical History* 44, pp. 389–404.

2 CMAC/WA/HSW/OR/L.1, p. 38. Evidence to the Royal Commission on National Museums and Galleries 1928–9. Typescript of written answers by Henry Wellcome.

3 Symons, J. 1998. '"These crafty dealers". Sir Henry Wellcome as a Book Collector' in Myers, R. and Harris, M. (eds), *Medicine, Mortality and the Book Trade.* Kent: St Paul's Bibliographies/ Oak Knoll Press.

4 Symons, J. 1991. 'The Benevolent Autocrat' in *Wellcome Journal* 6, no. 6.

5 Engineer 2000.

6 Syrie Wellcome to A. Chune Fletcher, 14 August 1910 (Wellcome Institute Archives).

7 Skinner, G.M. 1986. 'Sir Henry Wellcome's Museum for the Science of History' in *Medical History* 30.

8 Skinner 1986.

9 The Wellcome Historical Medical Museum, 1927, p. 99. A handbook which outlines 'the chief features and objects exhibited in the Museum'.

10 Skinner 1986.

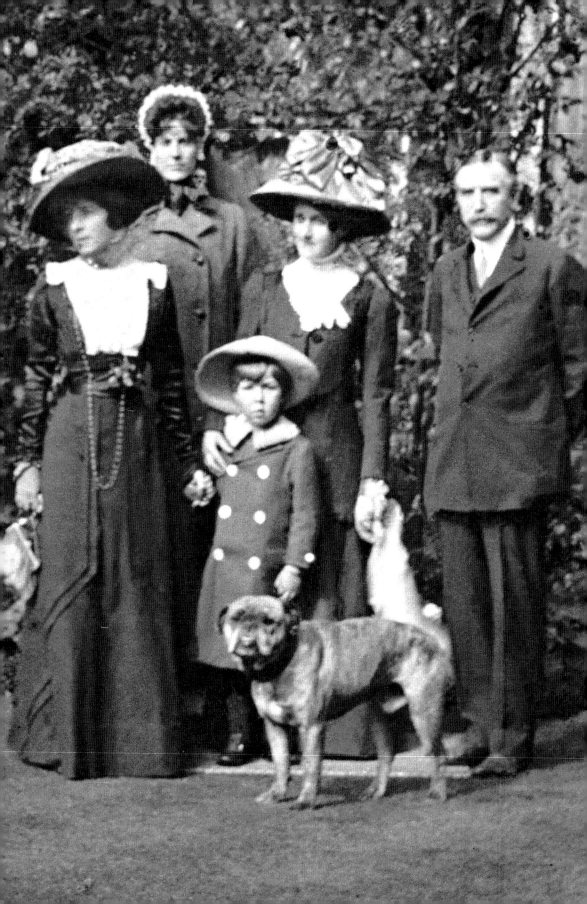

The Wellcome family outside
their home, The Nest, Hayes, Kent,
c. 1908. Syrie front left, Mounteney
front middle, Henry front right,
with an unknown woman and a nanny.

'Henry Wellcome was curiously
lonely. . . . It may be doubted
whether anyone knew him with
sufficient intimacy to do more
than speculate as to his real
feelings and motives.'

SIR HENRY DALE, OBITUARY TRIBUTE, *THE TIMES*, 1 AUGUST 1936.

Wellcome's Museum for the Science of History

Ghislaine Lawrence

'The study of anthropology comprehends
all human activities including the healing art'
(Henry Wellcome in *Great Britain, Royal Commission
on national museums and galleries*, London, HMSO, 1929)[1]

I have a sense of *déjà vu*. Sixteen years ago I wrote a paper with this
title and here I am doing it again. First time round, it was an attempt
to make sense of new circumstances. Transformed overnight from a
general practitioner into a museum curator, my new surroundings
were somewhat perplexing. The world for which I had chosen to leave
medicine was distinctly odd. Storerooms bulged with weird and apparently unrelated objects – African spears, slot machines, chamber pots
and the like (or unlike). Clearly, they had been brought together for a
reason – but what? Undoubtedly, the whole enterprise was sanctioned
by the state. Obviously it was a form of public service. My first job was
to help a visitor photograph the nineteenth-century stethoscopes. He
hadn't mentioned that he wanted to position them on a naked female
torso. Dispirited, I thought perhaps I should have been a brain surgeon after all. After a while I decided that there was nothing for it but
to dig more deeply into the reason for the bricolage. What follows is a
much-shortened version of my original paper.[2]

The science of history

By the early 1930s, Henry Wellcome had a hugely disparate collection of artefacts five times larger than that of the Louvre. He had first
conceived of an historical medical museum in the 1880s. It was to
embody a version of the history of medicine inconceivable before the
1860s, unconvincing to many during his lifetime, and almost incom-
prehensible after his death. Wellcome was a wealthy and somewhat
isolated amateur enthusiast who wrote little and pursued his con-
suming interests through paid employees. His place in the London

scientific community was earned through philanthropic support for scientific ventures. Convinced of the pre-eminent value of science to humankind, why did he create, as well as research laboratories, a historical museum? After all, Sir Henry Cole (1808–82), first director of the Victoria & Albert Museum, had expressed the hope that museums would furnish 'a powerful alternative to the gin palace'. Rational amusement for the working man, however, was not exactly what Wellcome had in mind.

In the decades following Cole's remark, the new disciplines of archaeology and anthropology had provided a much-needed rationale for museum practice. C.J. Thomsen (1788–1865) introduced his seminal Stone, Bronze and Iron Age classification in the guide to the Copenhagen Museum. The importance placed on the systematic arrangement of artefacts by archaeologists and anthropologists quickly led to museums being viewed in large part as places for research rather than relaxation, for edification of the scientist rather than education of the masses. By 1893, in Sir William Flower's presidential address to the five-year-old Museums Association, the first duty of museums had become 'without question to preserve the materials upon which the history of mankind and the knowledge of science is based'. A few years later Henry Balfour called them the 'laboratories of anthropologists'. Balfour (1863–1939), curator of the Pitt Rivers Collection, might be expected to stress this role, but Flower (1831–99), first director of the Natural History Museum, was addressing curators from all types of museum, and still felt able to prescribe 'history' and 'mankind' as the prime concerns. By the end of the nineteenth century, a 'museum' virtually implied an exposition of developmental history, rather than a cabinet of curiosities.

The scientific study of the history of mankind was precisely the goal which the evolutionist founding fathers of anthropology set themselves. 'Anthropology began as the science of history' – a 'scientific' history of man in all his aspects, perceived as an essentially regular progression through various stages of civilisation. The process was universal, and law-like. For the evolutionist school, unchallenged until the 1890s, anthropological enquiry consisted of the reconstruction of this sequential progress. Their conception of the generally regular nature of man's progression through various stages of civilisation – from savagery through barbarism to civilisation – made possible its reconstruction by means of a procedure known as the 'comparative method' to fill the gaps in the available knowledge of universal history. In this method, contemporary 'primitives' were taken to represent earlier, prehistoric stages of development. Enlightenment theories of progress, biology, eighteenth-century linguistics, and nineteenth-century geology have all been cited as sources. The British prehistorian, John Lubbock (1834–1913), for example, remarked that 'the van Diemaner and South American are to the antiquary what the opossum and the sloth are to the geologist'.

It was A.H.L.F. Pitt Rivers (1827–1900) who most vigorously applied the comparative method to material culture. 'Human ideas as represented by the various products of human industry' were capable of 'classification into genera, species and varieties, in the same manner as the products of the vegetable and animal kingdoms, and in their development from the homogenous to the heterogeneous they obey the same laws. If, therefore, we can obtain a sufficient number of objects to represent the succession of ideas, it will be found that they are capable of being arranged in Museums upon a similar plan'. This Darwinian conception of the evolution of man's material culture by minute changes (with 'utility' substituted for natural selection) was ideally suited to reconstructing and representing the progressive history of mankind, if the comparative method was used. 'The existing races, in their respective stages of progression, may be taken as the *bona fide* representatives of the races of antiquity . . . whose implements, resembling, with but little difference, their own, are now found low down in the soil.'

Such historical accounts of the development of culture facilitated the rearrangement of existing collections of antiquities, collected originally because they were very old, and ethnographic objects, collected because they were very curious, into a coherent reconstruction of the past in museums not directly related to centres of archaeological or anthropological research. No longer would 'the familiar "cannibal club from the South Seas" languish against its neighbour, as likely as not a stuffed "Egyptian ibis"' or 'the label drop from "the authentic Dagger which killed Captain Cook" henceforth to adorn the back of the unsuspecting "Turtle from the West Indies" below'. Museums would not remain 'mere scrap-heaps of curios'. The links between the museum world and the archaeologists and anthropologists who had

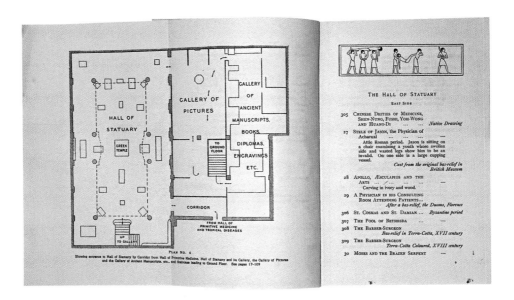

1 Handbook of the Historical
Medical Museum, organised
by Henry Wellcome, for the
XVIIth International Congress
of Medicine. London, 1913.
Partial floor plan and 'The Hall
of Statuary'.

2 OPPOSITE The Wellcome
Historical Medical Museum,
Wigmore Street, c. 1919.

provided it with a new mandate were never stronger than at the turn
of the nineteenth century. It is clear that Wellcome considered his
museum venture just as 'scientific' as his research laboratories. 'No
effort was being spared to bring the Museum into line with, or even
ahead of, the scientific institutions in London.'

The Wellcome Historical Medical Museum

Collecting began in earnest around 1903. Wellcome's first curator,
C.J.S. Thompson (1862–1943), made endless visits to dealers, auc-
tions, private vendors, museums, and libraries in Britain and abroad.
Wellcome controlled purchasing and was certainly aware that job lots
were often bought, sometimes containing large numbers of apparently identical objects. First exhibited in 1913 at the International
Congress of Medicine in London (fig. 1), the collection moved to permanent premises in Wigmore Street in 1914 (fig. 2), with the stated
intention of connecting 'the links in the chain of human experience
which stretch back from the present time into the prehistoric period of
the early ages'. Information was to be sought on 'folklore', 'items of
curious medical lore', 'early traditions' and 'quaint customs', and,
most of all, in ethnographic material. By 1926 this accounted for
almost three-quarters of the collection. The Hall of Primitive Medicine

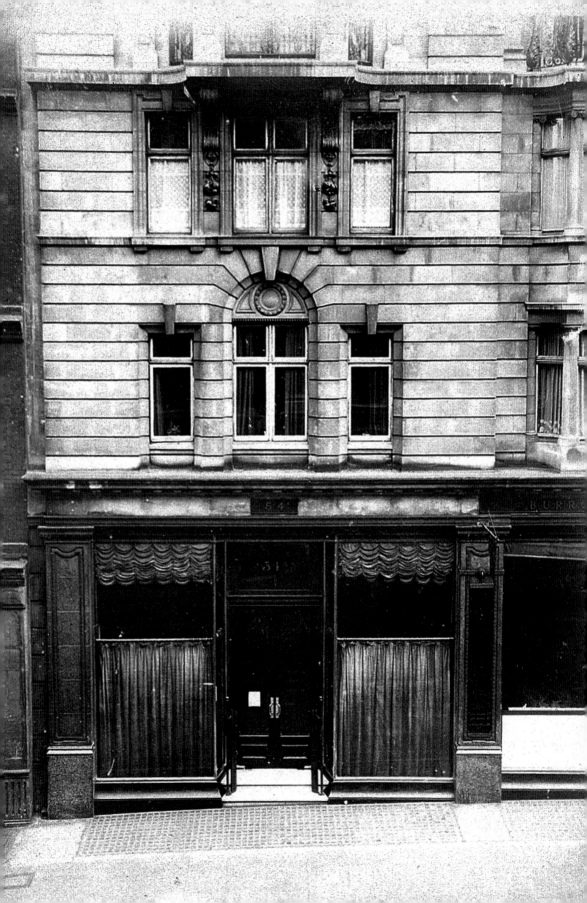

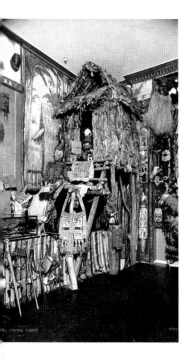

(fig. 3) occupied almost a quarter of the main floor of the Museum. Things were still not 'scientific' enough for Wellcome, however. In 1926 he replaced C.J.S. Thompson, essentially a writer and journalist, with L.W.G. Malcolm (1888–1946), a Cambridge anthropologist taught by A.C. Haddon (1855–1940) and W.H.R. Rivers (1864–1922). 'In future', instructed Wellcome, 'the Museum is to be run on strictly scientific lines.' Malcolm divided the museum into seven sections: Prehistoric archaeology, Classical archaeology, Antiquities, Folklore, Ethnology, and Racial development with Physical anthropology. Assistants for each section – four anthropologists and three archaeologists – were appointed in 1928.

The layout remained very much as Wellcome had first planned it before 1913 – a Hall of Primitive Medicine, Hall of Statuary (fig. 4), and Picture Gallery (fig. 5) occupied most of the main floor. Reconstructed pharmacies and other room settings were placed in the basement (figs 6 and 7). The major emphasis was firmly on primitive culture and representational art. The Hall of Primitive Medicine formed an obligatory introduction to the Museum. Other than this

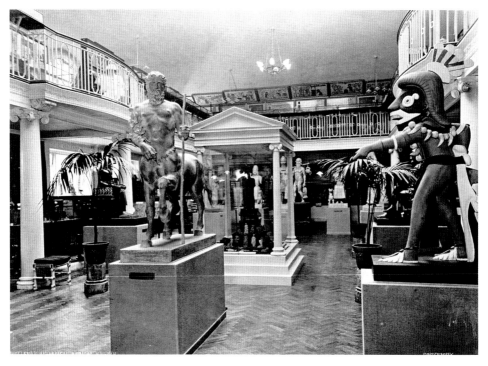

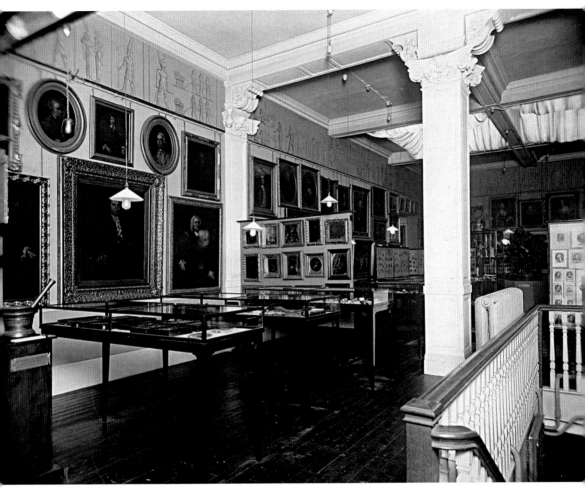

3 LEFT TOP A head-hunter's
hut, south-east New Guinea,
in the Hall of Primitive
Medicine, *c.* 1914.

4 LEFT The galleried Hall
of Statuary, *c.* 1914.

5 West wall of the Gallery
of Pictures, *c.* 1914.

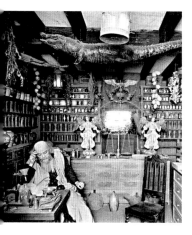

there was no attempt at an overall chronological arrangement or at grouping objects of the same period together. Within groupings of similar *types* of object, however, sequence was of paramount importance. Surgical instruments, for example, were arranged in sequences of single types – the trepan, the speculum, the dental forceps and so on (fig. 8). 'As far as possible the scheme is evolutionary and the series are so arranged that the history of each instrument may be studied separately.' 'The evolution of the lancet' showed the fingernail, the shell and sharpened flint as the earliest forms (fig. 9). A display of weaponry began with animal tusks and ended in the repeat firing musket. Similar hypothetical sequences dealt with, for example, the evolution of the surgical knife, the stethoscope, the toothbrush, the

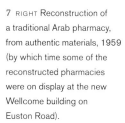

6 ABOVE Reconstruction of an apothecary's shop, London, seventeenth century, with model of an apothecary seated at table, *c.* 1914.

7 RIGHT Reconstruction of a traditional Arab pharmacy, from authentic materials, 1959 (by which time some of the reconstructed pharmacies were on display at the new Wellcome building on Euston Road).

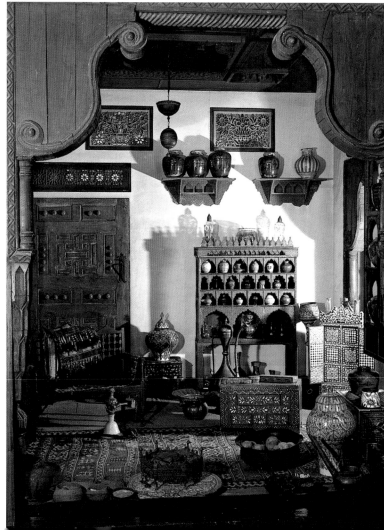

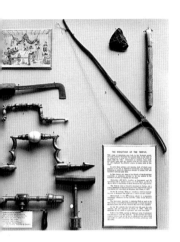

8–9 Displays from the Museum showing the sequential 'evolution' of the trepan and the lancet.

enema, and, later, 'the evolution of the gas mask'. Wherever possible, the earliest examples in each sequence were parts of the body, followed by natural objects. To complete the later parts of surgical instrument sequences, Malcolm removed hundreds of single items from eighteenth- and nineteenth-century boxed instrument sets.

There is ample evidence that all this was at Wellcome's instigation. In 1926 he instructed Malcolm to explain to an eminent visitor 'the plans on which we are working in the Museum to illustrate in our collection the whole story of life . . . that I have for many years been collecting for the purpose of demonstrating by means of objects that will illustrate the actuality of every notable step in the evolution and progress from the first germ of life up to the fully developed man of

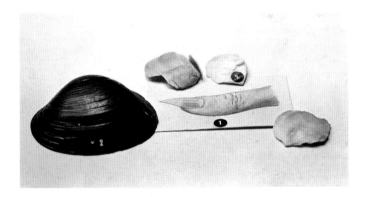

today. Furthermore, we aim to illustrate the continuous perils and ravages of disease encountered in the battle of life. Also the weapons to combat and the shields to protect'.

Several similar statements are to be found in Wellcome's evidence to the Royal Commission on Museums and Galleries of 1927. His adherence to Pitt Rivers' injunction that sequence was 'the funda-mental rule of the game' when dealing with material culture was complete. 'The one thing most desirable in a matter of this kind is to show from the beginning, the evolution and development throughout, the passing on from one stage of progress to another of particular objects . . . as far as possible to trace each step from the period of their origin throughout the whole course of development.' Indeed, he was unable to contemplate any disruption to universal, progressive sequences. Asked how he would illustrate the substitution of a piece of bottle glass for a flint arrowhead by 'the modern savage races' of the Magellan Straits, he unhesitatingly replied, 'I would put a thing like that down as a freak.' He also made clear the rather limited role, which he accorded, to archaeological material. It seems he regarded it very much as a 'prop' for anthropology, to be resorted to for filling in the early parts of object sequences but with a subservient role in elucidating history. 'Archaeology is practically in a different field', he told the Commission, who were surprised to hear that he would not advocate incorporating the British Museum's Stone Age collections in any proposed national ethnographical museum. 'Archaeology mainly

10 The Museum's visitors book. Opening beginning with Tuesday, July 28, 1914.

represents the higher cultures of antiquity. In the Historical Medical Museum anthropology represents the more primitive life from the earliest periods and traces the developments up to the present day.' Here Wellcome demonstrates that overriding concern with retrieving the most primitive origins that characterised evolutionist methods. The 'higher cultures of antiquity' had already 'advanced' too far.

The Commission pressed Wellcome on the matter of public access. He told them that 'A great many people visit museums simply as

stragglers'. A confusing discussion ensued with Wellcome describing
an ideal museum of two, or possibly three sections involving an educational research department, where laboratories were the 'special
features' and the promotion of 'scientific research' on each branch of
anthropology represented 'one of its first aims'. 'Intellectual people',
'those genuinely concerned and interested in the subjects represented
there who attend entirely for beneficial information', might be admitted to a 'Museum devoted to research purposes' such as he envisaged.
The Committee soon abandoned this line of enquiry, perhaps rightly
concluding that the concerns of the general public were not uppermost in Wellcome's mind. His Historical Medical Museum seems not,
in his lifetime, to have been open to them without prior written application, and certainly little effort was made to attract non-specialist
visitors or children. Not surprisingly, overall attendance figures were
low. In June 1926, for example, there were 104 visitors, the largest
figure for that month since 1919 (fig. 10).

One group of visitors for which Wellcome was prepared to cater,
however, were those guardians of the Empire whose duties brought
them into contact with the 'subject native races': 'Colonial and military officials, explorers, colonizers, planters, missionaries – would
find it invaluable'. He hoped the Museum would be 'the laboratory
where cultural and technological problems would be solved', echo-
ing, nearly sixty years later, the anthropologist Edward Burnett
Tylor's (1832–1917) famous conclusion that 'the science of culture
is essentially a reformer's science'. The usefulness of anthropology to
colonial administrators was frequently alluded to by those who
wished to promote the discipline in the late nineteenth and early
twentieth centuries.

Anthropological methods

If it is accepted that Wellcome saw the history of medicine as a part of
anthropology, then the collection which he amassed, and the methods
he used to acquire it, appear less extraordinary. Amateur collecting (in
Wellcome's case, by paid agents, missionaries, and museum employees) had respectable precedents. Large ethnographic collections were
built by this means in the nineteenth century, and often involved commercial considerations – the British Association for the Advancement

of Science compiled *Notes and queries on anthropology for the use of travellers and residents in uncivilized lands* in 1874, providing guidance on what to ask and what to collect. During the late 1920s, the Wellcome Historical Medical Museum produced a similar pocket-sized booklet entitled *Memoranda concerning the collection of information and material among primitive peoples*, with questions on deities, medicine men, disease, superstitions, poisons, family life and marriage, childbirth, burial, astrology, artistic workmanship, weapons, and currency. Several hundred unused copies remain in the archives. By the 1920s, when anthropologists had ventured into the field themselves, this method was old-fashioned, but it had been acceptable during the decades when they constructed theories at home, from data collected by others. Like them, Wellcome considered collecting of major importance. Neither exhibitions nor cataloguing were high priorities for his Museum, and he was generally unreceptive to suggestions that staff be engaged in sorting and identifying, rather than collecting. So long as sufficient data was gathered together, 'scientific' researchers would construct their theories from it at a later date.

In many other ways, the activities of the Wellcome Historical Medical Museum reveal an indebtedness to anthropology. The enormously wide range of items collected gave rise to subsequent speculation that Wellcome intended to create an additional ethnographical museum, and some of his public utterances support this view. However, the firm distinction between 'medical' and 'ethnographic' objects is largely one imposed by later writers. It was not one which Wellcome made easily, and was certainly not one made in the museum's everyday activities. Wellcome admitted that his 'collections of anthropological material, considered as such, are vastly greater than the strictly medical'. But it seems he shared the biologised definition of medicine still current amongst some anthropologists. As a fellow of the Royal Anthropological Institute put it when they met at the Museum in 1927, 'The distinctive attribute of all living creatures is the preservation of life, and the great majority of the activities of all living creatures are concerned unwittingly with this process. When man first became rational he attempted by the use of his reason to devise means of protecting his life from extinction.' 'The great central aim of this Museum is to illustrate the motive that underlies all these collections of objects.' Viewed in this light, as the result of an instinct for self-preservation, the practice of medicine was equated with the preservation of health and was hard to disentangle from the provision of food, a mate, and protection from the elements and enemies. As Wellcome put it, 'most . . . anthropological material possesses strong medical significance, for in all the ages the preservation of life and health has been uppermost in the minds of living beings'. 'Medical' artefacts were 'anthropological', and 'anthropological' or 'ethnographic' artefacts almost always possessed medical significance.

Although Wellcome was unstinting in financial support for the Museum, much of the collections lacked any great aesthetic or monetary value. In many ways the same criteria were applied to the collection of the material culture of literate, more recent societies as to that of primitive or ancient ones. Concerned to illustrate changes in the external morphology of objects, or the content of representational art, it is as though auction houses, market stalls, the columns of *Exchange and Mart*, and indeed existing museums were to him as much a part of 'the field' as the jungles of Borneo. They were to be scoured for objects in a similar way. As with ethnographic objects, information about their age, function, or place of origin was recorded if available. Yet the absence of such details was not a contraindication to acquisition, since, provided enough had been collected, the accurate position of each could subsequently be detected within an absolute progressive sequence – as the archaeologists were able to do. 'A stray fragment of carving without date or locality can be surely fixed in its place if there is any sufficient knowledge of the art from which it springs.' A large part of Wellcome's collections lacked any provenance at all. Soon, only estimates of the holdings were available. 'The more you can complete the various series . . . the more effectually the collections will visualize and demonstrate the characteristic features; thus you would be able to trace the evolution from A to Z in the development of any particular branch.' The collections of the Pitt Rivers Museum, assembled on a similar basis, became as large as Wellcome's. The evolutionists were committed to dealing with huge amounts of data, not only for the reconstruction of complete sequences on which a science of universal history depended, but to minimise error, hoping to balance out the effects of unreliable data by examining sufficient instances. Further impetus to collect came from the fear that the data was fast vanishing. Folklorists warned that the 'footprints in the sands of time' which they sought to record were 'fast being trampled out by the hurrying feet of the busy multitudes of the present'. The changes induced in 'primitive' societies by the proximity of 'civilised' ones – later to be areas of intense interest to anthropologists – were dreaded by many at the turn of the century, since they obscured the distant origins of culture they sought to recover.

In its exhibition galleries the Museum made no attempt to incorporate the chronology of written history. No use was made, for example, of

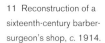

11 Reconstruction of a sixteenth-century barber-surgeon's shop, *c.* 1914.

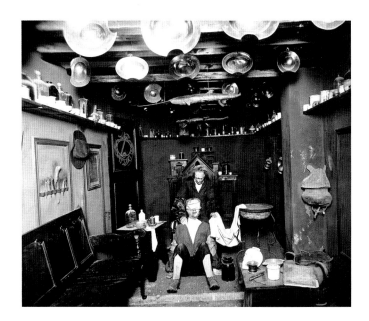

organising principles such as the Renaissance or the Enlightenment. This sacrificing of chronicled events to the 'grand scheme of comparative reconstruction' was precisely the fault which Franz Boas (1858–1942) and the accidentalist school were to perceive in the evolutionist anthropology they did much to discredit. The Museum's total lack of an overall chronological arrangement, apart from the obligatory beginning in the Hall of Primitive Medicine, was entirely consistent with the evolutionist approach – as was the use of reconstructed room settings (fig. 11).

The museum displays also made quite extensive use of replicas – a replica which could illustrate some sequential continuity was more useful than an unobtainable original. Representational art could easily be reproduced, and Wellcome used contemporary artists, including one known as 'Hayman the faker', to copy paintings with a 'medical' content. Others, who specialised in the genre of historical reconstruction, were commissioned to produce paintings of particular events where none existed. The scenes selected were often those for which there was little documented evidence. Wellcome seems almost to have been seeking a pictorial record of the mythology of Western Medicine to the present time. In similar vein, he fostered a cult of the eminent physician, going to great lengths to secure the academic robes of the eminent physician Sir William Osler (1849–1919) and many others, displaying personalia such as surgery door-plates and knobs and devoting a whole display case to 'doctors' walking sticks and canes', much in the same way that he exhibited the equipment of medicine men and shamans. By and large, however, his intense concern for the primitive led to a relative disregard for the contemporary. As founder of the country's first physiological and pharmacological research laboratories, Wellcome was in a prime position to collect the equipment used there. However, not even an association with notable discoveries or famous men tempted him to acquisition. The collection apparently contains no apparatus at all from the Wellcome research laboratories and only about 5 per cent of the 'non-ethnographic' items were twentieth-century, a tiny proportion of these being laboratory apparatus. In at least one instance the Museum considered selling modern instruments acquired as part of job lots. Modern material that might shed light on origins, however, was acquired. In 1915, for example, the Museum accepted a collection of charms removed from the bodies of fallen German soldiers, via the Folklore Society (see also fig. 12).

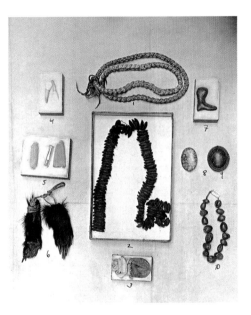

12 Collection of amulets and charms found in London, part of the Lovett Collection exhibited in the Museum.

Who used the Museum?

Although the Wellcome Historical Medical Museum aspired to 'scientific' anthropology, it was, by the late 1920s, increasingly out of touch with the academic discipline. Malcolm's appointment brought some contact, and the retiring A.C. Haddon offered his services. A major transitional figure in anthropology, opining that 'the comparative method is liable to lead the unwary into mistakes', that 'the chief danger to which [anthropology] is liable is that its fascination and popularity . . . tend to premature generalisations', and aware of the 'promising' methods of the French sociologists, Haddon might have preserved the Museum from an approach that was becoming distinctly old-fashioned, had Wellcome accepted his offer.

HISTORICAL MEDICAL EXHIBITION
LONDON, 1913

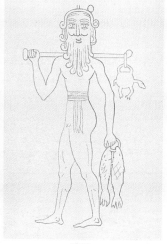

ADAPA
A SUMERIAN DEITY OF HEALING
About 6000 B.C.

Adapa is the earliest known personage directly associated with medicine. He was the human incarnation of Marduk, the divine Son of Ea, and was believed to possess the spells of life and death.
"Ea gave him wisdom,
So that his command was like unto the word of God.
To him also he gave deep knowledge;
With the healing spell of life and the spell of death he was made."
(Translated from a Babylonian Tablet)

13 An illustration from an advance publicity leaflet for the Historical Medical Exhibition of 1913 that was also used as the frontispiece of diaries and distributed to the medical profession.

For the tide was turning inexorably away from the study of material culture, this being firmly (though not necessarily) associated with the increasingly discredited evolutionist school. As early as the mid-1890s, a sense of crisis had been evident in evolutionary theory in Britain, and, by 1910, 'the theoretical malaise . . . was becoming acute'. In the United States, Franz Boas, finding anthropology a 'happy hunting ground for the romantic lover of primitive things', was to leave it radically changed by his criticism of the comparative method and insistence on exhaustive fieldwork. Boas did find some role for material culture studies that provided evidence for the diffusion of culture traits, and took issue with the curator Otis T. Mason (1838–1908) in 1887 for using Pitt Rivers' classification system at the American Museum of Natural History. Together, they rearranged the collections using the 'culture area' concept. But, overall, interest in material culture was waning even before Wellcome began to collect.

Nor did medical historians pursue significant research at the Museum. For some it was a source of illustrations, and in 1939 Max Neuburger (1868–1955) found refuge there. But only a handful of papers directly relating to objects in the collections have ever been published. In Wellcome's day, the eminent medical historian Charles Singer (1876–1960) was dismissive – 'It is no good laying out a lot of instruments and having a sort of Madame Tussaud's show and saying "This is the History of Medicine"'. Norman Moore (1847–1922), a future President of the Royal College of Physicians, intimated that the Museum was out of step with his own views. The 'two great branches', of the history of medicine were typified for him by two figures in the Museum – the black masked and feathered Mexican God Ixtlilton, and the Apollo Belvedere. Moore was in no doubt that Apollo, and his son, Asklepios, represented 'the true ancestors, the true observing predecessors of Hippocrates and Galen and Avicenna' – and doubtless himself.

This was not merely hubris restricted to men who were fashionable London physicians first and historians second. As the century progressed, historians of medicine of all persuasions were more concerned with the emancipation of medicine from magic. 'Folk medicine is a big hodge podge', wrote Henry Sigerist (1891–1957) in 1951, placing it at the end, not the beginning, of his projected magnum opus *A History of Medicine*. 'The chief source of medical history is literature' he concluded – a view from which subsequent historians have not dissented. While the Museum mounted exhibitions such as

14 Front cover to and spread from an advance publicity leaflet for the Historical Medical Exhibition.

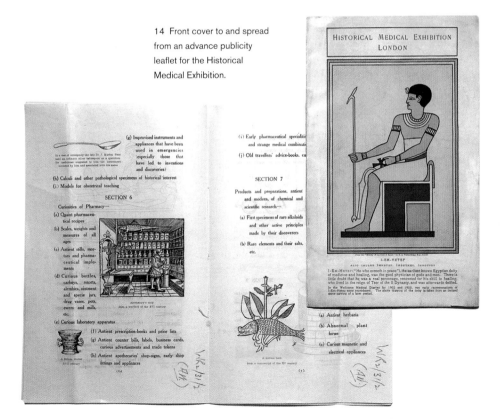

'The Folklore of London', or 'Japanese Amulets and Charms', and commissioned publications dealing with Celtic medicine, doctors suggested 'Objects of Shakespearean Interest', celebrations of the Henry Hill Hickman centenary, and publications on pre-Vesalian dissection. It would not be surprising if, at a time when the General Medical Council was decorating its new building with bas-reliefs of ancient Greece, medical men were a little discomfited to find 'Adapa, the Sumerian fish deity' fronting the professional diaries they received from Wellcome (fig. 13). The Museum's friezes and logos, however, from the sketch of 'Marduk, a Chaldean deity of medicine, about 5000 BC', which had accompanied the first circular, to 'Phenuka, an Egyptian Priest physician of the Fifth Dynasty', on the frontispiece of the 1927 Guide, remained, if not prehistoric, very ancient indeed (fig. 14). If anything, Malcolm's appointment in 1925 further entrenched the Museum in Tylorian anthropology of the 1880s. Although trained at the 'revolutionary' Cambridge school, he was pliable and not particularly innovative. His own field was physical anthropology, traditionally a conservative area that continued to rely on the serial arrangement of specimens, deriving its methods from comparative anatomy.[3]

If the Museum was isolated from contemporary anthropologists and out of step with medical men, it also had little connection with any other 'medical' museum. When Sir William Osler commented that 'nothing like it has ever been put together before', he was essentially accurate. Of the forty-six 'medical museums' known to be in existence in the British Isles in 1913, only six included any 'historical' material, and it is clear that the prime function of all of them was to teach anatomy and gross pathology. The Royal College of Surgeons had begun a historical collection of instruments in 1910, but this served largely as a repository for those instruments with which the Fellows felt they had contributed notable advances, or which were part of the personalia of eminent surgeons. The Museum of the Royal College of Surgeons of Edinburgh had a similar collection, dating from 1883. The British Museum had acquired between two and three hundred Greek and Roman instruments by 1925, of which an indeterminate number were medical. Abroad, the Medico-Chirurgical Museum in Ravenna had, since its foundation in the first half of the eighteenth century, collected examples of surgical instrumentation, as well as anatomical specimens, but these were expressly for teaching surgical practice. The medical museums of Europe were founded largely for teaching purposes at the university medical schools or to commemorate these, or other, institutions. The Museum of the Val-de-Grâce in Paris, for example, which opened in 1916, was intended to commemorate 'the actions of the French military medical services in the Great War, and to instruct future officers of the *Corps de Santé*'.

The Smithsonian Institution in Washington, first showing significant numbers of medical exhibits in 1921, adopted another approach. Amulets and charms were displayed not as indications of the 'roots and foundations of things', but 'to warn the public against the perils of quackery and the faults of folk medicine'. This museum saw its role in pointing out the evils of the past rather than reconstructing cultural history. The Smithsonian had a traditional role in evaluating and patenting inventions and innovations not shared by European museums, and in 1929, American medicine was still a 'paradise for quacks'. Their medical exhibits in the Smithsonian's 'Hall of Health' were reminiscent of the sanitary and hygiene exhibitions held in Europe and the United States from the 1870s onwards. None of these attempted historical exposition.

Wellcome's amateur interest in anthropology had of course been shared by some of his countrymen – those industrial tycoons who embraced the Spencerian doctrines of Social Darwinism. Attracted to a progressive 'science of society', they gave substantial financial backing to anthropological research. American anthropologists 'had educated their millionaires', and, liberally endowed by bodies such as the Rockefeller Foundation and the Carnegie Trust, were the envy of their English colleagues. It has been suggested, however, that the adoption of anthropology as a prescriptive science by United States reformers and politicians at the turn of the century contributed to the depressed state of the discipline there during the 1910s and 1920s. Historians of anthropology describe a mediocre milieu of amateur theorisers from which only Boas, trained as a physicist and an immigrant member of an ethnic minority, stood apart. Returned to his country of origin, Wellcome might have merged perfectly into this milieu – a successful self-made business man, a philanthropist who held commonplace Spencerian views of nature and positivist conceptions of science and found them perfectly blended in a pre-scriptive 'science of history'. His involvement with museums had several parallels with the activities of Americans such as Andrew Carnegie (1835–1919), John Pierpont Morgan (1837–1913), and

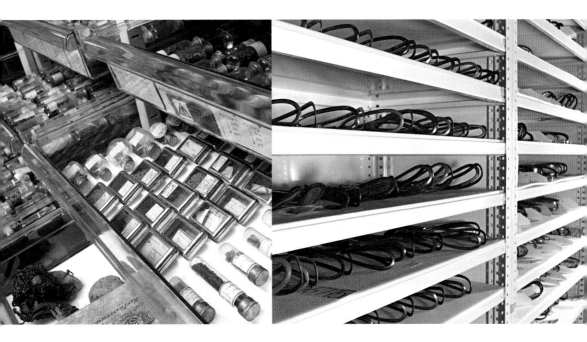

15–17 Although considerably reduced in size since Wellcome's day, the collections today remain vast. Among over 100,000 items there are multiple examples of such artefacts as materia medica specimens, obstetric forceps and medical glassware.

Henry Ford (1863–1947). The connections that could be drawn between past and present could and did serve political aims, Pitt Rivers' Farnham museum being a case in point.

There remains no comparable venture to the Wellcome Museum of the History of Medicine. Relocated, not in the national ethnographical collections, but in the National Museum of Science and Industry, the re-display of the collections also attempts a comprehensive coverage of the history of medicine. The reconstruction of cultural history, however, is no longer the peculiar province of anthropologists. Their involvement in museums not specifically devoted to non-literate cultures has greatly decreased since they abandoned their claims to universal history. Wellcome's collections, never again under the direction of an anthropologist, were greatly reduced by those subsequently responsible for them (figs 15–17). Not sharing his preoccupation with origins, they dispersed many thousands of ethnographic and

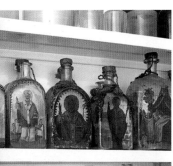

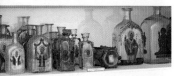

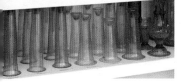

prehistoric items between 1936 and 1976. Not sharing his biologised definition of medicine as an extension of the instinct for self-preservation, they dispersed many more that now seemed unrelated to the subject. Material culture in 'non-ethnographic', 'historical' museums has come to be displayed as illustrative of textual history – an uneasy but often unprobed relationship. The Wellcome collections at the Science Museum illustrate the account of modern, textual, historians. Focusing primarily on 'society' rather than 'man', and attempting to apply the same scrutiny to present and past alike, the anthropological mode of enquiry is simply one amongst several others utilised and has ceased to predominate. A section on ethnographic medicine runs neutrally down the centre of an otherwise chronological arrangement, which takes the literate River Valley civilisations as its starting-point. There are no progressive typological sequences of objects, different artefacts from particular periods being grouped together under subject headings, such as 'Paris Medicine', which reflect an indebtedness to the constructs of modern textual historians and to the more sociological perspectives they now embrace. No historian, one suspects, would now agree with Wellcome's assertion that 'anthropology takes us from the beginning of the beginning and covers all'.

NOTES

1 'Oral Evidence, Memoranda and Appendices to the final report'. London: HMSO, p. 10.

2 Skinner, G.M. 1986. 'Sir Henry Wellcome's Museum for the Science of History' in *Medical History* 30, pp. 383–418. References for all my quotations can be found in this paper.

3 Examination of the Visitor Books reveals, however, another group of users. Artists featured quite prominently. This is surprising at first sight but it is well known that 'ethnographia' inspired several avant garde painters in the pre-war years, including Picasso and the school of Die Brücke. See Lawrence, G.M., 'Every Phase of Life and Art: The Wellcome Museum between the Wars'. Monkton Copeman Lecture, 1988, Society of Apothecaries, unpublished typescript.

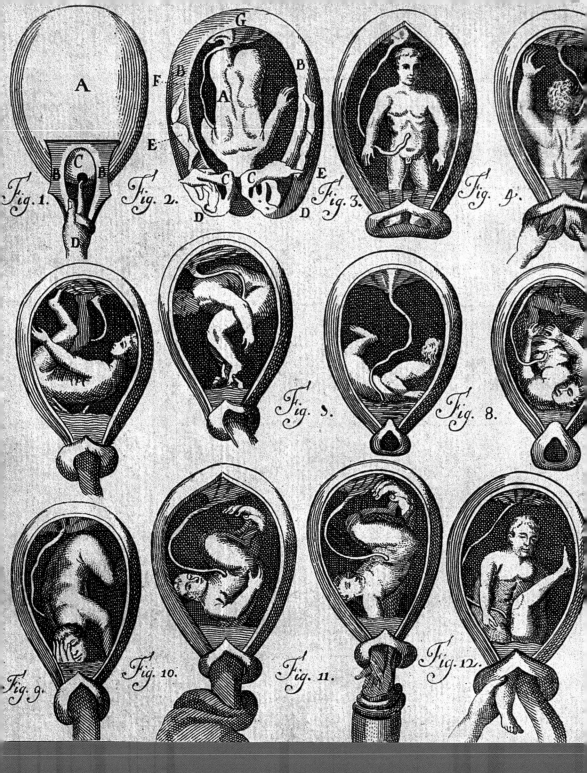

Thirteen diagrams of a child in the womb
in various positions, two obstetrical chairs
and several obstetrical instruments.
Etching by Francesco Sesone. Italian, 1749.
WL. 17074i

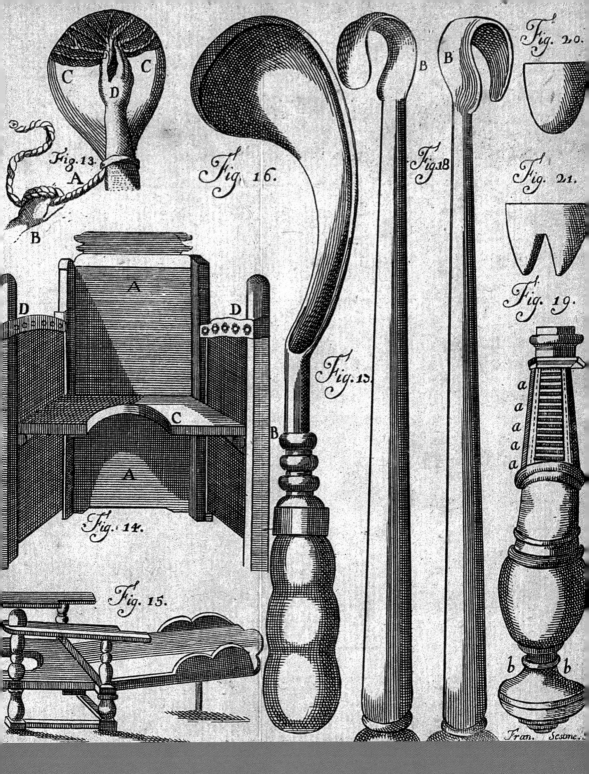

The beginning of life

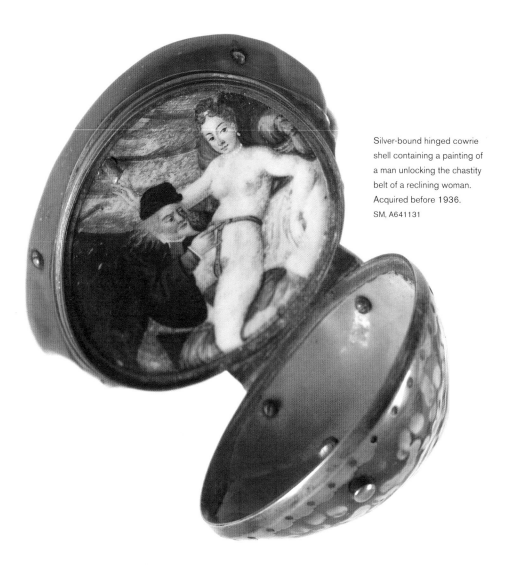

Silver-bound hinged cowrie shell containing a painting of a man unlocking the chastity belt of a reclining woman. Acquired before 1936. SM, A641131

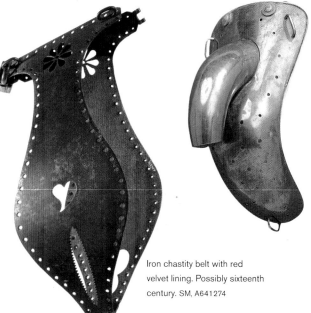

Anti-masturbation device. A metal guard shaped to cover the penis and testicles with a hole to allow for urination and metal loops for the attachment of a waistband. British, late nineteenth century. SM/SSPL, A641285

Iron chastity belt with red velvet lining. Possibly sixteenth century. SM, A641274

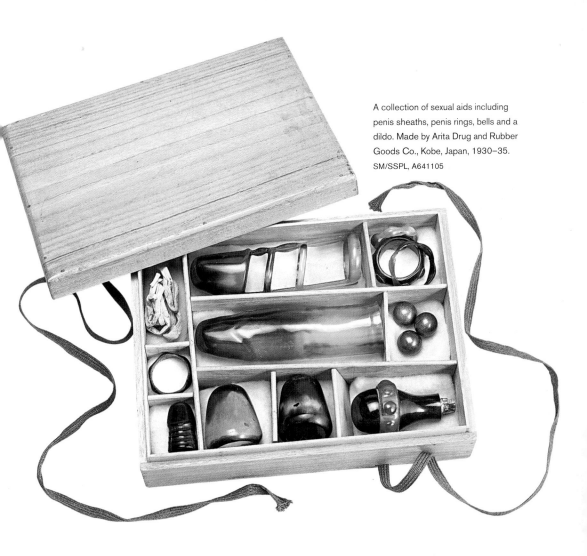

A collection of sexual aids including penis sheaths, penis rings, bells and a dildo. Made by Arita Drug and Rubber Goods Co., Kobe, Japan, 1930–35. SM/SSPL, A641105

Ivory statue in the form of a man and woman engaged in sexual foreplay. Chinese. Acquired in Paris. 1929. SM. A77274

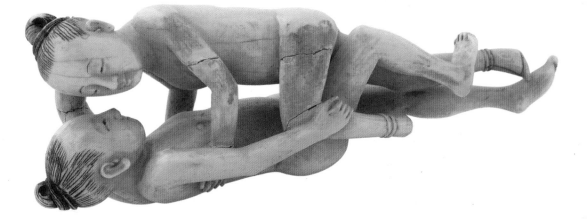

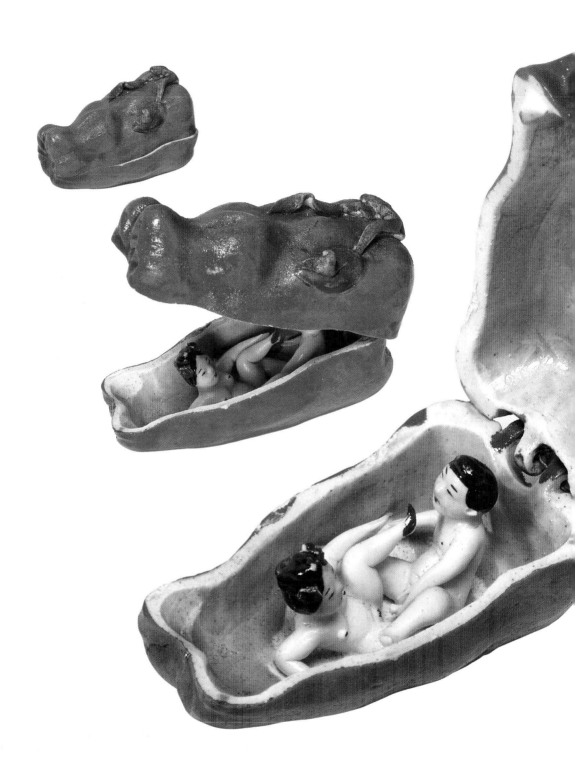

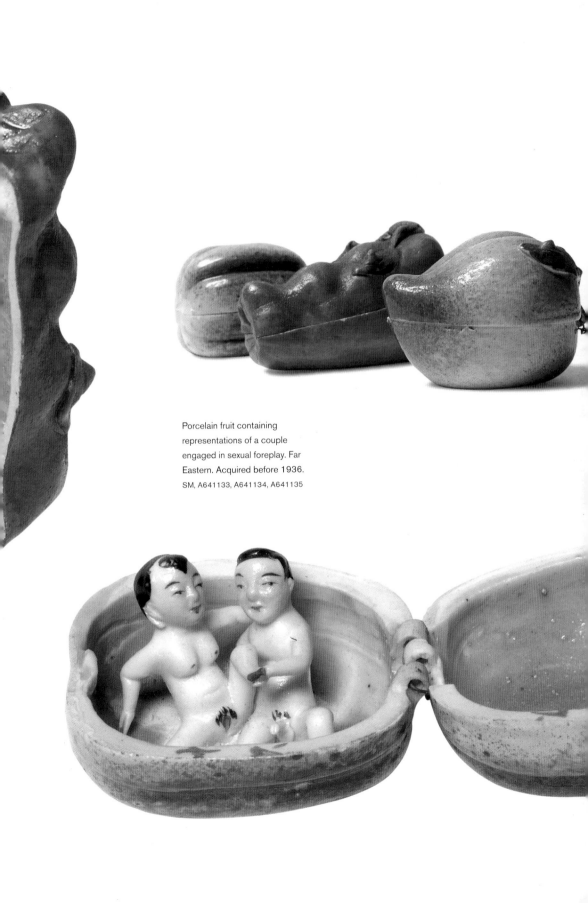

Porcelain fruit containing
representations of a couple
engaged in sexual foreplay. Far
Eastern. Acquired before 1936.
SM, A641133, A641134, A641135

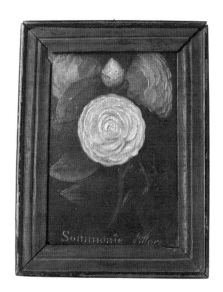

Still life of roses with concealed
erotic scenes. Oil painting by
Sommonte. Italian, nineteenth
century. WL, 47297i

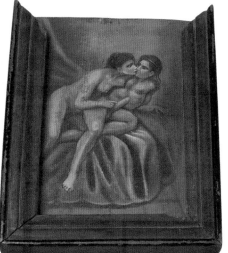

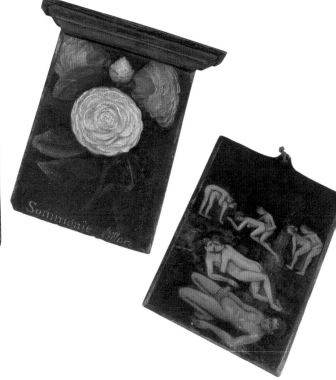

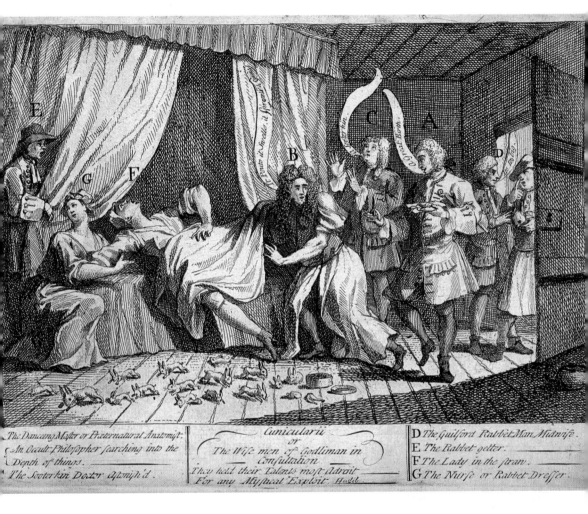

Mary Tofts duping several distinguished
surgeons, physicians and male midwives
into believing that she is giving birth to a litter
of rabbits. Etching by William Hogarth
(1697–1764). British, 1726. WL, 17342i

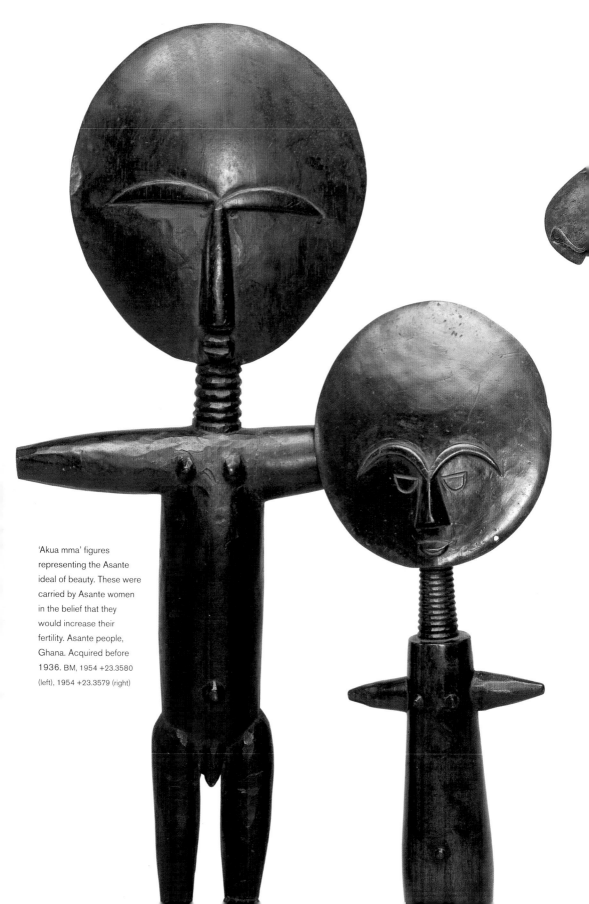

'Akua mma' figures
representing the Asante
ideal of beauty. These were
carried by Asante women
in the belief that they
would increase their
fertility. Asante people,
Ghana. Acquired before
1936. BM, 1954 +23.3580
(left), 1954 +23.3579 (right)

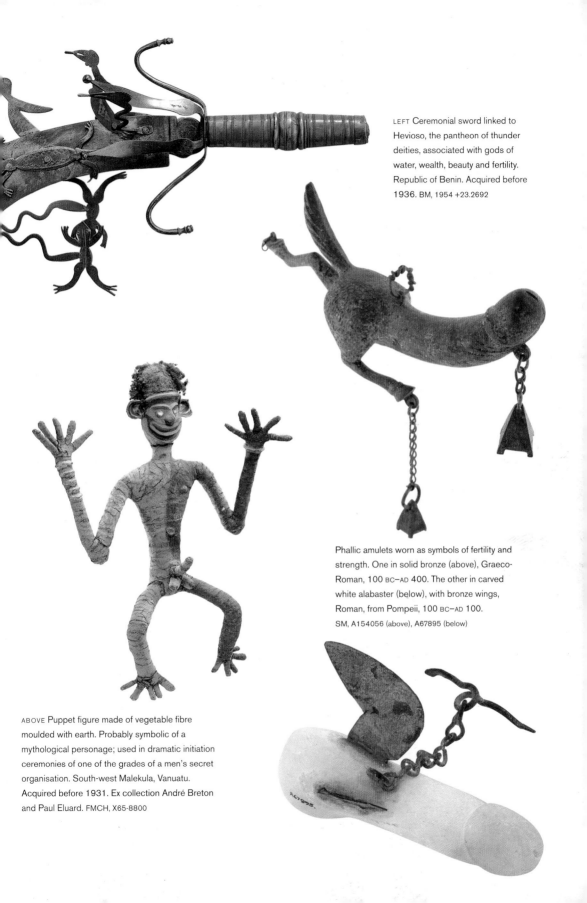

LEFT Ceremonial sword linked to Hevioso, the pantheon of thunder deities, associated with gods of water, wealth, beauty and fertility. Republic of Benin. Acquired before 1936. BM, 1954 +23.2692

Phallic amulets worn as symbols of fertility and strength. One in solid bronze (above), Graeco-Roman, 100 BC–AD 400. The other in carved white alabaster (below), with bronze wings, Roman, from Pompeii, 100 BC–AD 100. SM, A154056 (above), A67895 (below)

ABOVE Puppet figure made of vegetable fibre moulded with earth. Probably symbolic of a mythological personage; used in dramatic initiation ceremonies of one of the grades of a men's secret organisation. South-west Malekula, Vanuatu. Acquired before 1931. Ex collection André Breton and Paul Eluard. FMCH, X65-8800

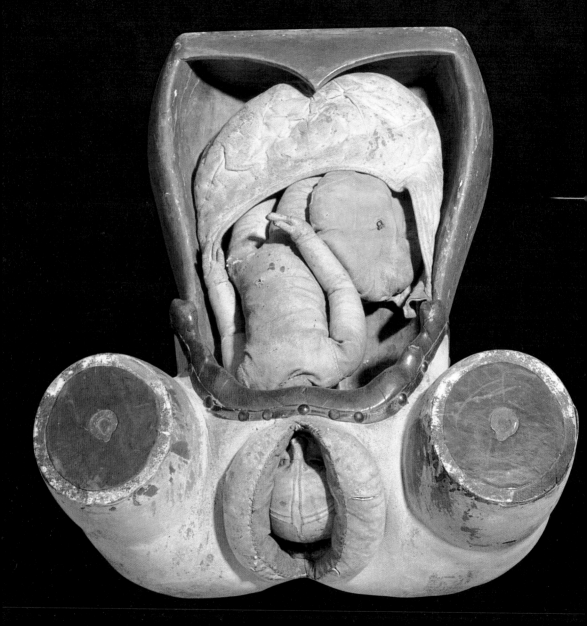

Eighteenth-century obstetric
phantom, used for teaching the
rudiments of childbirth, from the
Hospital del Ceppo in Pistoia, Italy.
It contains a doll-like foetus and is
made from leather and wood.
SM/SSPL, A600052

RIGHT Foetus in presentation
position from William Hunter's
*Anatomia uteri humani gravidi
tabulis illustrata* (*The anatomy of
the human gravid uterus exhibited
in figures*), Birmingham, 1774.
WL, EPB F.438a

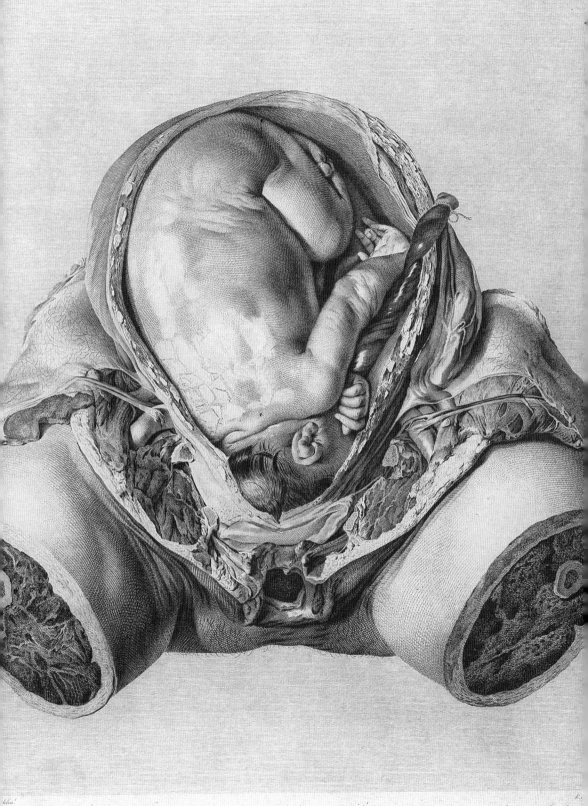

TAB. VI. *Fœtus in utero, prout a natura positus, rescissis omnino parte uteri anteriori,*
ac Placenta ei adhærente.

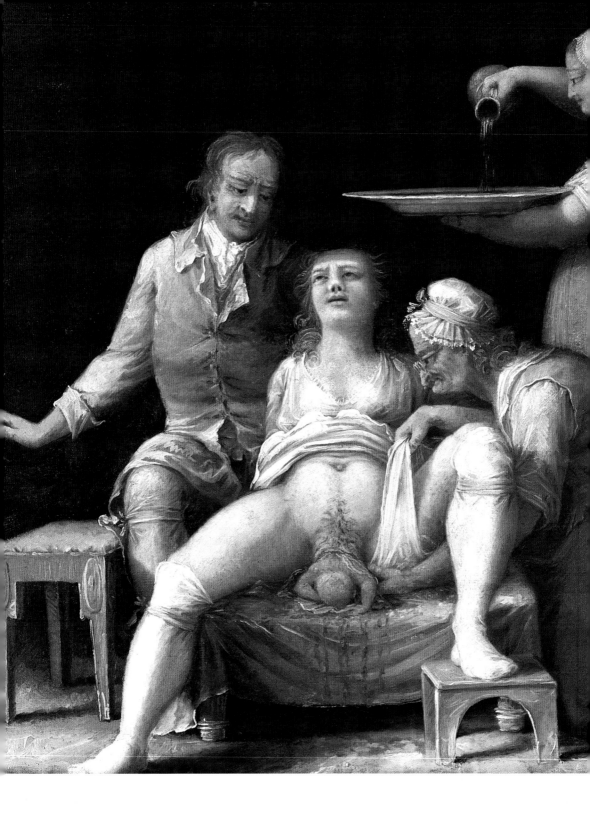

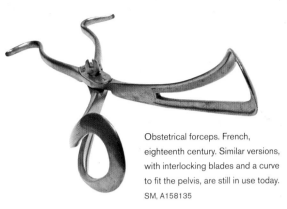

Obstetrical forceps. French, eighteenth century. Similar versions, with interlocking blades and a curve to fit the pelvis, are still in use today.
SM, A158135

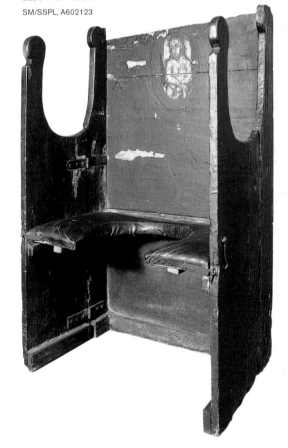

Folding birthing chair. Called the 'Miraculous Chair of Palermo', it reputedly comes from Sicily and has an image of Christ on the back. 1701–1830.
SM/SSPL, A602123

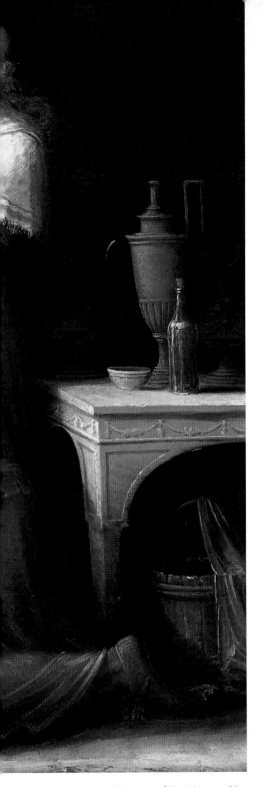

A birth scene. Oil painting, possibly by a French painter, 1800. Acquired in Åbo, Sweden (now Turku, Finland).
WL, 44694i

LEFT A pregnant
woman depicted in
a fifteenth-century
English anatomy
text. Pseudo-Galen.
WL, Western MS 290

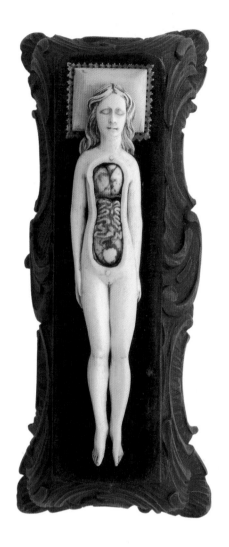

Ivory anatomical models
of pregnant females,
with removable parts.
These would have been
of little use for detailed
instruction but may have
been used by obstetric
specialists or midwives
to provide reassurance
for pregant women.
Possibly German,
c. seventeenth century.
SM, A127699 (right),
A642631 (below)

OVERLEAF The position of the
heavens at the moment of
Iskandar's birth on 25 April
1384. Iskandar ruled in Fars,
south-west Iran, from 1409
to 1414. This horoscope
predicts that he will lead a
long life of good health; he
was however deposed and
blinded by a rival and died
in prison. Kitāb-i vilādet-i
Iskandar (Horoscope of
Iskandar-Sultan ibn Umar-
Shaykh), 1411.
WL, Persian MS 474

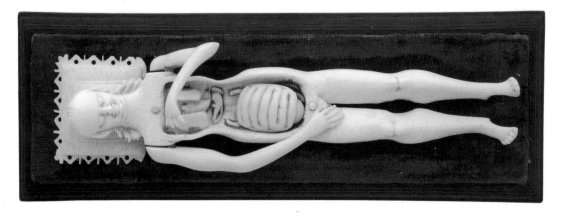

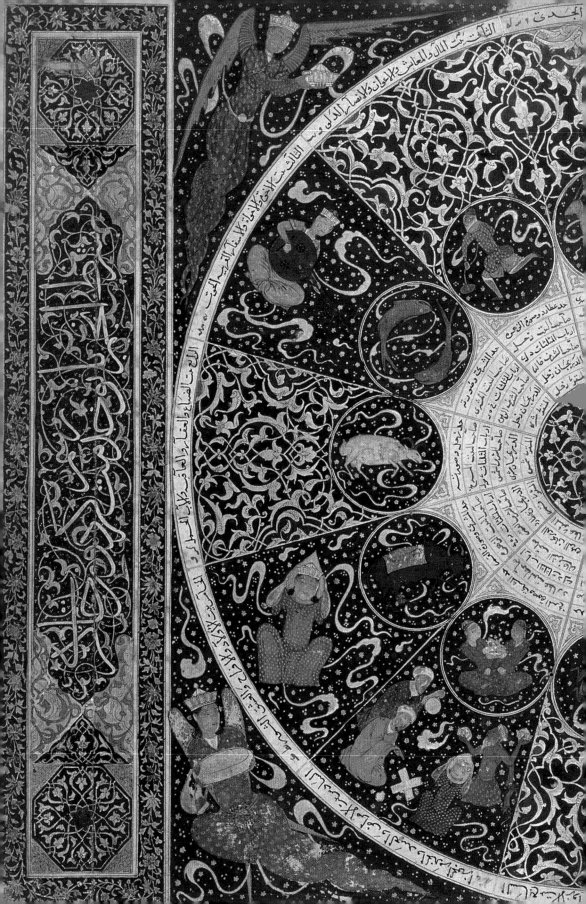

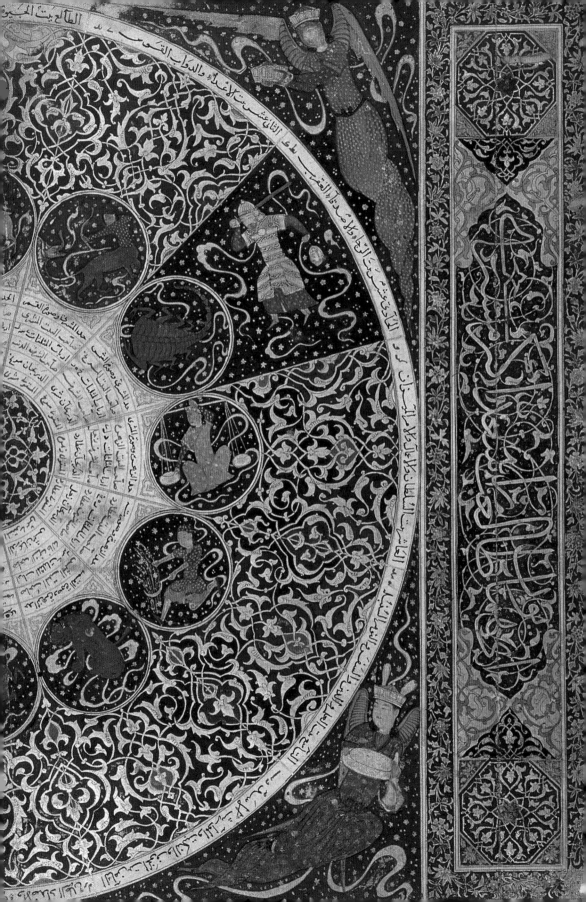

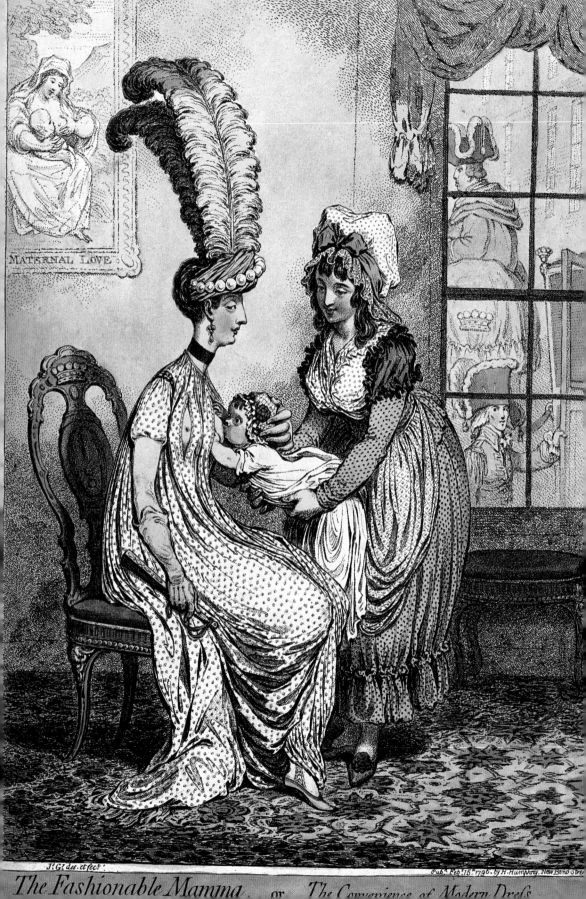

MATERNAL LOVE

The Fashionable Mamma, — or — The Convenience of Modern Dress.

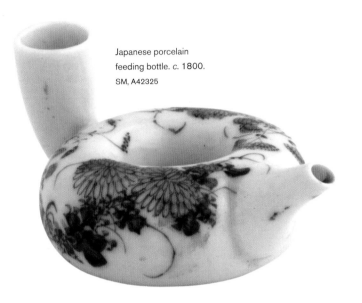

Japanese porcelain
feeding bottle. c. 1800.
SM, A42325

Sterling silver, ivory and glass
nipple-shields. The silver one is
hallmarked with the maker's initials
and George III's head, and has
been dated to 1786–1821. British.
SM, from left to right: A641255,
A606830, A606829

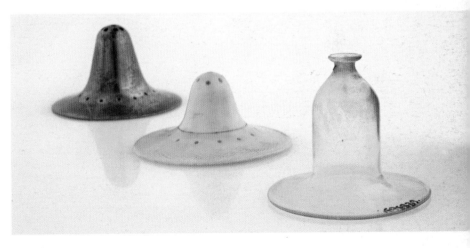

LEFT A fashionable mother wearing
a dress with slits across the
breasts in order to feed her baby
before she dashes off to the
carriage waiting outside.
Coloured etching by James Gillray
(1756–1815). British, 1796.
WL, 17465i

OVERLEAF Footprint of a baby
being taken in a hospital
to be used for identification.
Photograph, c. 1936.
WL, V31303

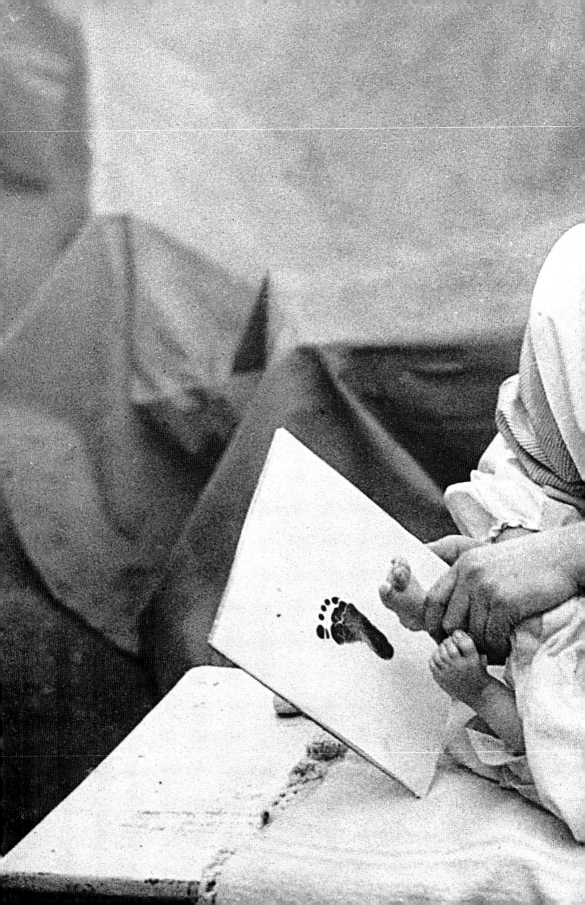

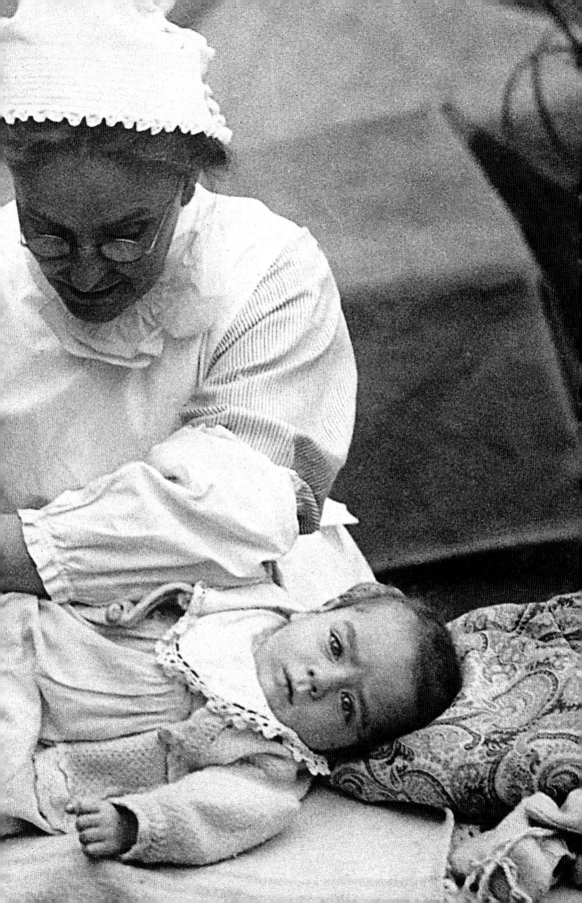

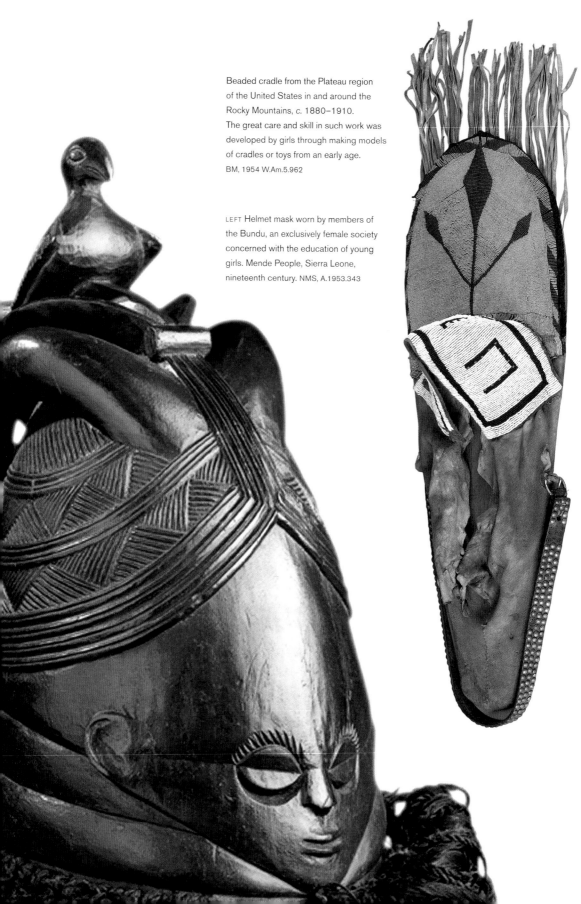

Beaded cradle from the Plateau region of the United States in and around the Rocky Mountains, c. 1880–1910. The great care and skill in such work was developed by girls through making models of cradles or toys from an early age. BM, 1954 W.Am.5.962

LEFT Helmet mask worn by members of the Bundu, an exclusively female society concerned with the education of young girls. Mende People, Sierra Leone, nineteenth century. NMS, A.1953.343

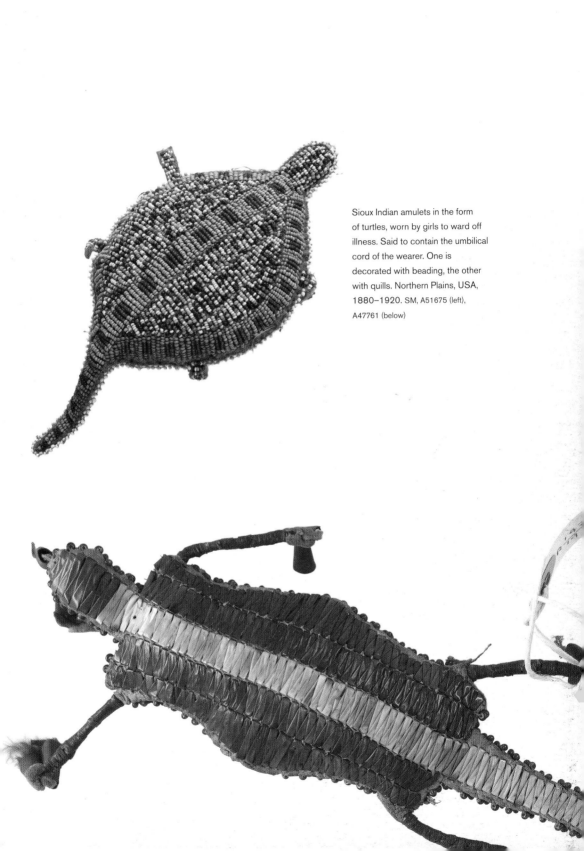

Sioux Indian amulets in the form
of turtles, worn by girls to ward off
illness. Said to contain the umbilical
cord of the wearer. One is
decorated with beading, the other
with quills. Northern Plains, USA,
1880–1920. SM, A51675 (left),
A47761 (below)

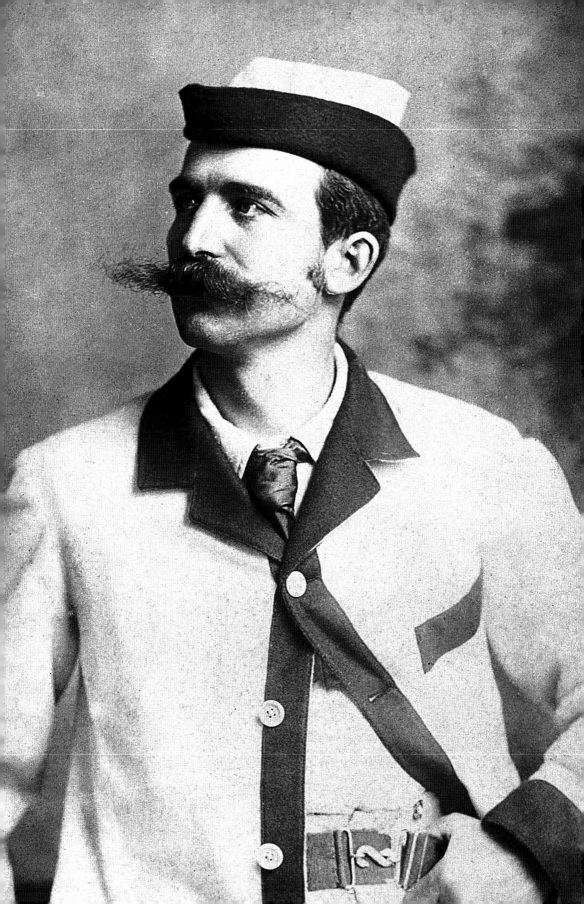

Henry Wellcome in
canoeing costume, *c.* 1884.]

‘My plans exist in my mind
like a jig-saw puzzle,
and gradually I shall be able
to piece it together.’

HENRY WELLCOME, QUOTED BY GEORGE PEARSON,
WELLCOME'S DEPUTY AND GENERAL MANAGER, 12 DECEMBER 1940.

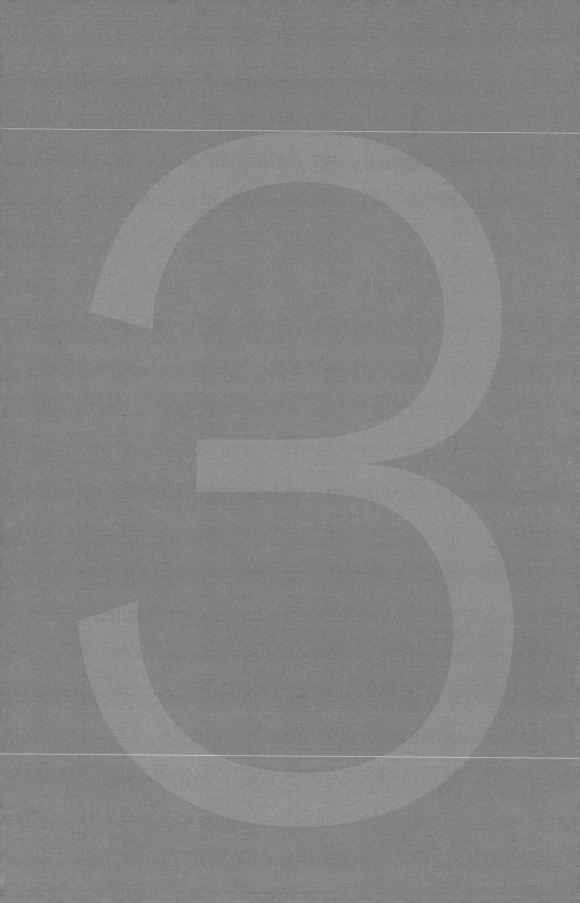

Exploring the Wellcome Library

Frances Knight

'Man alone, of all the animals, possesses the graphic instinct, and that faculty he appears to have developed from a period which is lost in the mists of antiquity. It is in the exercise of this gift that we find the genesis of journalistic record, as it is clearly evident that the earliest form of recording and disseminating news was the illustrated chronicle which prehistoric man depicted on such primitive media as horns, bones, rocks, and the walls of caves.'

(Henry Wellcome writing in the introduction to *The Evolution of Journalism. Souvenir of the International Press Conference, London, 1909*. Burroughs Wellcome & Co.)

Today the Wellcome Library brims with students of all ages who share an interest in the history of health and wellbeing. The reading rooms exist as a haven of quiet and learning hidden away on the second floor of the building Henry Wellcome himself founded on Euston Road. For me, as a student, working to piece together some of the stories which shaped Wellcome's vast historical medical collection, it is thrilling to be able to consult first-hand the material he gathered over a hundred years ago. Visitors to the Wellcome Library can still leaf through thousands of the books, prints and manuscripts, and study many of the paintings and photographs that Wellcome bought and preserved. The library has become the enduring archive of a spectacular museum collection long since scattered.

It is fitting, then, that it was the hunt for books and manuscripts which dominated Wellcome's initial forays into large-scale collecting. Although he had amassed a considerable personal collection already, the first recorded purchase made by one of Wellcome's collecting agents was that of a single book. *Receits of phisick and chirurgery* by Lady Ayscough (fig. 1) was bought in late 1897 by C.J.S. Thompson (fig. 2), a journalist and pharmacist who had been employed by Wellcome as a researcher a year previously. Indeed, discussions over book sales monopolise the earliest correspondence between Wellcome and Thompson, who later became the first curator of the Historical Medical Museum. By the time the Museum opened, however, Wellcome's financial status and personal ambitions had grown to the extent that he was employing numerous people to collect a huge variety of historical material.

The immense scale and breadth of Wellcome's collecting project has challenged curators and researchers alike since the Historical Medical Museum opened in 1913. The wealth of the Library's collections alone is staggering. From ancient Egypt's earliest herbal to Edward Jenner's *An inquiry into the causes and effects of the variolae vaccinae* (fig. 3); from an etching by Rembrandt (fig. 4) to Tibetan gouache paintings on cloth (fig. 5); from the horoscope of Iskandar Sultan, grandson of Tamerlane the Great (fig. 6) to Robert Hooke's *Micrographia* (fig. 7), the range of objects Wellcome gathered is constantly awe-inspiring. The graphic arts are variously depicted on parchment, paper, palm leaves, papyrus, vellum, ivory, metal, porcelain, glass, silk, silver, bamboo, tree bark, canvas, wood, skin and bones (figs 8 and 9). At times it seems as though Wellcome's interests showed no limits whatsoever. One of the necessary and extremely difficult processes involved in the dispersal of the collections during the middle of the last century was dividing the material up into manageable heaps for redistribution to suitable institutions. And,

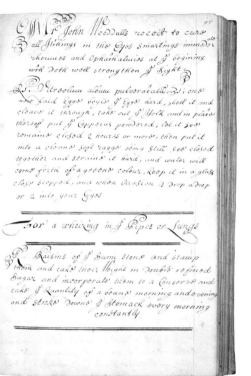

1 A page from *Receits of phisick and chirurgery*, Lady Ayscough, 1692.
WL, Western MS 1026

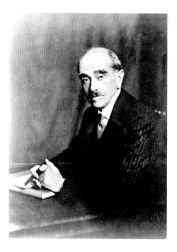

2 Portrait of Charles John Samuel Thompson (1862–1943).

most recently, the question of how to convey the scale of Wellcome's venture to the wider public has been a constant concern of the curators working on the *Medicine Man* exhibition.

Wellcome's scheme may appear incoherently inclusive but his collecting was purposeful and directed: he simply believed that all material culture could hold the key to understanding humankind. Many of his contemporaries used their collections to illustrate preconceived theories of history and evolution, making their desire for objects more directed and explicit. In contrast, Wellcome was constantly learning about the world through the collecting process. History's narrative was unfolding around him as his collection grew. This meant that his criteria for acquisition were more flexible than most, a characteristic that has caused his reputation to suffer subsequently. But Wellcome *did* decline sales if he already owned a similar piece, thought an object lacked medico-historical importance, or felt that the asking price was too high given the object's intellectual worth. His active interest in the collection's developing historical narrative is clear from the minutely explicit reports he demanded from his staff when he was abroad – detailing every purchase, every missed opportunity, every sale attended and object met with – and the care and effort he took to respond to each of these reports despite the many demands upon his time.

Although discerning, Wellcome felt that his museum collection should be as comprehensive and all-inclusive as possible since each link in the chain of knowledge was equally weighted and momentous

3 Edward Jenner's *An inquiry into the causes and effects of the variolae vaccinae*, London, 1798. WL, EPB 30385C

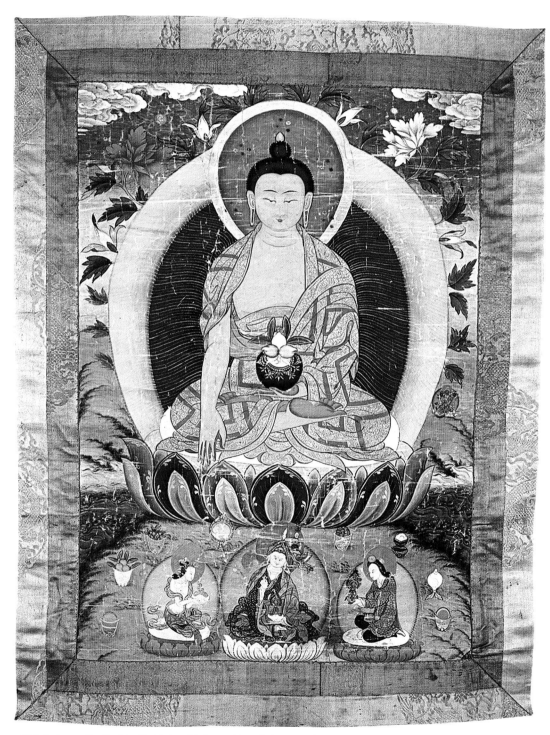

5 Bhaisajyaguru (the Medicine Buddha) and Padmasambhava (below, centre) with his two disciples.
Gouache painting by a Tibetan painter. Acquired in 1920. WL, Thanka No. 10

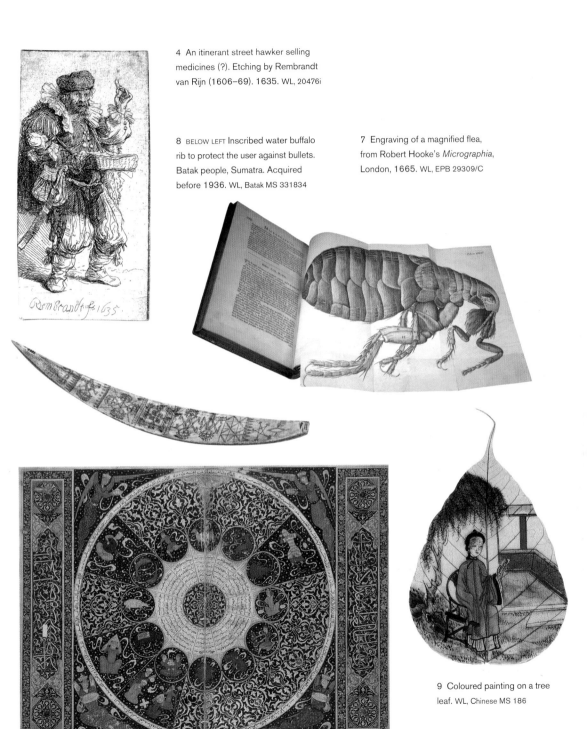

4 An itinerant street hawker selling medicines (?). Etching by Rembrandt van Rijn (1606–69). 1635. WL, 20476i

8 BELOW LEFT Inscribed water buffalo rib to protect the user against bullets. Batak people, Sumatra. Acquired before 1936. WL, Batak MS 331834

7 Engraving of a magnified flea, from Robert Hooke's *Micrographia*, London, 1665. WL, EPB 29309/C

9 Coloured painting on a tree leaf. WL, Chinese MS 186

6 *Kitāb-i vilādet-i Iskandar* (*Horoscope of Iskandar-Sultan ibn Umar-Shaykh*), 1411. WL, Persian MS 474

in reconstructing the correct path of human history. In this respect he was certainly a man of his time, in an age when collectors were 'committed to dealing with huge amounts of data' so as to minimise historical error.[1] In an early leaflet publicising the planned Historical Medical Exhibition,[2] Wellcome writes requesting donations of objects for the growing collection:

> 'Even though the items be but small, they may form important connecting links in the chain of historical evidence . . . Every little helps, and as I am desirous of making the Historical Medical Exhibition as complete as possible, I shall be grateful for any communication you may be able to make.'[3]

It was crucial for him to gather together as many varied objects as possible, to ensure that the overall picture was undiminished. Only when all the relevant material was arranged in sequence would a clear picture of the history of human health be possible.

A place for the graphic arts

Despite the breadth of his curiosity Wellcome envisaged all his objects under the same roof. Each artefact, whether book or painting, weapon, drug or costume, tool or relic, was destined to play a part in his endeavour to chart and understand the history of the earth. The graphic arts took their place alongside all manner of other objects in the Historical Medical Museum. When it opened in London in 1913 the Museum included a Gallery of Pictures, a Corridor of Photography and a Gallery of Ancient Manuscripts and Printed Books. A display of reproductions of illustrations from early manuscripts adorned the staircase to the Museum's gallery. These displays were not intended as isolated exhibits; instead they formed part of a Museum which explored the cultures of the world, from Africa, Asia, and the Pacific to ancient Greece, early Egypt and contemporary London, weaving them into a single thread of linear history. Likewise, the objects themselves were perceived as links in a common historical chain.

The Wellcome Library was part of this desire for completeness in museum documentation. The Library existed before the Museum but was subsumed into it in 1913. When asked to outline his ideal ethnographic museum for the Museums and Galleries Commission in 1928,

Wellcome included a reference library, but the Museum was itself to be, in many ways, a reference library, with an 'index series' of objects on display and a second 'comparative series' in accessible storage for additional examination by researchers. Wellcome's ambitions for this all-inclusive museum never came to fruition but his Library remained administratively linked to the Wellcome Historical Medical Museum, except for a brief period between 1961 and 1964, until the 1970s. The chief collecting agents who gathered material for Wellcome abroad – men like Louis Sambon, Paira Mall, Peter Johnston-Saint and C.J.S. Thompson – while retaining their own personal interests, collected written works, artworks and other medico-historical material concurrently.

The Wellcome collection teaches us not to be too hasty in sectioning off different types of object. Books and paintings share a special ability to mesmerise us into forgetting their physicality: we are too wrapped up in their descriptive qualities to realise the many ways that they shape our lives as *objects* which surround and frame us. As the opening quotation from Wellcome's introduction to *The Evolution of Journalism* suggests, he saw writing, printing, drawing, engraving and painting as evidence of the genesis and development of man's 'graphic instinct', and as such they found their place at the heart of the Historical Medical Museum. However, it is true to say that once absorbed into the museum the message a piece could give was limited to its particular place in the evolutionary narrative. Each artefact was lodged as a link in the historical chain, and if it expanded or broke away from that discrete chain of knowledge it would become useless and obsolete. The story of mankind as a whole was emphasised. The subtle ways in which a single artefact can act in the world were not appreciated.

Only in the last decades of the twentieth century have scholars begun to realise that objects, like books and paintings, which find their way into collections, form vital links in many, varied and ongoing chains of human interaction. They constantly bring people together – producers, collectors, curators, cultural groups, political movements, professionals and the public – and define the social interactions by which these people understand the world. Objects have many stories to tell and the hundreds of thousands of books and paintings in the Wellcome collection are no exception. At the turn of the twenty-first century, when information is increasingly transmitted

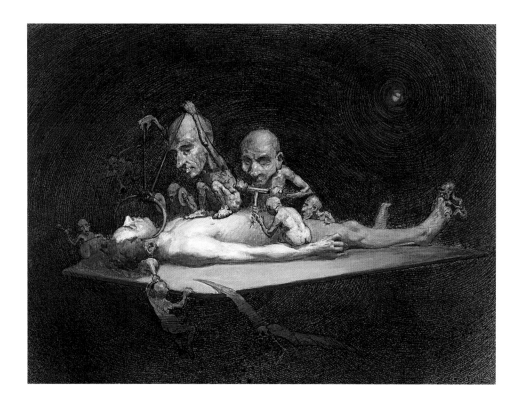

10 An unconscious naked
man lying on a table being
attacked by little demons
armed with surgical
instruments, symbolising
the effects of choloroform on
the human body. Watercolour
by R. Cooper. *c.* 1912.
WL, 24004i

in virtual form, it is worth pondering the varied layers of understanding a book or painting can give. Scientists today live in a world where images and text are forever in flux, but when printed or painted, ideas begin to shape and influence people through their physical characteristics, giving future generations a series of links into the past. A closer look at a tiny handful of Wellcome's acquisitions throws light on the business of buying, negotiating and commissioning objects for the collection in the early decades of the twentieth century. Each gives further insight into the desires of Wellcome and his employees to document and illustrate the history of humankind.

Collecting stories

Over fifty thousand of Wellcome's paintings, prints and photographs have been catalogued at the Wellcome Library. Although the total number is not known, it is estimated at over one hundred thousand. Selections are made regularly to be hung in corridors and public rooms

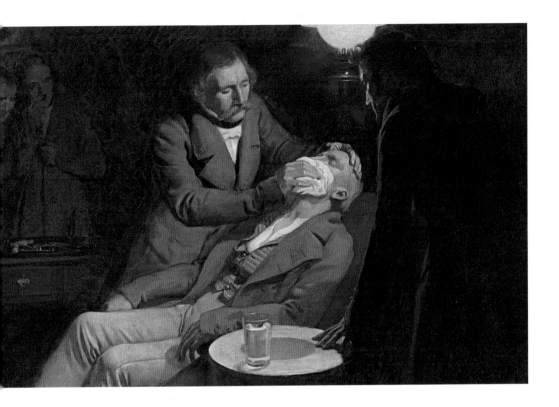

11 The first use of ether in dental surgery, 1846. Oil painting by Ernest Board. WL, 45904i

of the Wellcome Trust's Euston Road buildings. At the time of writing two oil paintings by Ernest Board are hanging in a corridor on the first floor: *Joseph Priestley, the discoverer of oxygen* and *Sir Patrick Manson experimenting with filaria sanguinis-hominis on a human subject in China.* Wellcome commissioned these works towards the end of the first decade of the twentieth century, as part of a series depicting critical moments in the history of science and medicine. He paid another illustrator, Richard Tennant Cooper, to depict the history and attributes of diseases and medical discoveries. As they worked, Board and Cooper kept Wellcome updated on their projects, but he was often abroad on business and so it fell to C.J.S. Thompson to check their progress. In fact, Thompson regularly suggested changes to the artists' compositions. His monthly reports record his alterations to Cooper's piece *The Plague* (to which he suggested the addition of more rats) and his sketches for *Anaesthesia* (fig. 10).[4] Indeed, Thompson suggested so many 'improvements' for Board's *Lavoisier, explaining the results of his experiments on air to his wife* that the artist 'has practically painted the greater part of the

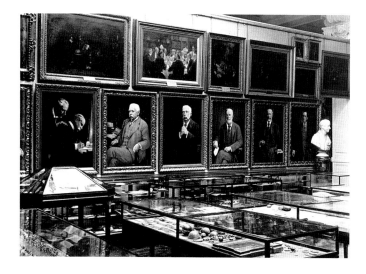

12 The Wellcome Historical Medical Museum, Wigmore Street, London: east wall of the Gallery of Pictures, c. 1914.

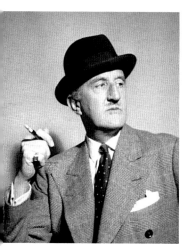

13 Captain Peter Johnston-Saint (1886–1974).

old study out'.[5] Other works were deemed more successful. Thompson wrote of Board's depiction of the first operation conducted under ether that 'the figures are well grouped and the portraits are excellent, and, beyond a few trifling alterations, I think it is the best thing he has done for us' (fig. 11).[6] What these pictures record, then, is not simply a solitary artist's impression frozen in time, but an intensive collaboration between a group of men nearly a hundred years ago.

Wellcome also commissioned H.H. Salomon to produce a series of oil portraits, from photographs, of leading men in science at that time. Salomon's works can be clearly seen in an early photograph of the Historical Medical Museum and, although not always individually inspiring, they make an impressive group when hung together (fig. 12). One of the portraits hanging today at the Wellcome Trust is of Albert Nachet, son of the microscope-maker Camille Sébastien Nachet. Wellcome actually bought the famous Nachet collection of microscopes in the late 1920s. Peter Johnston-Saint (fig. 13), who joined the Museum as Secretary in 1920 and started collecting for Wellcome in 1926, visited Albert Nachet in Paris in May 1927 to see his 'extremely important collection of old microscopes' and books on microscopy.[7] Wellcome himself felt that this collection was 'of great interest to us and should be watched very vigilantly in case it is offered for sale'.[8]

Initially, Johnston-Saint procured a handful of duplicates from Nachet, but in October of that year he began to negotiate for a larger

14 Two telegrams from Johnston-Saint to the Wellcome Museum, sent whilst he was on a collecting tour in Paris.

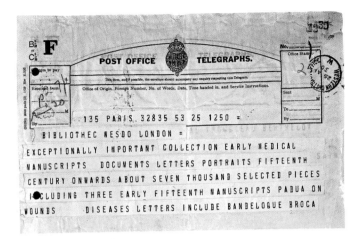

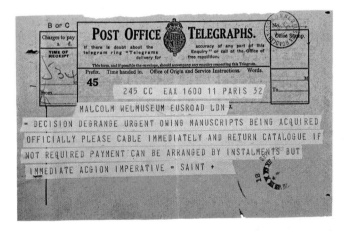

portion of the collection. His report highlights one of the problems the Museum's agents constantly struggled with: Wellcome never allowed expensive purchases to be made without his definite authority. This could stifle negotiations, especially when Wellcome himself was abroad and all correspondence had to be passed through the firm's London offices. Often discussions were conducted via telegram and it was quite a skill compressing vital information about acquisitions into just a few words (fig. 14). On this occasion, Johnston-Saint wrote from Paris:

'If I were given power to negotiate on the spot for odd instruments, I could whip them up or get off with them before he had time to change his mind. At present I cannot clinch with him

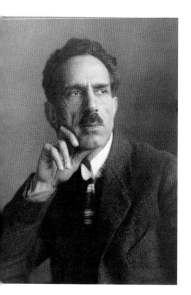

15 Paira Mall (1874–1957).

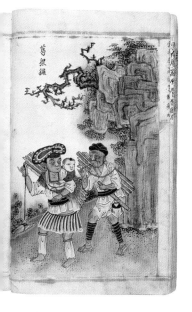

17 Yun-nan ying chih Miao-Man t'u ts'e. Result of the author's tour of inspection through Yunnan province, vol. 1.
WL, Chinese MS 103

when I get him red hot. I can only say I must come again. If it should be left to my discretion, I think I could manage things for the benefit of the Museum. At present his mind is like a balance, first it is yes, next minute it is no, and so on.'[9]

Eventually Johnston-Saint closed the deal and acquired thirty-nine microscopes 'all of the highest importance, many of them being of the 17th century', and a collection of twenty-one telescopes and spy-glasses from the same period.

Other collecting agents shared Johnston-Saint's frustrations. Cyril Barnard was working as a young librarian for Wellcome in 1919 and much of his time was spent scouring bookshops and dealers' catalogues for potential acquisitions. On one occasion he wrote to Thompson in embarrassment: 'It places me in rather an unpleasant position if I am always going into the shops and looking at books, and yet never buy anything, especially as I am not allowed to say where I come from'.[10]

When Wellcome's agents were working further afield, his exacting demands for information about purchases could be even more agonis-ing. Paira Mall (fig. 15) collected for Wellcome in India during the First World War, and in September 1919 he cabled Thompson about a valu-able collection of 1,200 manuscripts he had found at a Jain temple in Maliva. Mall considered them a bargain, since the young disciple who was in charge of the collection was willing to sell without the knowl-edge of his superiors who would never have parted with it, and the price worked out at less than five shillings per manuscript. Thompson immediately requested more information on the periods and subjects covered by the manuscripts, but having heard little by early October he decided to authorise the purchase. He later wrote to Mall: 'You will understand it is impossible for me to judge or form any idea of such a collection unless I know the approximate *period* in which they *were written*, the *subjects*, and whether illustrated by diagrams and draw-ings or not'.[11] He added that he considered the price high unless the manuscripts were of medical or surgical interest.

Notwithstanding the difficulties of communicating while abroad, Paira Mall collected thousands of manuscripts for Wellcome while in southern Asia between 1911 and 1921. The library's Oriental collec-tions are unparalleled and include such treasures as an eighteenth-century *Ketubbah* (marriage contract) (fig. 16) and a seventeenth-century report on the minority races of Imperial China (fig. 17).

16 Ketubbah (marriage contract) between
Baruch, son of the late rabbi Daniel Luzzatto,
and Hannah, daughter of the late Baruch
Kaprilis. Venice, 31 May 1754.
WL, Hebrew MS A1

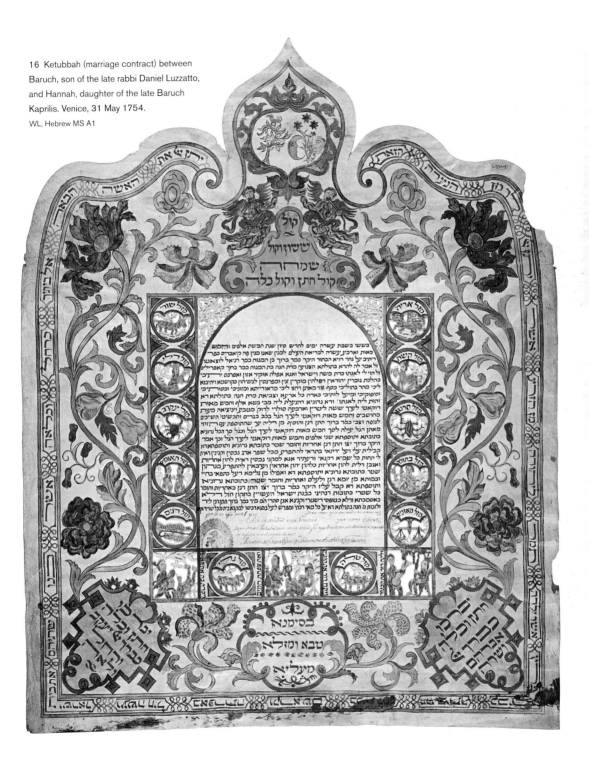

Collections within collections

Two important early acquisitions for the library were portions of the Morris Library and the Payne Library. Both were bought in the London sales rooms, which were a regular haunt for Wellcome's buyers from the late 1890s onwards. A large part of the William Morris library, which had been bought at Morris's death by a Manchester collector called Richard Bennett, came up at Sotheby's in

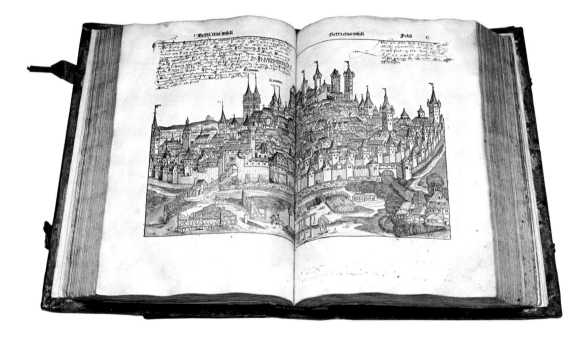

18 Hartmann Schedel, *Liber chronicarum*, Nuremberg, 1493. WL, EPB 5822

December 1898. About a third of the lots came to Wellcome, 482 in all, including a number of incunabula which were to form the foundation of his own collection.[12] Bennett was not inclined towards large folios, and this enabled Wellcome to buy many, including Schedel's famous *Liber Chronicarum*, also known as the Nuremberg Chronicle (fig. 18). This beautiful work divides the history of the world into six ages: the first five spanning the time of Creation to the birth of Christ, and the sixth and longest stretching through to the fifteenth century. A brief seventh age predicts the Last Judgement. Throughout his work, Schedel emphasised the story of the most important cities of Germany and the Western world, and it is the predominance of the illustrations and city portraits which make this Chronicle so fascinating.[13] It is estimated that only 400 copies of the Latin version (of which Wellcome's is one) and 300 copies in German survive today.[14]

A large part of the medical historian Dr J.F. Payne's library was purchased by Wellcome, again from Sotheby's, where it was offered as a single lot in 1911 (fig. 19). William Osler, a rival bidder, remembered the occasion: 'A more rapid sale I never saw! The bidding began at £2,000, and within a minute it was knocked down to an unknown bidder at £2,300'.[15] Wellcome's agent, recorded as 'Tobin', has never been identified, although it may have been Thompson himself: the cancelled cheques for payment of the Payne collection have recently been found amongst some of his personal papers. If he did indeed keep these as a memento for the rest of his life, he obviously considered the purchase a major triumph.[16] The acquisition of the Payne collection, which was an excellent general library of medical history, 'gave Wellcome's library a much improved coherence'.[17]

Perhaps the largest medical collection acquired by Wellcome was that of Evangelista Gorga, and a selection of Gorga's Italian ex-voto paintings have been selected for the *Medicine Man* exhibition (figs 20–23). Gorga was based in Rome, and his negotiations with the Wellcome Museum win the prize for the most protracted and difficult throughout the history of the Museum. Gorga met and dealt with at least four of Wellcome's staff over a sixteen-year period. His collection was first mentioned in early 1912 by Louis Sambon, a specialist in tropical diseases who worked for Wellcome during the run-up to the Museum's opening in 1913. It is rather fitting that Sambon wrote to Thompson that, 'in Rome there is an antiquarian Signor Gorga who has a splendid collection of Medical Antiquities he will not sell',[18] because it took Thompson twelve years to secure a portion of this collection for the Museum. Although approaches were made in 1912, eventually the War stalled negotiations. Then, in 1919, Thompson visited Rome to view the collection for the first time. Gorga, 'a wily and cunning-looking type of Italian' was in perpetual financial difficulties, but from the start Thompson could see that he was 'evidently going to be most difficult to deal with'.[19] One of the Museum assistants, Arthur Amoruso, visited Gorga in late 1915 – it was rather handy for Thompson that Amoruso was stationed in Naples at the time, serving in the army of his native Italy – and wrote back that

'Unfortunately, besides his own particular vices, he has also those of most collectors who wish to sell their precious ware. As a consquence his conception of prices is fabulous and not seldom exaggerates the importance and age of the objects'.[20]

Everyone who visited the Gorga collection was stunned by its vast size. It included thousands of Greco-Roman antiquities, early drug jars and mortars, ancient pharmaceutical apparatus and surgical instruments, statues, furniture, books and diplomas, charms and votive offerings, medicine chests, even a room full of 'articles of infusion' including tea pots and cups.[21] In 1921, Sambon noted that he was occupying 'no less than eight apartments merely as warehouses'.[22] It took Thompson three days to complete his inspection of the Gorga material in 1919, and by 1922 he noted that the 'medical collection alone . . . occupies eight rooms as well as the corridors in between which are full of objects'. In 1923, after continuous wranglings over price and selections, Thompson became concerned that Gorga might start playing off interest in his collection from American collectors and this may have prompted Wellcome's offer of £8,000 for a portion of the collection later that year. Negotiations continued into early 1924 when Thompson finally visited Italy to supervise the packing and transport of the antiquities into storage in Milan.

Wellcome's project was directed on such a vast scale that it would be surprising not to find a significant number of replicated objects in his collections. Some groups of similar acquisitions are particularly striking and can give us insight into his intellectual motivations. For instance, there are around seventy-five oil paintings currently held at the Wellcome Library, which are often referred to as 'alchemist' paintings, depicting alchemists or early physicians in their laboratories. (This number is not representative of the number Wellcome actually collected since many duplicates were dispersed following his death.) Initially, it is surprising that Wellcome should want so many similar works, until one remembers the intellectual framework within which he created his museum. Here is an extreme example of his desire for 'completeness'. Similarly, in April 1917 Thompson wrote informing Wellcome that he was 'endeavouring to get together photographs of all the known portraits of William Harvey in collections, both public and private throughout the country . . . to make our collection as perfect as possible'. Wellcome replied that this was a 'good plan for all *important*

19 Dr Payne's collection gave Wellcome a ready-made medico-historical library and included such classic printed books as the first edition of *De humani corporis fabrica*, by Andreas Vesalius, Basle, 1543. WL, EPB 6560

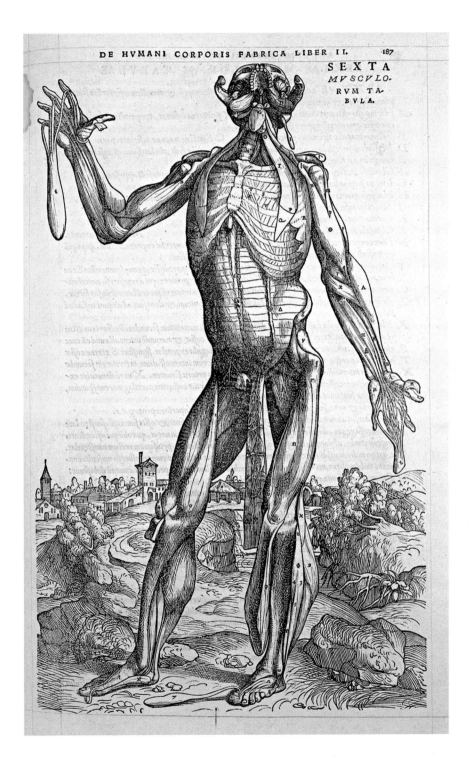

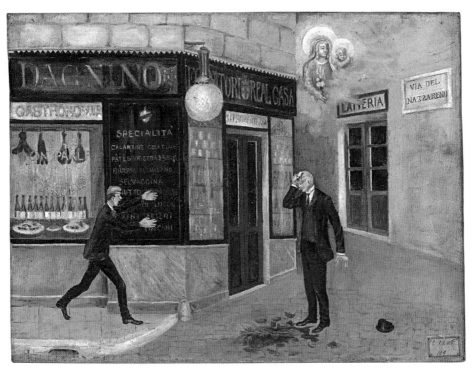

20 A man hit on the head by a falling flowerpot in Rome. Oil painting. Italian, *c.* 1890. WL, 44873i

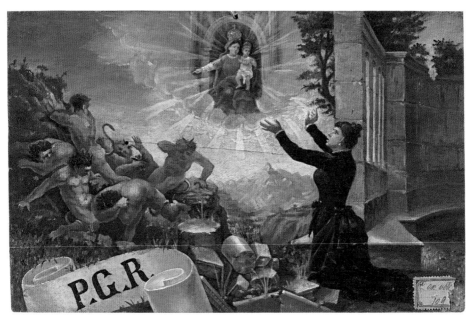

21 A woman thanking the Madonna del Parto for curing her of insanity. Oil painting. Italian, nineteenth century. WL, 44882i

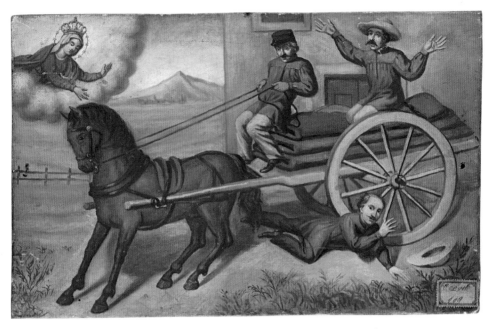

22 A man praying to the Virgin as he is run over by a horse-drawn cart. Oil painting. Italian, nineteenth century. WL, 44887i

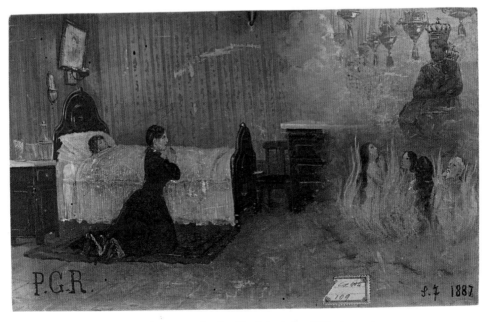

23 A woman praying for a child, with intercessors in a fire. Oil painting. Italian, 1887. WL, 44883i

figures in Med. Surg. Science' (italics in original).[23] A successful collection for Wellcome and his contemporaries meant procuring, copying or photographing every known example of a material type. Hence the extraordinary number of 'alchemist' paintings bought in sales rooms and abroad throughout the first decades of the twentieth century.

Documenting science

One aspect of this collecting criterion, which is especially apparent in the iconographic collections, is the sacrifice of aesthetic quality in favour of subject matter. While other collectors competed for the highly esteemed artworks of the day, Wellcome constantly avoided dealers who were selling rare etchings by Rembrandt and Whistler, or full-length portraits by artists such as Reynolds and Romney.[24] Despite his impressive purchasing power, there are very few pictures in the collection which would be considered 'star' pieces in the art world, and those that do exist were bought for their medical or anthropological associations. The famous van Gogh etching of Dr Paul-Ferdinand Gachet is one such example (fig. 24). In 1927, Johnston-Saint was in touch with Gachet's son, Paul-Louis. He knew of Gachet père's expertise in homeopathy, the treatment of melancholia and electrical therapeutics, and was interested in procuring any effects associated with the doctor. Amongst a variety of Gachet's apparatus and surgical instruments, he secured a print by van Gogh, *L'Homme à la Pipe*, for £5.16s.8d. This, the artist's only etching, was initially printed on Gachet's private press.[25] Gachet, who was an artist himself, had befriended van Gogh and, whereas previous doctors had diagnosed his psychotic illness as epilepsy, Gachet suggested it was due to too much sun and turpentine poisoning. Although his diagnosis was almost certainly erroneous, he later pronounced van Gogh cured and, in turn, the artist produced three studies of his doctor: the etching along with two works in oil.[26] One of the paintings, developed from the etching, broke all records when it sold at auction for $82.5 million in May 1990.

Wellcome was driven by a desire to document the history of mankind, hence the works by Board and Cooper, and illustrators like them. Even when artists were commissioned to produce works it was always the need to document over and above aesthetic criteria which

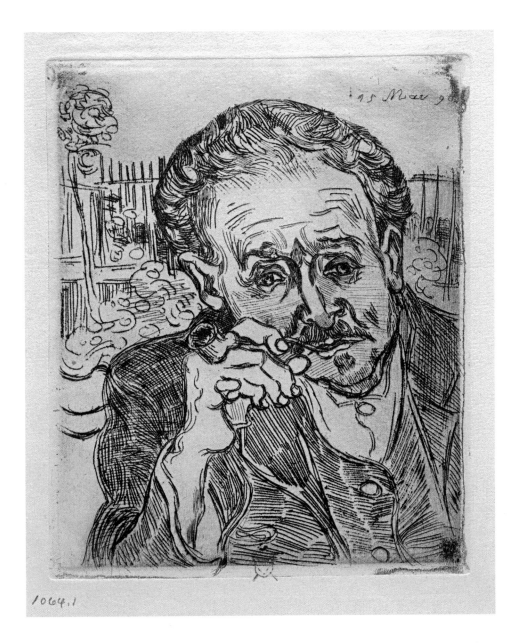

24 *L'Homme a la pipe: portrait du Docteur Gachet.* Etching by Vincent van Gogh (1853–1890). Dutch, 1890. WL, 3418i

motivated Wellcome. Edward S. Curtis, the photographer and anthropologist, is another artist whose works now reside in the Wellcome Library (figs 25–6). Curtis is famous for his ethnographic project *The North American Indian*. These twenty volumes of illustrated text and accompanying portfolios of large-size photogravures took him nearly

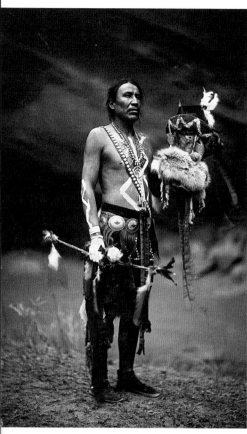

25 A Navajo man in ceremonial dress
representing the Yebichai god Za-Ha-
Bol-Zi. Photograph by Edward S. Curtis,
1904. WL, 559067i

26 RIGHT Navajo war gods.
Photograph by Edward S. Curtis, 1904.
WL, icv 39041

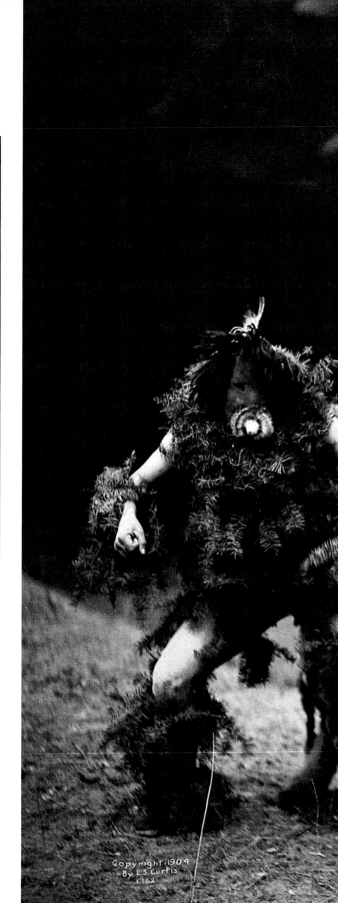

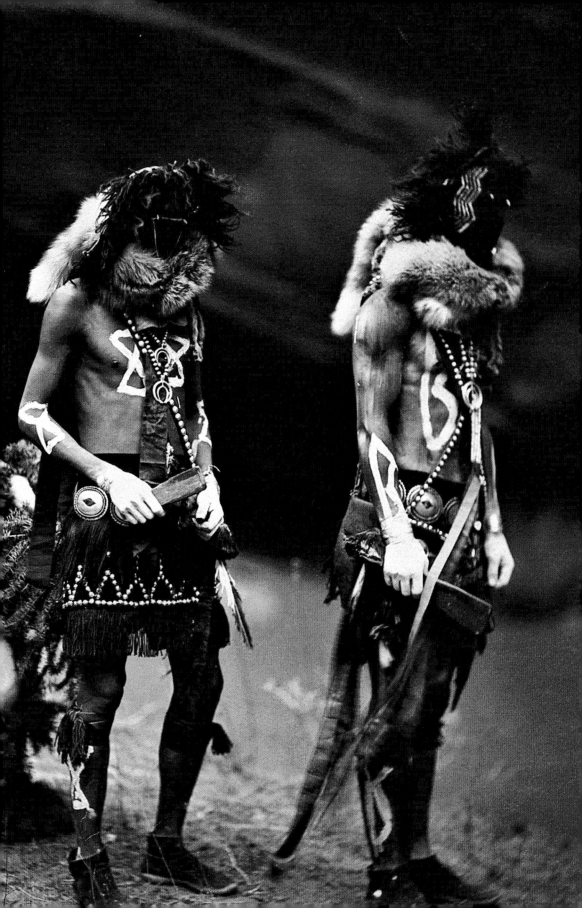

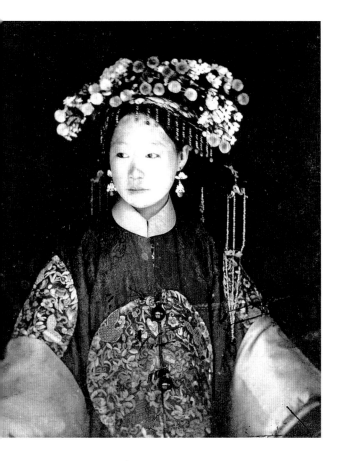

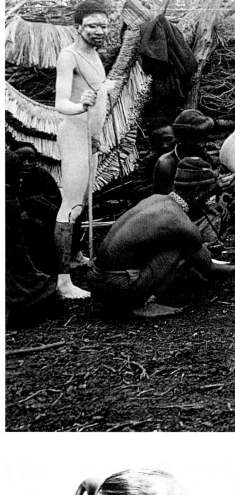

27 Manchu bride, Peking, China. Photograph from a negative by John Thomson, 1871/2. WL, 19685i

28 RIGHT Old woman, Canton, China. Photograph from a negative by John Thomson, 1869. WL, 19579i

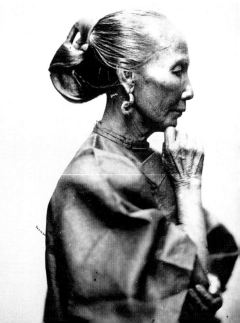

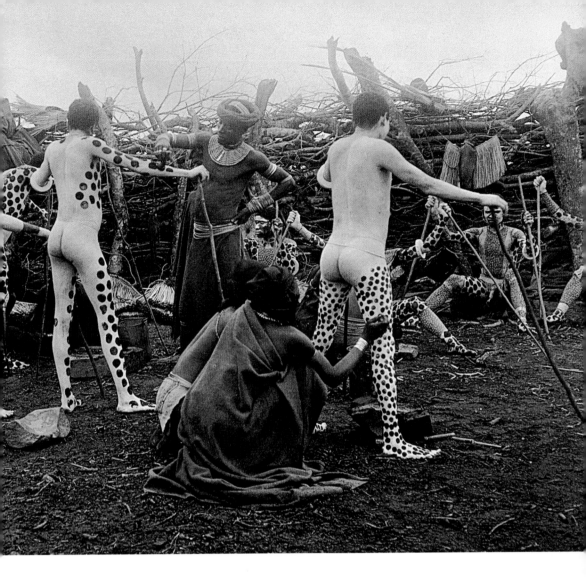

29 AmaBomvana tribe
members being painted,
South Africa. Photograph
by Alfred M. Duggan-Cronin,
early twentieth century.
WL, 541220i

thirty years to complete and were published between 1907 and
1930.[27] He intended them to be the most comprehensive compendium possible, and to present the very essence of the Native
American peoples. It has been argued that 'the documentary and
aesthetic impulses are inextricably expressed to perfection in Curtis's
works',[28] which makes the presence of his photographs in Wellcome's
collection appropriate, especially in the light of Wellcome's own personal investment in the welfare of the Native Americans. Other
countries are also represented in the photographic collections at the
Wellcome Library, which include John Thomson's photographs from
China (figs 27–8) and A.M. Duggan-Cronin's images of South Africa
and its peoples (fig. 29).

Wellcome's role in the production of the Burroughs Wellcome
souvenir book *The Evolution of Journalism* (fig. 30), which was brought

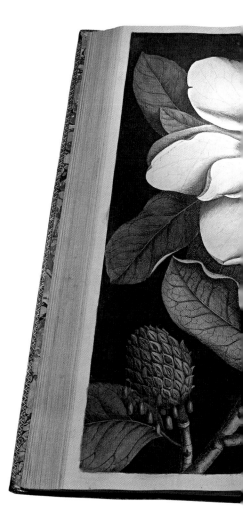

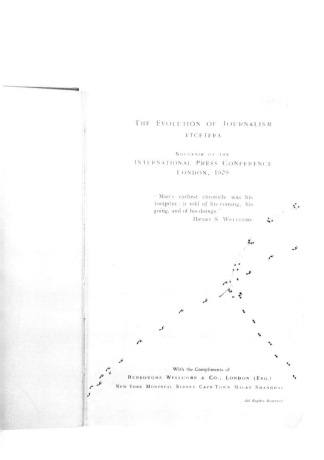

THE EVOLUTION OF JOURNALISM
ETCETERA

SOUVENIR OF THE
INTERNATIONAL PRESS CONFERENCE
LONDON, 1909

"Man's earliest chronicle was his
footprint ; it told of his coming, his
going, and of his doings."
HENRY S. WELLCOME

With the Compliments of
BURROUGHS WELLCOME & CO., LONDON (ENG.)
NEW YORK MONTREAL SYDNEY CAPE TOWN MILAN SHANGHAI

All Rights Reserved

30 *The Evolution of
Journalism, etcetera: Souvenir
of the International Press
Conference*, London, 1909.
WL, Wellcome Coll. 223

out to accompany the International Press Conference held in London
in 1909, is a clear reminder of his belief that print and pictures were
vital links in the chain of history, and should be thought of as historical evidence. This book, which is predominantly pictures, outlines the
historical progression of print journalism from prehistoric times to
the present day. Wellcome's interest in pictures and print as historical
documents draws us back to some of the gems of his book collection.
Staying, for the moment, with the American theme, Wellcome would
have admired the remarkable artworks in Mark Catesby's book *The*

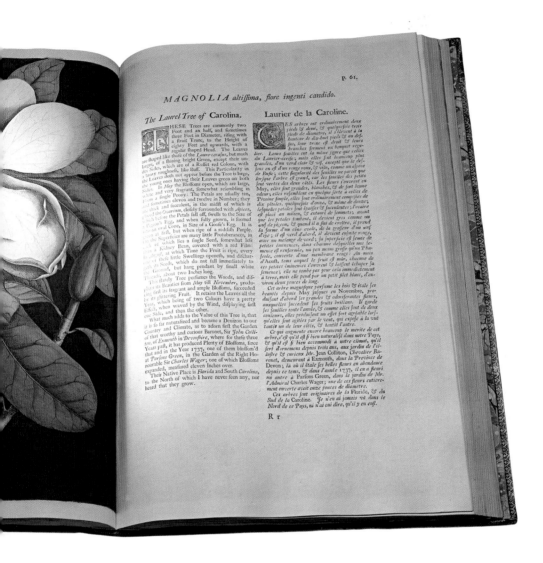

31 Mark Catesby, *The Natural History of Carolina, Florida and the Bahama Islands*, vol. 1, London, 1731–43. WL, EPB F.963

Natural History of Carolina, Florida and the Bahama Islands which was completed in 1747 (fig. 31). One commentator has observed that 'It is impossible to convey to a reader who has not seen the original editions of Catesby's masterpiece the full splendor of his hand-coloured, meticulously detailed engravings, all of which he had cut himself'.[29] Perhaps Wellcome admired Catesby's belief that his art was not merely illustration, but 'presented American nature as it really was'.[30]

Another landmark work of natural history, Georges Buffon's *Histoire Naturelle*, also resides in the Wellcome collections. Buffon, 'one of the

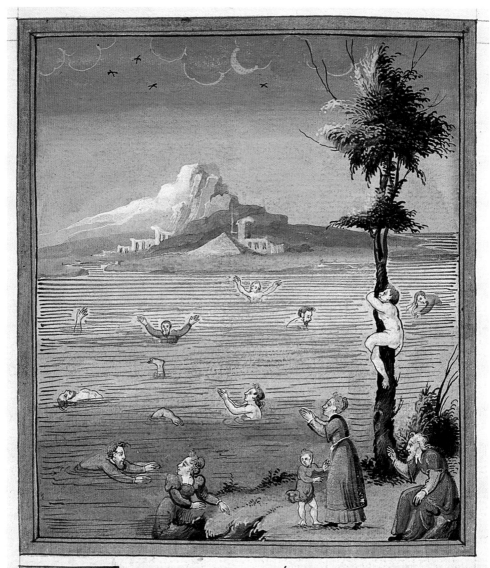

LANTIQVITÉ *a tant experimenté de*
chaſtimens de ſeau, que ſi ie les voulois tous
recenſer par ordre, ſa parolle me deffaudroit
plus toſt que le ſubieƈt. Le premier, & le plus memora=

32 LEFT Different regions
and provinces submerged
and drowned by deluges
and inundations of water.
Illustration from the manuscript
Histoires Prodigieuses
by Pierre Boaistuau.
French, 1560.
WL, Western MS 136

giants of the French Enlightenment'[31] and a contemporary of
Catesby, completed his vast work in fifteen volumes over a twenty-year
period. In it, he touched on the history and theory of the earth, the
formation of the planets, and a study of man which covered physiology, psychology and ethnology. He went on to describe and classify all
species of animal and plant. The last volume, a *History of Quadrupeds*,
was completed in 1767 when Buffon was sixty years old. Both enthu-
siastic and unrealistic, the scale of Buffon's project in many ways
reflects Wellcome's own. Incidentally, Johnston-Saint was promised
the very important Buffon microscope by Albert
Nachet during negotiations for his collection in
1928. An inscription on the microscope records
that it was presented to Buffon by his pupils.

A rather more fantastical, but equally impressive, work of historical documentation is that of
Pierre Boaistuau's manuscript version of *Histoires
Prodigieuses* (fig. 32). This manuscript was produced by the Frenchman Boaistuau as a forerun-
ner to the printed version, and was presented in
person to Queen Elizabeth I by the author in 1559.
Wellcome bought it for £95 in 1931 when it was
put up for sale at Sotheby's as part of the library of
the late John Thomas Adams, a discerning book
collector based in Sheffield.[32] The later, printed version of the work – a popular anthology of marvels
including Siamese twins, ghosts, floods, superstitions and multiple births – contains a note by
Boaistuau recounting his reception by the Queen
of England, 'who, despite the fact that she was
not well when I arrived, and that she had every
reason not to be accessible to persons of such

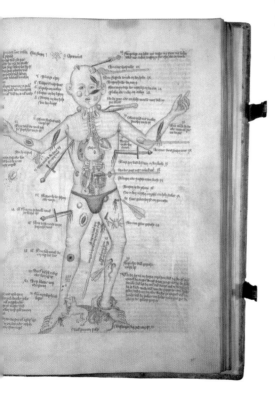

33 'Wound Man' illustration
from the German Wellcome
Apocalypse. *c.* 1420.
WL, Western MS 49

little quality as myself, did me the very great honour of having me
summoned before her Majesty, where in the presence of several
great lords and ladies, she began to speak on several lofty and difficult subjects'.[33] Another of the Library's most prized possessions,
the fifteenth-century German manuscript known as the Wellcome
Apocalypse (fig. 33), was bought at the same sale in 1931. Wellcome spent £2,300 on this single work: it was a purchase that

attracted much press attention, no doubt to Wellcome's personal annoyance because he always resented publicity.[34]

Recent reflections

It is appropriate to end with some commentary on the relevance of Wellcome's legacy today. The value of his collection is particularly evident to me as I have been working on my doctoral thesis in the archives of the Wellcome Library for the past two years. When I started my project it was easy to get the impression in academic circles that Wellcome was seen as something of a hopeless eccentric: a social recluse in his later years, who spent too much money on objects which were of little research value. His vast collection has been seen variously as purposeless, indiscriminating and even misguided. But, rather than having too much money and not enough sense, I think of Wellcome as a man who had too *little* money to carry though his ambitious intellectual purpose. Similarly, Wellcome – ever the perfectionist – ran out of time. An employee, William Britchford, remembered: 'one of the things about Sir Henry was that he never thought he would die. [Even in old age] he would talk about things he wanted done in five years time and ten years time'.[35] Wellcome's aspirations may have been somewhat unrealistic, but his ideas were not misguided. A handful of recent developments in today's world of art, books and culture will illustrate that, on the contrary, Wellcome was a man ahead of his time. I leave them with you as a reminder, for want of a better phrase, not to judge a book by its cover.

In 2001 the National Portrait Gallery unveiled its first entirely conceptual portrait. Mark Quinn's work is called *A Genomic Portrait: Sir John Sulston* and it was jointly commissioned by the Gallery and the Wellcome Trust. Sulston was director of the Sanger Centre which has spearheaded the UK's contribution to the Human Genome Project and the portrait consists of Sulston's DNA. It seems, then, that Wellcome's criteria for commissioning works on the basis of their subject matter is not as alien to the modern art world as one might expect. Indeed, the National Portrait Gallery also makes subject choice a high priority in its current acquisitions policy.

In April 2000 Re:source, The Council for Museums, Archives and Libraries, was launched as a new government body replacing the previous Museums and Galleries Commission, and the Library and Information Commission. It includes for the first time historical archives within its portfolio. On its website, Re:source is described as 'the strategic body working with and for museums, archives and libraries, tapping the potential for collaboration between them', and one of its aims is to establish a single database for the nation's collections. The manifold links between different types of object, more usually kept apart in libraries, museums and art galleries, are being prioritised in a way Wellcome himself would have appreciated. While disciplinary divisions bring strengths and insights, Wellcome always understood that it was equally important to appreciate, and try to understand, the ways in which various cultural artefacts are part of an altogether larger whole.

Perhaps the most apt modern development to finish on is that of computer power. The computer may be the only 'storehouse' large enough and flexible enough to accommodate the Wellcome collection for future researchers. All the documentation relating to the Wellcome Historical Medical Museum has recently been fully catalogued on to a computer database, and is accessible via the Internet.[36] This is a development which makes the groundwork for research like mine beautifully simple when before it would have been much slower and more complicated. Wellcome himself looked forward to a museum designed specially to house his collection for scholars and students, but in reality the scale of his collecting project was too vast for human hands to deal with. His staff were simply unable to keep up with the rate of acquisition and rooms full of packing cases and boxes lay untouched for years until they were redistributed to other institutions decades after his death. The computer has revolutionised the accessioning and cataloguing process for museums and libraries.

Computer power also raises new problems. A conference hosted by the Wellcome Trust in February 1999 – *A Healthy Heritage: Collecting for the Future of Medical History* – brought to the fore many new issues that curators are having to address. For example, it is thought that two million articles are published every year in biomedical science alone, and this excludes all the information to be found on the Internet. In fact, electronic modes of publication are now so dominant that 'some academic scientists never enter the traditional research library'.[37] Medical Libraries are having to work together to keep up with the floods of current scientific research and publication. Such changes in the world of information are bringing new challenges for librarians and curators, which might even have outdone a man as fervent and ambitious as Henry Wellcome, but the power of the computer is surely a resource he would have embraced. It might even have helped him get a little closer to his elusive, all-inclusive research museum.

NOTES

1 Skinner, G. 1986. 'Sir Henry Wellcome's Museum for the Science of History' in *Medical History* 30, p. 404.

2 Possibly dated to 1904; see Symons, J. 1993. *Wellcome Institute for the History of Medicine: A Short History*. London: The Wellcome Trust, p. 6.

3 WA/HMM/PB/Han/1. The prefix WA/HMM refers to the Wellcome Historical Medical Museum Archives, one of nine collections which make up the Wellcome Archives kept at the Wellcome Library.

4 WA/HMM/RP/Tho/4 and 6.

5 WA/HMM/RP/Tho/4.

6 Ibid.

7 WA/HMM/RP/Jst/B.1.

8 Ibid.

9 WA/HMM/RP/Mal/3.

10 Symons, J. 1998. '"These crafty dealers". Sir Henry Wellcome as a Book Collector' in Myers, R. and Harris, M. (eds), *Medicine, Mortality and the Book Trade*. Kent: St Paul's Bibliographies/Oak Knoll Press, p. 119.

11 WA/HMM/CO/Ear/566.

12 Symons 1993, p. 4.

13 Schedel, H.; introduction and appendix by Füssel, S. 2001. *Chronicle of the world: the complete and annotated Nuremberg chronicle of 1493*. Köln and London: Taschen, p. 8.

14 Ibid., p. 32.

15 Symons, J. 1997. 'Illustrations from the Wellcome Institute Library: Wellcome and Osler' in *Medical History* 41, p. 215.

16 John Symons (personal communication).

17 Symons 1993, p. 10.

18 WA/HMM/CO/Ear/844.

19 WA/HMM/RP/Tho/13.

20 WA/HMM/ST/Ear/A.2.

21 WA/HMM/RP/Jst/B.2.

22 WA/HMM/CO/Ear/844.

23 WA/HMM/RP/Tho/10.

24 William Schupbach (personal communication).

25 Prescott, G.M. 1987. 'Illustrations from the Wellcome Institue Library: Gachet and Johnston-Saint: the provenance of Van Gogh's *L'Homme à la Pipe*' in *Medical History* 31, pp. 219–20.

26 Aronson, J. 1990. 'Coloured Vision?' in *New Scientist* 30, p. 80.

27 See Gidley, M. 1998. *Edward S. Curtis and the North American Indian, Incorporated.* Cambridge: Cambridge University Press.

28 Gidley, M. 1976. *The Vanishing Race: selections from Edward S. Curtis' 'The North American Indian'.* London and Vancouver: David and Charles, p. 20.

29 Irmscher, C. 1999. *The Poetics of Natural History: From John Bartram to William James.* New Brunswick, New Jersey, London: Rutgers University Press, p. 163.

30 Ibid., p. 190.

31 Roger, J.; trans. Bonnefoi, S.L. 1997. *Buffon: A life in Natural History.* Cornell University Press, p. vii.

32 Bamforth, S. 2000. *Histoires prodigieuses: MS 136 Wellcome Library by Pierre Boaistuau.* Milan: Franco Maria Ricci, p. 15.

33 Ibid., p. 14.

34 Symons 1998, pp. 117–19.

35 WA/HSW/PE/C.23.

36 Http://archives.wellcome.ac.uk.

37 Lowood, H.E. and Rider, R.E. 2000. 'The scientific book as a cultural and biographical object' in Hunter, A. (ed.), *Thornton and Tully's scientific books, libraries, and collectors: a study of bibliography and the book trade in relation to the history of science.* London and Vermont: Ashgate, p. 1.

INTERNET REFERENCES

Re:source http://www.resource.gov.uk

A Healthy Heritage: Collecting for the future of Medical History 1999 Symposium
http://www.wellcome.ac.uk/en/1/hompreher.html

ACKNOWLEDGEMENTS

My thanks to Danielle Olsen, William Schupbach, David Pearson and Charmian Knight for all their help and advice, and to Chris Gosden and John Symons for reading and commenting on this paper.

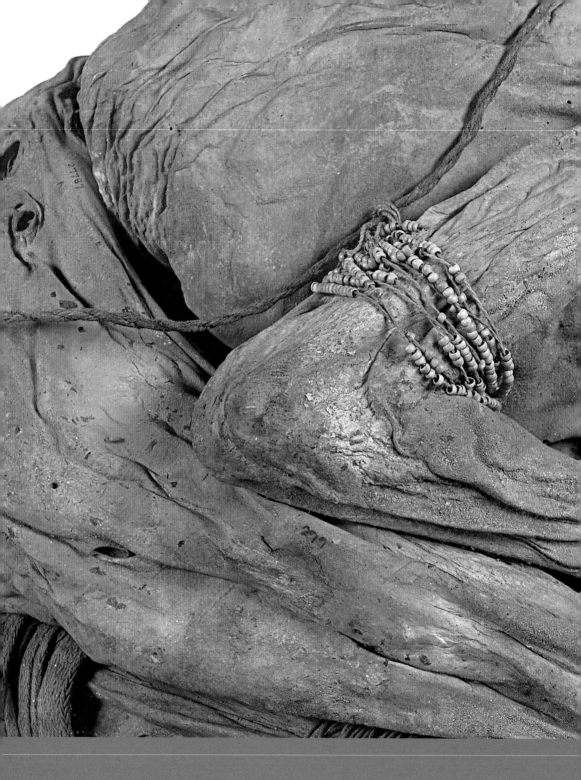

Peruvian mummified male. Typical of such
mummies, the body has bound wrists and ankles
and has been placed in a tightly flexed position.
c. 1200–1400. SM, A31655

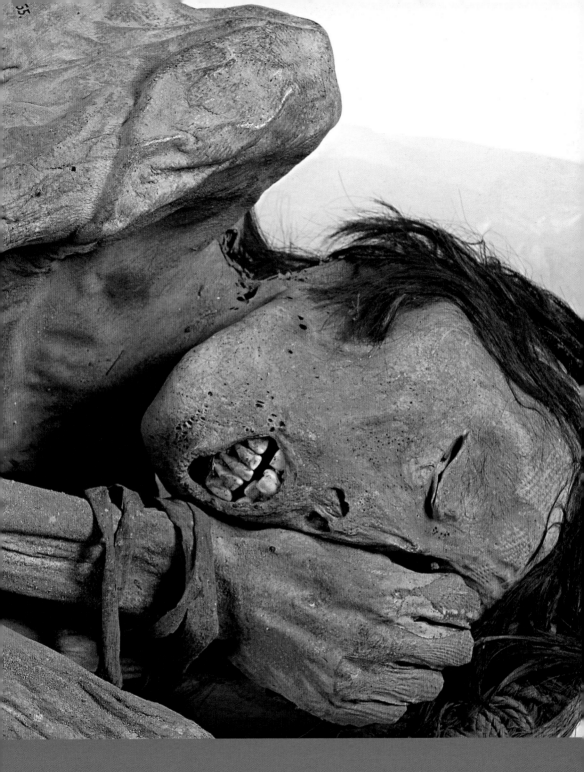

The end of life

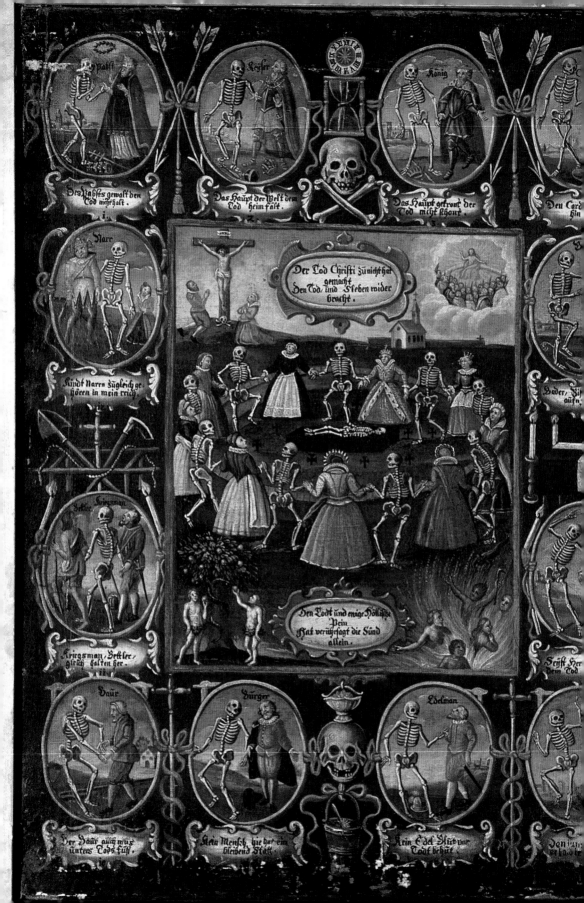

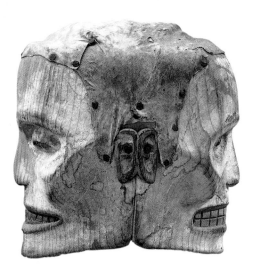

This painted wooden double-faced mask was worn by a follower of the Ghost Dance religion whilst performing songs and dances to bring back the dead. Tsimshian people, British Columbia, Canada, c. 1900. FMCH, X65-8554

OVERLEAF The death of Rachel after giving birth to Benjamin. Oil painting after Francesco Furini. Italian, seventeenth century. WL, 44819i

LEFT Oil painting of the *danse macabre* in which Death as a skeleton holds a dialogue with all classes of society. Dance of Death iconography has been traced back to the plague epidemics of the fourteenth and fifteenth centuries. German, 1750–1850. WL, 45066i

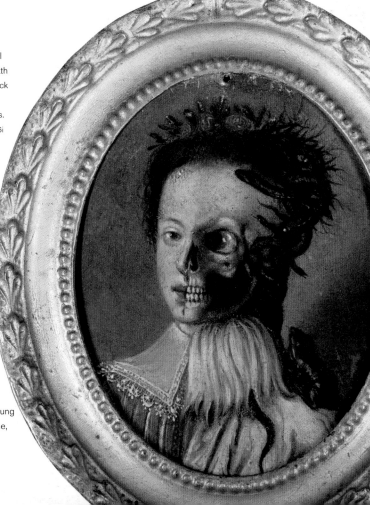

RIGHT Miniature oil painting contrasting life and death in a young woman's face. Possibly Florentine, eighteenth century. WL, 45064i

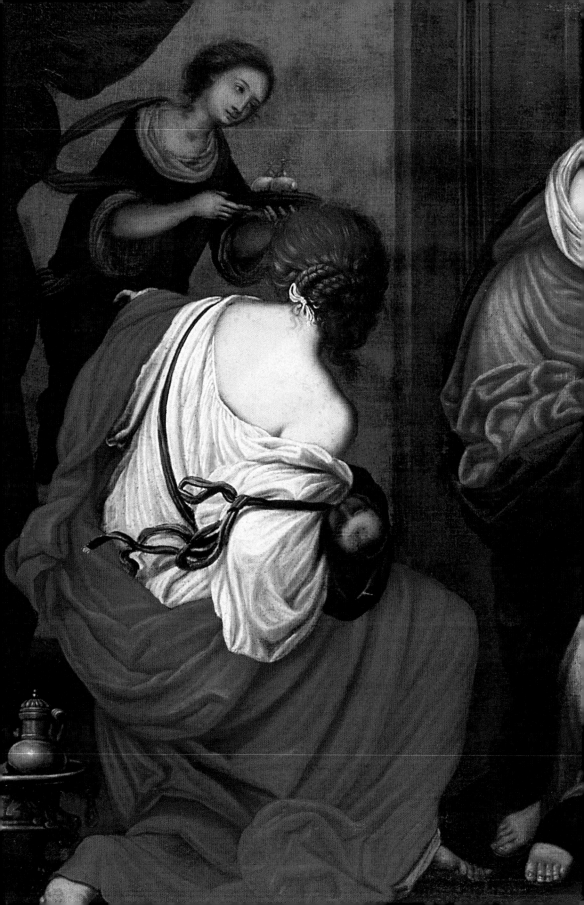

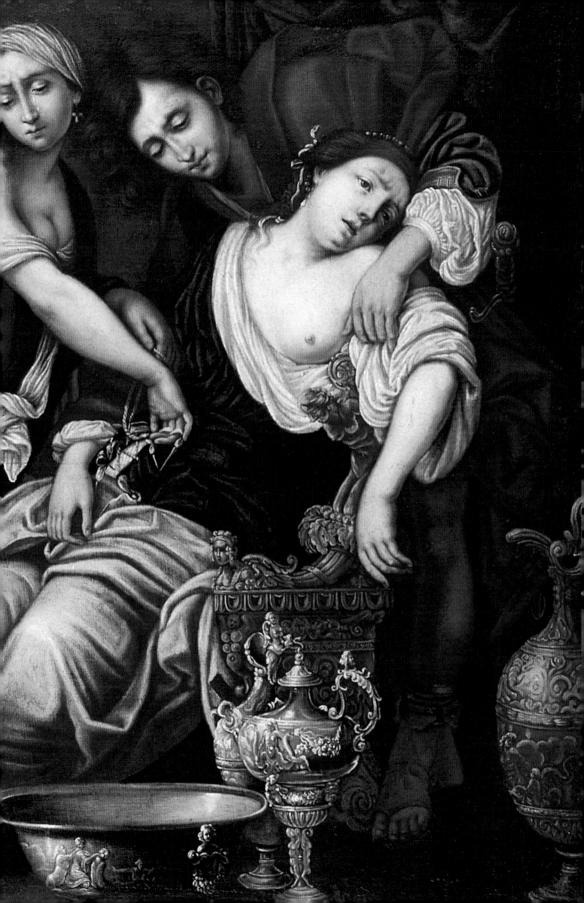

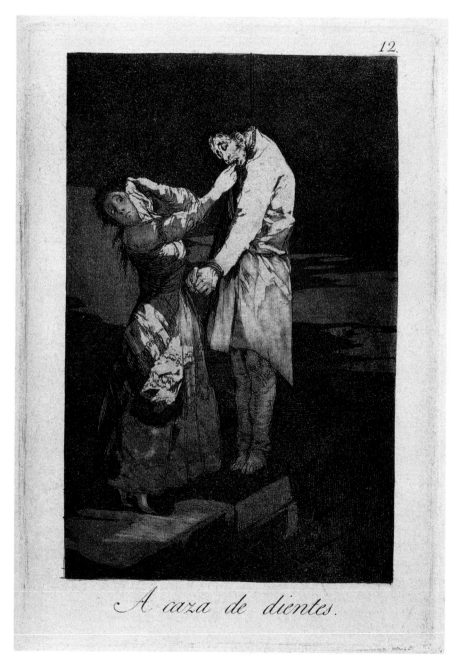

12.

A caza de dientes.

A woman covers her eyes as she steals the teeth of a hanged man.
Aquatint with etching by Francisco Goya (1746–1828). Spanish, c. 1797. WL, 18059i

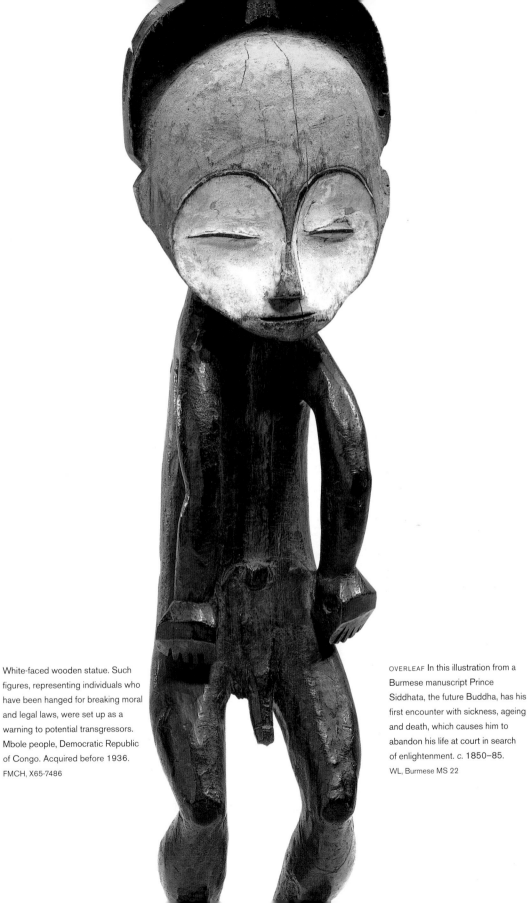

White-faced wooden statue. Such
figures, representing individuals who
have been hanged for breaking moral
and legal laws, were set up as a
warning to potential transgressors.
Mbole people, Democratic Republic
of Congo. Acquired before 1936.
FMCH, X65-7486

OVERLEAF In this illustration from a
Burmese manuscript Prince
Siddhata, the future Buddha, has his
first encounter with sickness, ageing
and death, which causes him to
abandon his life at court in search
of enlightenment. *c.* 1850–85.
WL, Burmese MS 22

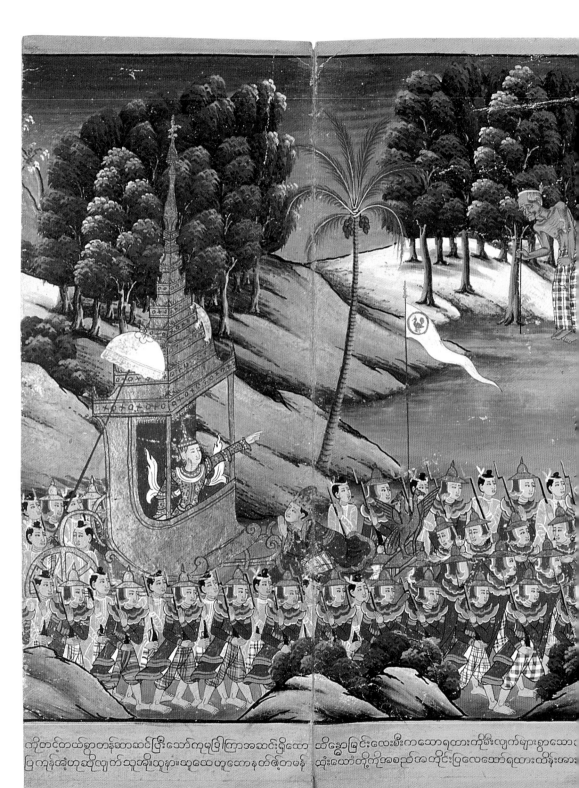

ကိုကင်တယ်ဇွာတန်ဆာဆင်ပြီးသော်ကုဗုဒ္ဒိကြာအဆင်းရှိသော ထိုဆွေဉာမြင်းလေးစီးကသောရထားကိုမိုးလျက်များစွာသော
ပြကုန်အံ့ဟူဆိုလျက်သူအိုးထူးနုး။သုလေဟူသောနတ်ဖိဘကဗန် သုံးဒယာ်တို့ကိုအစဉ်အ‌တိုင်းပြလေသော်ရထားထိန်းအား

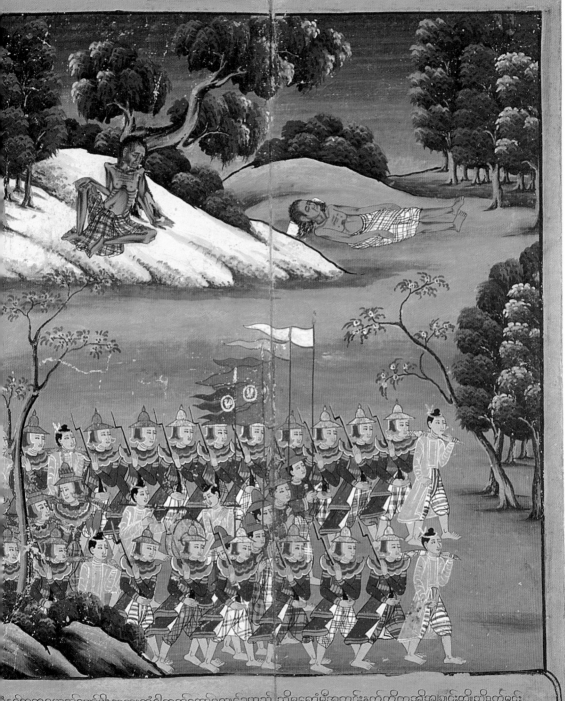

ဒဲ့နှင့်ကွ၌ဥယ္ယာဉ်ဖျောင်ပါး ကစားအံ့ငှါတွက်တော်မူလျှင်ဥယ္ယာဉ် သို့မရောင်မီအတွင်းနတ်တို့ကအရိအာလျှင်းတိုးတို့၌တ်မင်း
ယံဝေဂဖြစ်လျှက်မသာသေနသူးလုံးဖြင့်နန်းတော်သို့အသောကက လျှင်ပြန်သွားဟန်ပြီး။

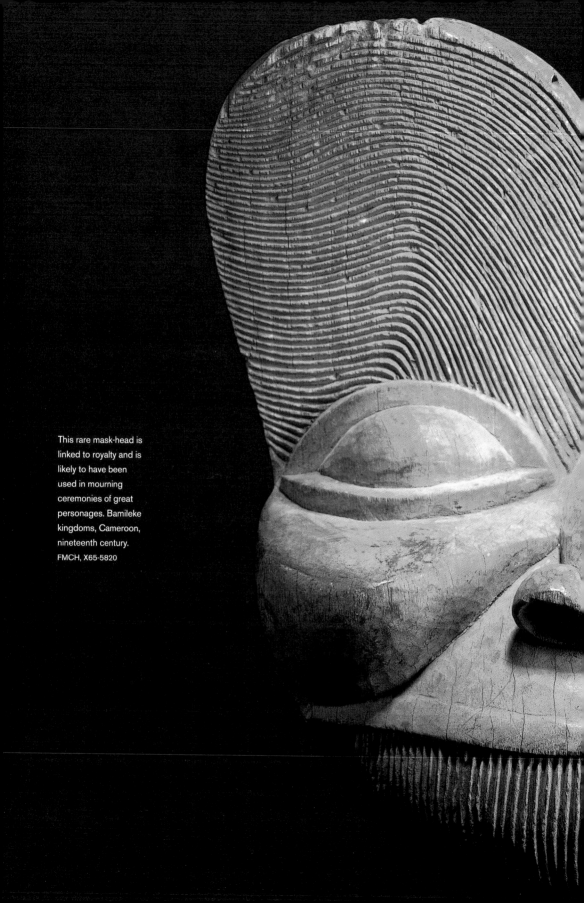

This rare mask-head is linked to royalty and is likely to have been used in mourning ceremonies of great personages. Bamileke kingdoms, Cameroon, nineteenth century. FMCH, X65-5820

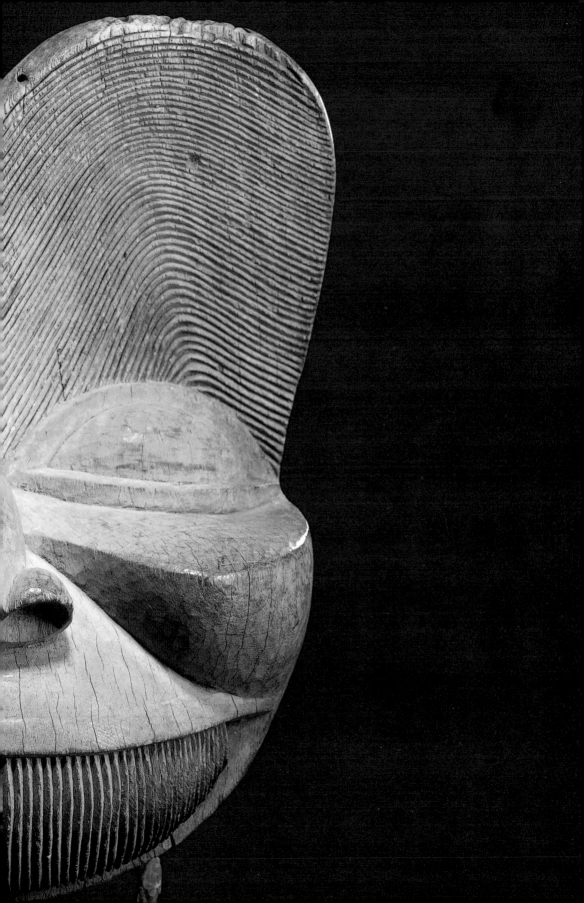

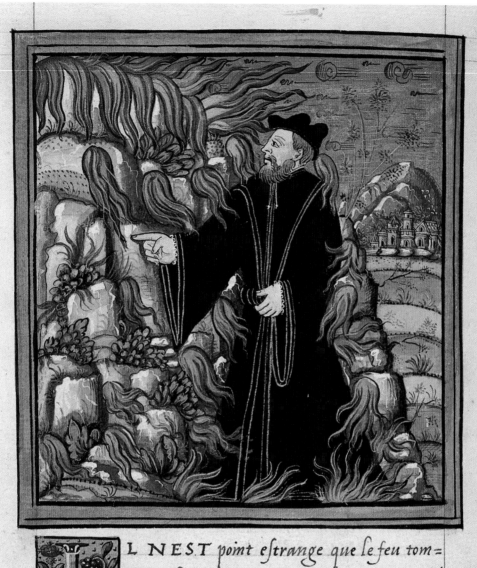

 L NEST point eftrange que le feu tom=
bant du ciel bruſle les lieux qu'il attaint
mais il eſt monſtrueux de ſe voir yſſir
de la terre, ſans ſcauoir dou il prent ſa nourriture, ori=
oine

Pliny, who ventured too close to the volcanic flames of Mount Vesuvius and was reduced to cinders.
Illustration from the manuscript *Histoires Prodigieuses* by Pierre Boaistuau. French, 1560. WL, Western MS 136

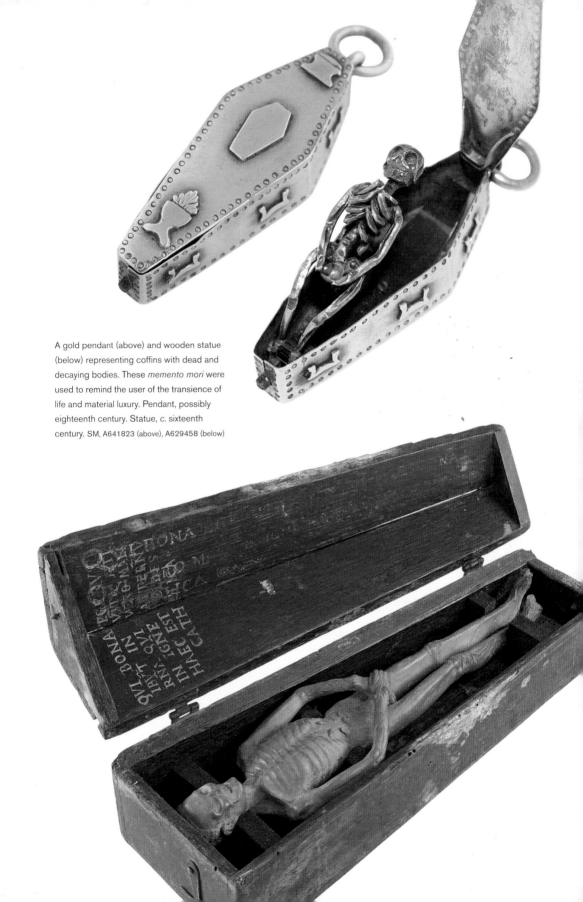

A gold pendant (above) and wooden statue (below) representing coffins with dead and decaying bodies. These *memento mori* were used to remind the user of the transience of life and material luxury. Pendant, possibly eighteenth century. Statue, *c.* sixteenth century. SM, A641823 (above), A629458 (below)

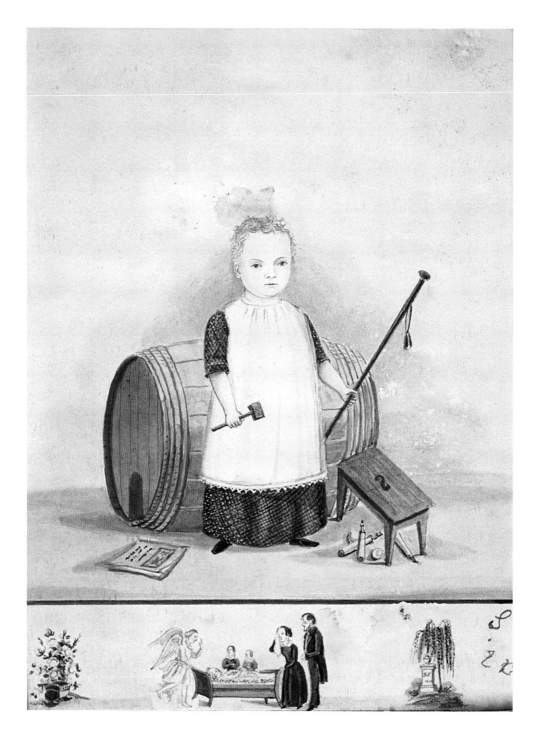

A memorial portrait of a dead
child with deathbed scene below.
Watercolour, 1846. WL, 45065i

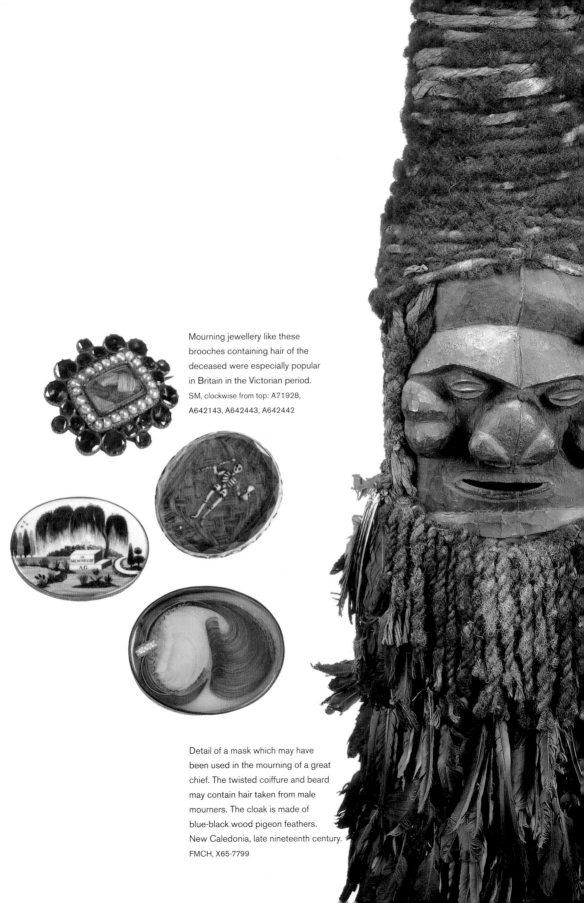

Mourning jewellery like these brooches containing hair of the deceased were especially popular in Britain in the Victorian period. SM, clockwise from top: A71928, A642143, A642443, A642442

Detail of a mask which may have been used in the mourning of a great chief. The twisted coiffure and beard may contain hair taken from male mourners. The cloak is made of blue-black wood pigeon feathers. New Caledonia, late nineteenth century. FMCH, X65-7799

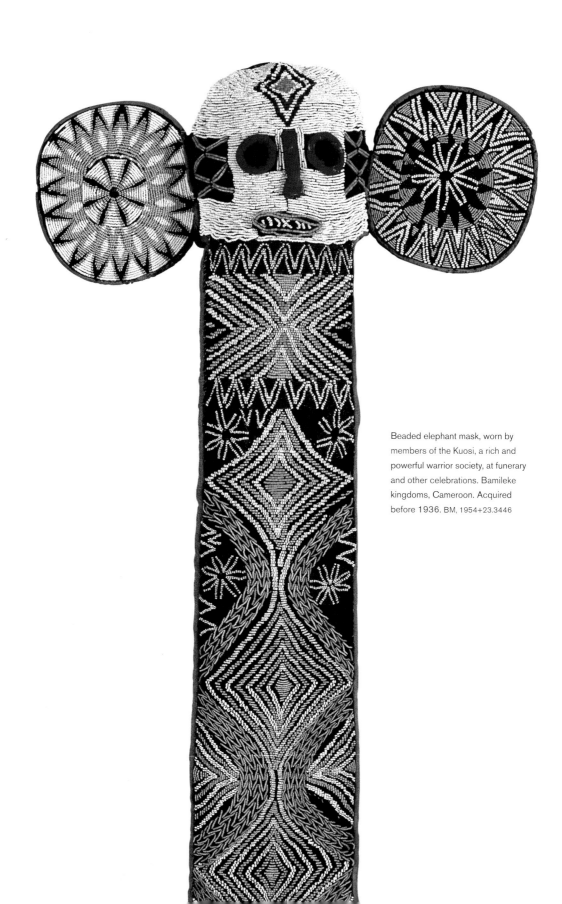

Beaded elephant mask, worn by members of the Kuosi, a rich and powerful warrior society, at funerary and other celebrations. Bamileke kingdoms, Cameroon. Acquired before 1936. BM, 1954+23.3446

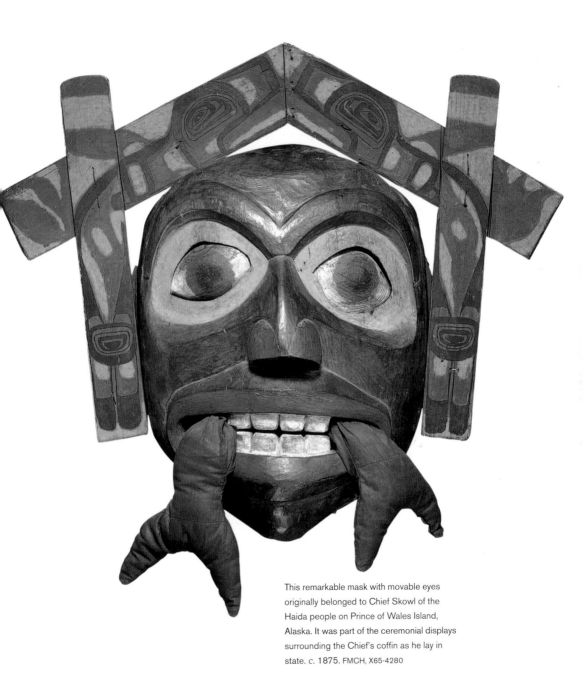

This remarkable mask with movable eyes
originally belonged to Chief Skowl of the
Haida people on Prince of Wales Island,
Alaska. It was part of the ceremonial displays
surrounding the Chief's coffin as he lay in
state. c. 1875. FMCH, X65-4280

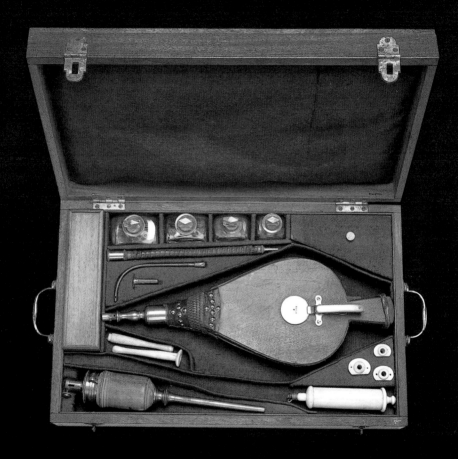

Tobacco resuscitator kit, used to
revive the 'apparently dead' by
either blowing smoke up the rectum
or through the nose or mouth. The
Royal Humane Society provided
such kits at various points along the
Thames for reviving victims of
drowning accidents. English, 1774.
SM/SSPL, A640992

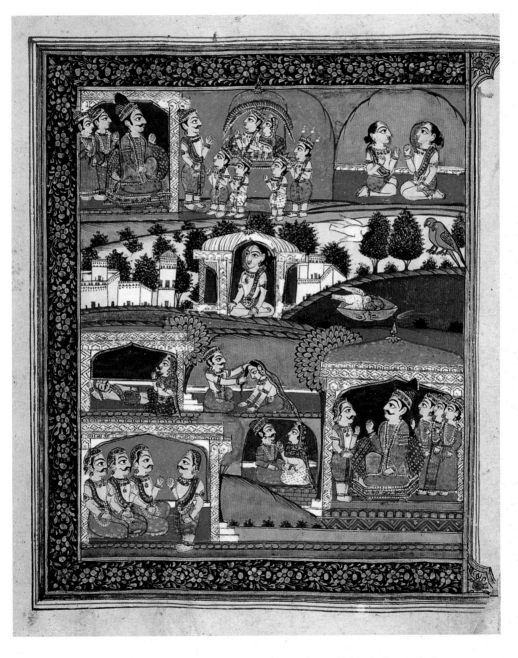

Painting depicting the life of a Brāhman and his wife who are reborn as birds and subsequently given new divine bodies. Illustration from a copy of Kiśordās's vernacular translation and commentary of the Sanskrit *Bhagvadgītā*. Indian, *c.* 1820–40. WL, Panjabi MS 255

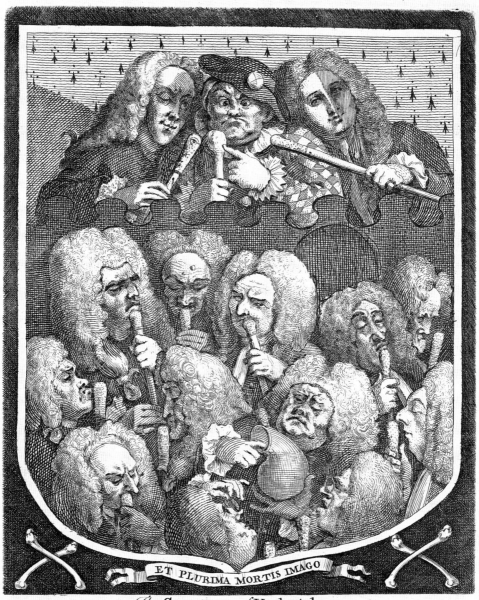

A Company of Undertakers or a Consultation of Physicians. Represented within a satirical coat-of-arms:
the engraving is bordered in black, like a mourning card. Beneath it is a pair of ominous crossbones and the motto,
'*Et Plurima mortis imago*' – 'And many an image of death'. Etching by William Hogarth (1697–1764). British, 1736. WL, 10756i

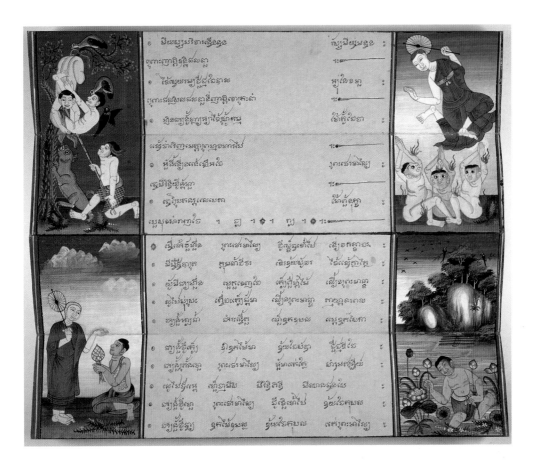

Thai manuscript illustrating the Buddhist story of the monk Phra Malai and his journeys to Heaven and Hell. The top left scene depicts adulterers in Hell being punished on a thorn tree. *c.* 1860–70. WL, Thai MS 1

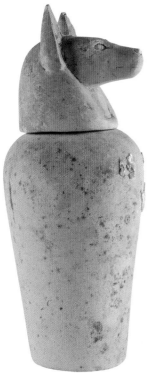

Limestone jackal-headed canopic jar. Such vessels were part of the Egyptian mummification process and were used to store the removed stomach, liver, lungs and intestines. Each organ was assigned to a different jar. Excavated between 1850 and 1894. SM, A635038

OVERLEAF Line engraving by Cornelius Huyberts, 1709. A plate to Frederick Ruysch's *Thesaurus anatomicus octavus*, Amsterdam, 1709. Ruysch, a Dutch anatomist and pioneer in techniques of preserving organs and tissue, constructed tableaux such as this from body parts including foetal skeletons, gallstones and kidneystones, veins and arteries. The actual foetuses shown here are now in the Academy of Sciences, St Petersburg. WL, icon. anat. 202

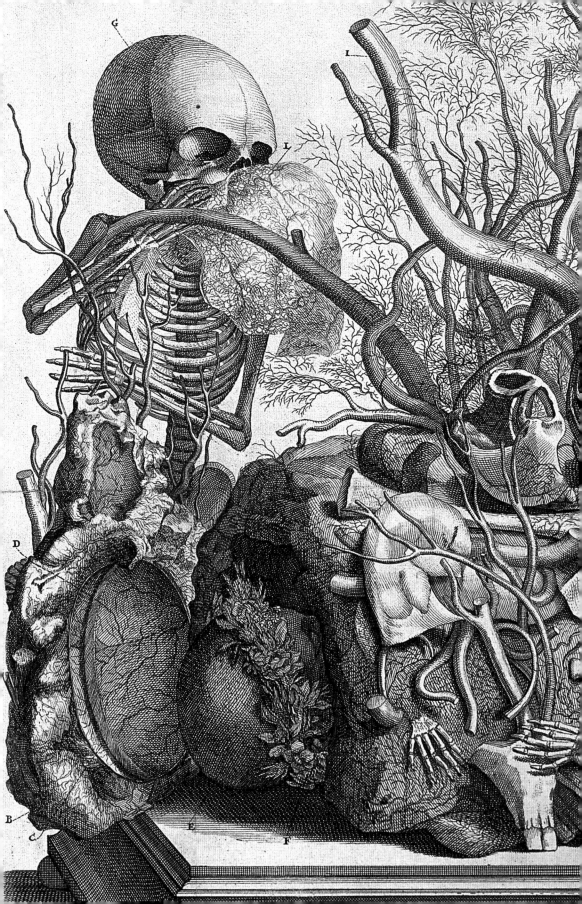

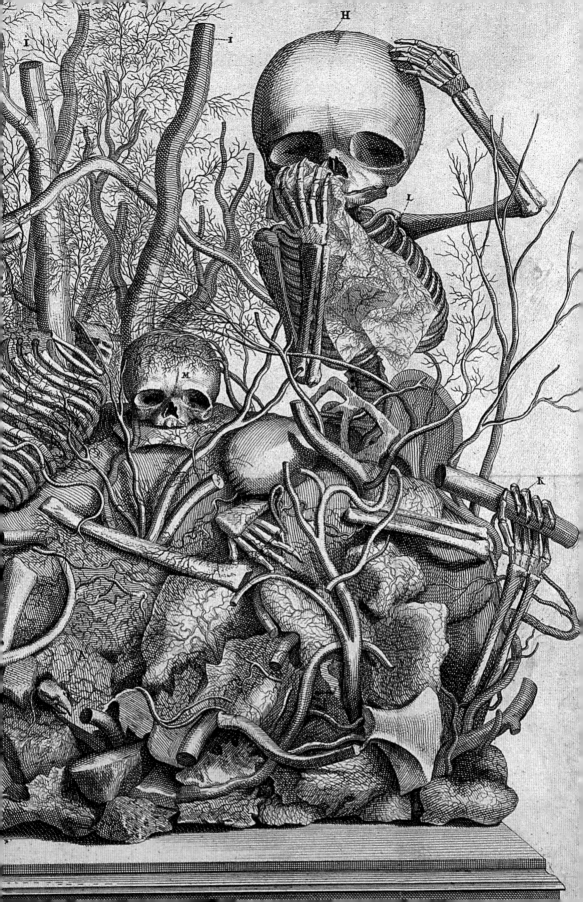

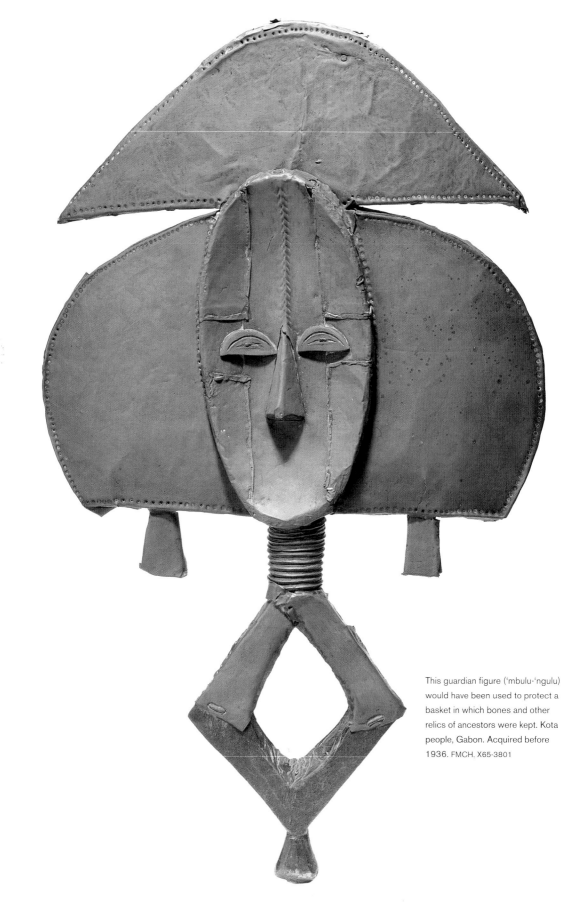

This guardian figure ('mbulu-'ngulu) would have been used to protect a basket in which bones and other relics of ancestors were kept. Kota people, Gabon. Acquired before 1936. FMCH. X65-3801

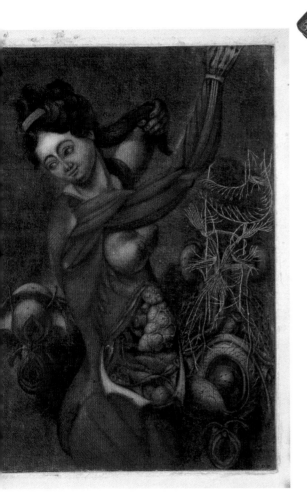

A woman with the muscles of her upper body
and viscera exposed. On each side of her is a
figure of part of the urogenital system.
Coloured mezzotint attributed to Jacques-
Fabien Gautier d'Agoty (c. 1717–85)
who worked directly with anatomists and
eventually performed dissections himself.
French. WL, 225i

Fragment of skin of the eminent
English philosopher and jurist
Jeremy Bentham (1748–1832),
with a handwritten inscription.
Bentham 'bequeathed his body for
anatomical purposes' and was
dissected in 1832. SM, A44694

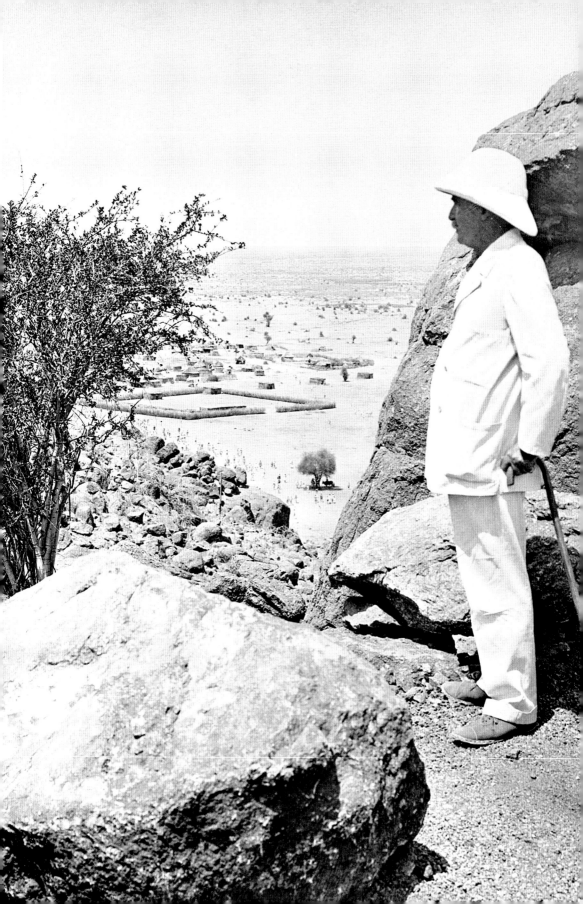

Henry Wellcome on the north-west
terrace at Jebel Moya, *c.* 1913.

'When I was four years old, I got

my first object lesson from a

Neolithic stone implement which

I found; and my father explained

to me the different periods of the

Stone Age. . . . That excited my

imagination and was never

forgotten. It made me an ardent

student of prehistoric periods.'

HENRY WELLCOME, EVIDENCE TO THE ROYAL COMMISSION

ON NATIONAL MUSEUMS AND GALLERIES, 14 DECEMBER 1928.

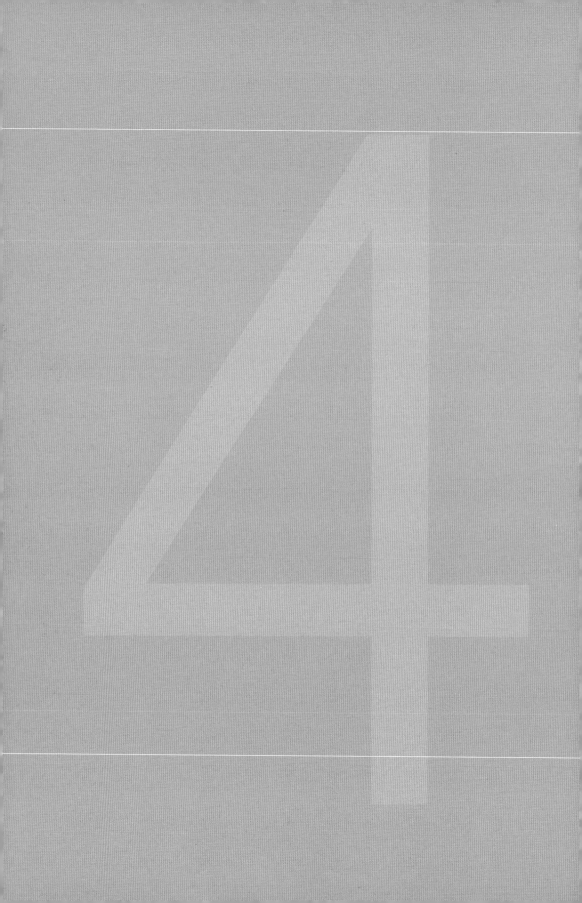

Object Lessons
and Wellcome's Archaeology

Chris Gosden

Prehistory is the period before written records, when the only evidence
we have for human action is the objects people left behind. Henry
Wellcome published so little that understanding his thoughts, motives
and actions is almost an exercise in prehistoric reconstruction. Fortunately we can learn a lot from objects and their relationships with
people, so that a dearth of words does not preclude understanding. The
gargantuan scale of Wellcome's collections and excavations have left
us with an embarrassing richness of material through which to consider Wellcome's intellectual endeavours; this I feel may have been
more systematic and interesting than some have given him credit for.

Small but sharp observations may have left their mark on the
young Wellcome. His biographer, Robert Rhodes James, records that
in later life Wellcome retained little memory of his childhood, but one
of his few remembrances was the discovery, when he was four, of an
arrowhead: '[My father] explained to me that the perfecting of that
late Neolithic implement meant more to those ancient peoples for
their protection and as a means of gaining their livelihood than the
invention of the electric telegraph or the steam railway engine meant
to us' (fig. 1). Wellcome later wrote that this 'stimulated a babyish
interest [in history] that lasted through my life'.[1] Wellcome's interests
in things, in inventions and in origins are all captured here, to be reinforced later in his life by his inventiveness which he must have seen as
part of his own contribution to human history.

People and objects

Before looking in more detail at Wellcome himself, let us think a little
about objects and what they can tell us about people, starting with origins. Thirty years ago the idea of 'Man the Toolmaker' was current – that
only humans make and use tools and that technology has been the
motor for human history. From studies of chimpanzees and other primates it has become obvious that in their search for food they often use

sticks to fish termites out of their mounds or rocks to crack nuts. The mother chimpanzees teach their children how to make and manipulate tools which often require considerable manual dexterity and skill to use, and different groups of chimpanzees have their own forms of technology. Some of the apparent uniqueness of human culture has been eroded through such studies: we can see that chimps have cultural differences of their own, and that their histories slightly differ from group to group.

The social life of primates is also crucial in determining their intelligence. Physical anthropologists Robin Dunbar and Leslie Aiello have

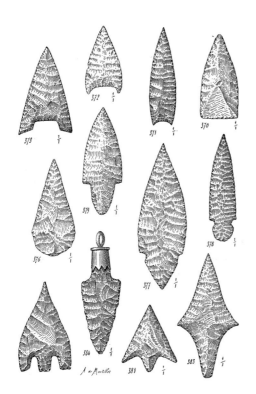

plotted primate brain size (or, more precisely, the ratio between brain and body size) against the average size of social group and found that the bigger the group, the bigger their brains relative to body size. This has led to the 'social brain' hypothesis which holds that the most complex element of any primate's life is its social relations (rather than food-gathering, for instance) and that the development of intelligence is directly related to keeping track of the multiple nature of links with other individuals. Primate sociability is expressed in direct physical forms, such as grooming, fighting or sex, so that there are limits to the numbers of intimate contacts any one individual can keep up. Human beings, they argue, are freed from some of these physical constraints through language, so that we can maintain links with a greater range of significant others through speech (and later writing). Human brains have expanded to

1 Selection of Neolithic and Bronze Age arrowheads from Gabriel and Adrien de Mortillet's *Musée Préhistorique*. Paris, 1903. WL, ZC/MOR

cope with the demands of extra sociability, with language both being a cause and a result of increased brain size and complexity.

The concentration on sociability and its demands on the growth of intelligence has led to a lessening of emphasis on material culture, so that the 'Man the Toolmaker' hypothesis has been replaced by the idea of the 'social brain'. Yet I would argue that this is somewhat premature. Many primates (and other species) have tools. No other primate, as Dunbar and Aiello demonstrated, uses material culture to create its social relations. By contrast, all human social relations are created through the medium of objects.

It takes no great act of imagination on my part to conjure up a picture of you, the reader of this book. You are probably reading sitting down, in your own chair and own room, or on a bus, train or plane. You are most likely reading silently to yourself and engaged in some sort of dialogue with the authors of these pieces. A book is designed for an individual, not a group experience. The act of private reading might seem to represent the very absence of social relations, but much social and material effort has gone into maintaining our privacy and creating our own individuality. Reading alone is part of a spectrum of social and material practices that emphasise the individual in a manner that is historically recent. Beds are designed for one or two, but rarely more. When we sit down to eat we expect our own knife, fork and spoon, crockery and glasses. Food is designed with individual portions in mind. In the early modern period new techniques of butchery were developed to produce cuts of steak and chops for individual consumption to complement the stews and joints of the medieval period. In this earlier more communal time, people did not expect tables, chairs and their own place settings but lived and ate in close proximity to other people and to animals.

The objects that surround us contain within them a series of taken-for-granted assumptions as to appropriate forms of use and consumption. I remember, after a long walk in the Papua New Guinea rainforest, arriving at a house where we were to stay the night and, being exhausted, going off to a bedroom to sleep. I woke up the next morning to find my three New Guinean companions all asleep on the floor of one room, even though there were bedrooms for all of us. I had been tired and wanted to collapse into a bed, and it never occurred to me to do anything other than find my own room. It never occurred to them that they might sleep on their own: a strange place has ghosts and spirits at night that one would not want to meet alone.

We think of objects as external to us, with our 'real' life contained in our private thoughts or dealings with others. But material culture is not just the stage-setting against which the dramas of life are played out; objects are as much social actors as people. We shape the material world, but equally that world shapes us, making us the human beings that we are. Different cultures, by definition, give a different shape to social life, employing a variety of objects to do so. Material culture is a prosthesis, a means of extending our bodies in a social sense and helping to define us as social beings. A long period of time and a wealth of experience separates the first human ancestral use of material culture and our obsession with the individual today, but basic to human history has been the changing use of material culture in creating groups of different social structures and with more or less emphasis on the individual. Our attempts to create ourselves as autonomous, yet socially responsive, individuals is just one form that prosthetic uses of material culture takes.

Material culture can extend the social effects of a person beyond the limits of the body and its position in space and time, leading to the idea of extended personhood. Our social lives are not made up solely or mainly through face-to-face contacts, but are also composed of things that we have made, used or given to others. All the things connected to us that are out there in the world somewhere carry the traces of our social effects and efficacy. Indeed, the book that you are holding is part of the combined authors' social impacts, although it is also true that the authors lose control of the meanings of their writings once they are handed to the publisher and it is up to the reader to make what they can and will of the writings of others. Much effort goes into maintaining the integrity and impact of people over time and space, even after death.

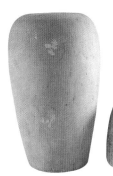

2 Limestone human-headed Egyptian canopic jar.
SM, A635039

Wellcome was fascinated by the ancient Egyptians (looking for the origins of Egyptian civilisation may have been one of the things that led him to dig in the Sudan). The Egyptians, in turn, were fascinated by bodies, objects and the integrity of the individual, and the best insight we get into this obsession is how they dealt with the problem of death. Egyptian funeral preparations were animated by a complex series of emotions, ranging from fear of the corpse and spirit of the dead person, to hopes for the spiritual and physical integrity of that person in the next life, mixed with hopes that the spirits of the dead might intercede with the gods on behalf of the living at times of crisis. A poignant sense of the transience of life pervaded preparations and funerals, making all present conscious that they needed to live life to the full. Egyptian funerary rituals (which were supposed to last up to seventy days in the case of important people) transformed the body of the deceased into a series of

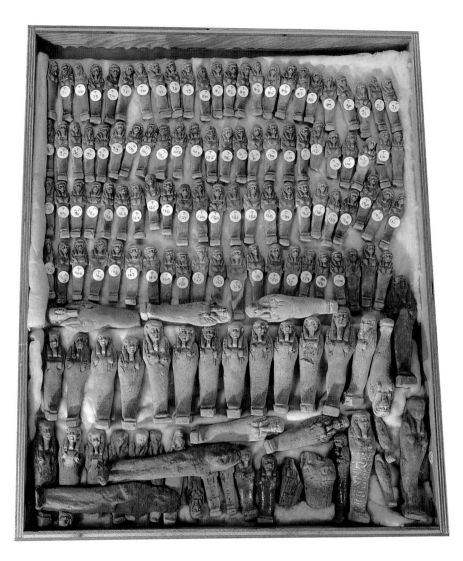

3 Ushabti figures originally placed in Egyptian graves.
UWS, uncatalogued

objects, whilst also transforming the living community into a new form whereby they could operate, live and work without the deceased. In cases of mummification the embalmers used the body to make a life-like image of the person, because it needed some continuing integrity to enjoy a full afterlife. The body was transformed from an animate state in the living world to an object in the form of a mummy, then an animate object in the world of the dead. Vital organs were removed and placed in canopic jars, which often took the form of people or gods (fig. 2). People were provided in the form of objects, as *ushabti* figures (fig. 3). These had a variety of significances and functions, one of the main ones being to act as servants to the deceased. Made of baked clay, stone or faience, they were considered to be animate in the next world, along with the mummified body, which needed food, furniture and other personal possessions in the tomb to equip it for the next life. Thus, an Egyptian tomb contained a number of objects which were viewed as objects, and a number of objects viewed as people, clustered round the body of a person made

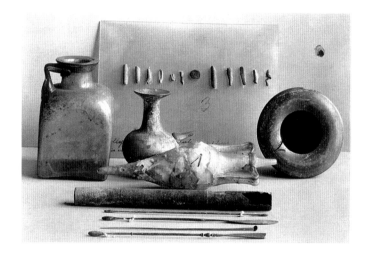

4 The equipment of a Greek aural doctor, consisting of scoops, spoons, a syringe and unguent jars. *c.* AD 300. WL, L10628

into an object. The process of mummification, it was hoped, would allow this person to be active in the next world. Our simple distinctions between active human subject and inanimate physical object obviously do not work well here. Nor were these reworkings of relationships between people and objects merely formulaic: we should not forget that death was a time of danger and high emotion. The depictions of funerals in elite tombs give us some glimpse of the people and the feelings lying behind what we have come to view as archaeological evidence, and we should imagine 'the garlands and incense, the weeping of the mourners, the pouring of water offerings, and the recitation of prayers'.[2] Given Wellcome's own interests in life, death, spiritual and physical health it is easy to see why Egyptian objects became such a part of his collection.

Other cultures used objects to work through concerns about the human body, blurring the distinctions between bodies and objects in the process. The usual role assigned to the Greeks and Romans in the

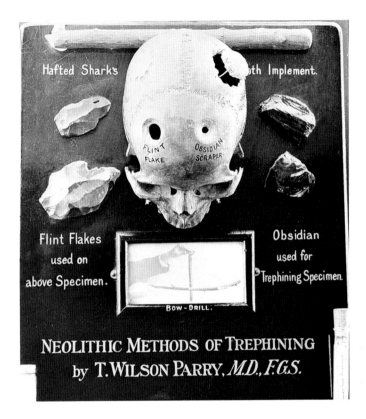

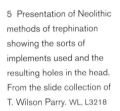

5 Presentation of Neolithic methods of trephination showing the sorts of implements used and the resulting holes in the head. From the slide collection of T. Wilson Parry. WL, L3218

history of Western traditions and thought is that they developed modes of rational thought and empirical investigation directly ancestral to our own; the Renaissance represents the rediscovery of Classical reason after a dark period of medieval mysticism. Consider the equipment of the Greek ear doctor (fig. 4), which is reassuringly specialised – the syringes, ear spoons and medicine bottles all indicate a long tradition of investigation into the workings of the ear and the possibility of a calm and knowledgeable response to problems of hearing or balance. This contrasts with the pain and doubt of Neolithic trephination where holes were made in the skull to reduce pressure (possibly seen as the removal of spirits), a drastic and agonising response to head wounds or other pain (fig. 5). Wellcome no doubt considered it remarkable that primitive people, whom he would have considered to lack any empirical traditions, should be able to undertake such relatively sophisticated interventions. Nevertheless, the vital growth in knowledge represented by the gap between the flint

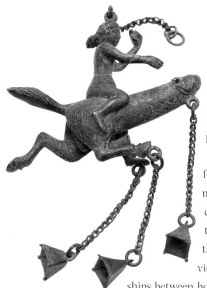

and obsidian trephining tools, and the range of specialised medical equipment of the Greeks, must have seemed to him a crucial indicator of progress in thought and treatment.

However, history is not quite that straight-forward in creating a linear progress towards our modern forms of science and medicine. There is no doubt that the Greeks and the Romans developed traditions of rational thought and action, but these maintained a complex coexistence with other views about the body, well or ill, and the relation-ships between bodies and things. Take, for instance, a rather con-fusing object in bronze, acquired by Wellcome on 10 July 1931 and now in the Science Museum in London (fig. 6). Let me quote from the catalogue entry on this object[3] to give a sense of our present need to codify objects in a neutral language – 'solid bronze amulet in form of nude female mounted on a priapus which has hindquarters of gallop-ing horse, itself with tumescent genitalia'. All museum professionals have written labels of this kind and we all respect the need to provide systematic information for those searching our catalogues for the

6 Graeco-Roman bronze phallic pendant. 100 BC–AD 400. SM, A97578

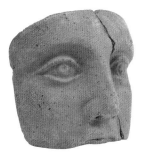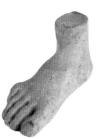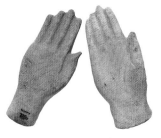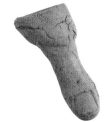

7 Terracotta Roman votive offerings.

purposes of research. Even in the act of writing, however, we are often aware of the gap between measured description and the strangeness of the material in our care.

This bronze amulet is an extraordinary object and was worn as a piece of jewellery. Part-horse, part-phallus with a woman rider and extra pyramidal pendants, the amulet defies classification. Was it an erotic object? The answer must be partly 'yes', but it might also have played some amuletic role to maintain the sexual powers of the wearer, or their attractiveness. And what of the combination of phallus and horse, which shows that human sexual powers and enjoyments were in some way linked to the strength and potency of animals? We lack a precise date and provenance for this enigma, but it may have overlapped in time with the aural doctor's equipment which conversely makes sane, good sense to us. Nevertheless, the combination of the two items hints at the complexity of Greek experience and identity, challenging us to rethink them as rational ancestors. And what of Wellcome himself? Did he acquire this object through some sort of prurient interest in the erotic? Or was he alert to the range of human experience, willing to be puzzled by some of its forms? My feeling is that Wellcome had a broad range of interests in both the odd and the mundane, giving each equal weight in his attempts to think through and collect world history. No wonder that he never came up with a final scheme or synthesis through which to display his collections.

The Romans had a difficult cultural relationship with the Greeks and, although they incorporated Greece into their empire, Romans always felt in awe of Greek cultivation, learning and science. And, like

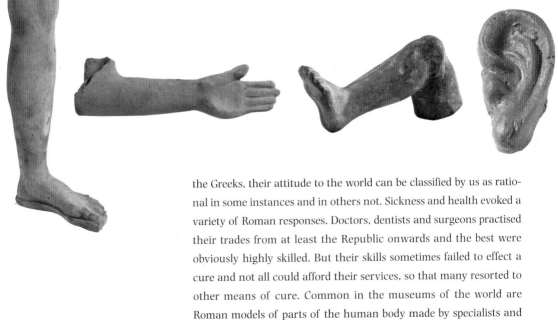

the Greeks, their attitude to the world can be classified by us as rational in some instances and in others not. Sickness and health evoked a variety of Roman responses. Doctors, dentists and surgeons practised their trades from at least the Republic onwards and the best were obviously highly skilled. But their skills sometimes failed to effect a cure and not all could afford their services, so that many resorted to other means of cure. Common in the museums of the world are Roman models of parts of the human body made by specialists and deliberately thrown into water (fig. 7). The part of the body giving trouble was modelled in terracotta or wood, then deposited with suitable imprecations to the gods. Can we see in the model of an ear someone who couldn't afford the services of the aural doctor, or who distrusted them, or who felt that they had been the victims of a curse or sorcery so that only supernatural help would work? We don't, of course, know the motivations behind individual cases, but the range of motives just outlined existed alongside others, which helped to blur distinctions between bodies and objects.

I have been thinking about these matters recently as, by chance, I have been excavating a Romano-British site at Marcham in south Oxfordshire. It has a temple at one end and a large circular feature at the other end, which we thought until recently might be an amphitheatre, but now are starting to wonder whether it might not be a sacred pool of the type designed for votive offerings (and other objects like lead curses, intended to harm through supernatural means, rather than cure). At the time of writing, interpretations of our site are still fluid (pardon the pun), but by the time you read this we will have excavated some of the centre of the pool/amphitheatre and might be closer to an answer. Wellcome, of course, similarly engaged in excavation on a grand scale, which also took him close to the material world and the sense we try to make of it.

Origins and objects: probing early social life

'Burrow and welcome' wrote the Military Governor of the Sudan on Wellcome's excavation permit and burrow Wellcome did on a grand scale. His hopes for the age and importance of his main site, Jebel Moya, were misplaced, but the excavations were important nonetheless. In a presentation to the British Association for the Advancement of Science in Scotland in 1912 Wellcome said, 'It has been suggested that here also we should seek the veritable birthplace of human civilisation itself. Do the sands of this land of enigmas still hide within their depths an answer to the eternal enigma of man's beginnings and a record of his first steps upon the pathway to knowledge?' We would now place Jebel Moya some time early in the first millennium BC in a continent for which the earliest evidence of human ancestry goes back around six million years. So Wellcome's hopes were laughably

8 General view of the
1910–11 excavations at
Jebel Moya. WL, M15954

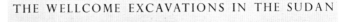

THE WELLCOME EXCAVATIONS IN THE SUDAN

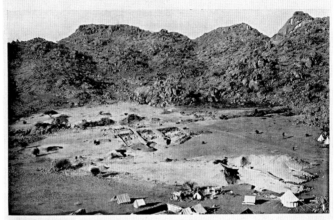

JEBEL MOYA

exaggerated, although the links he made between civilisation and knowledge would not have been emphasised by all at this time, when most archaeologists were fascinated by cultivation and power. However, in quite a different sense, his excavations represented a number of original points which were to have a lasting, although largely unacknowledged, effect on the development of archaeological fieldwork.

Wellcome excavated at Jebel Moya and other adjacent sites for four seasons between 1910 and 1914 (fig. 8). He intended to return but the First World War caused a hiatus that turned into a permanent cessation of excavation, even though he kept renewing his permission to excavate in southern Sudan until his death, to the annoyance of others who wanted to dig in the region. Wellcome's excavation may well have been the largest anywhere in the world at that time and few digs since would have approached this scale. Size is not everything and the numbers of people involved derived from Wellcome's mixture of motives: 'Mr. Wellcome regarded his enterprise from its inception as one undertaken primarily for the benefit of the natives of the Sudan, and not solely as an archaeological expedition'.[4] 'Wellcome's father had been a missionary amongst the North American Indians, and Wellcome himself must have spent his early years in an atmosphere of

moral uplift. One of his hobbies was teetotalism . . .'[5] Crawford's
agnostic bias notwithstanding, Wellcome obviously did see his excavations as some form of moral crusade, especially against the perils of
drink. No local person who wanted to work was turned away (fig. 9),
as long as they agreed to stop drinking *merissa*, the local millet-seed
beer. Anyone who managed to remain sober for six weeks was made a
member of the Order of the Peacock's Feather into which he was
inducted with due ceremony and given a peacock's feather. Over
2,000 men were made members and peacocks were brought out from
London to show the Sudanese what kind of bird the feathers came
from. As Crawford wrote, 'What is the use of being a nabob if one
can't indulge a whim?'.[6]

The result of Wellcome's philanthropy was that by April 1914, 4,000

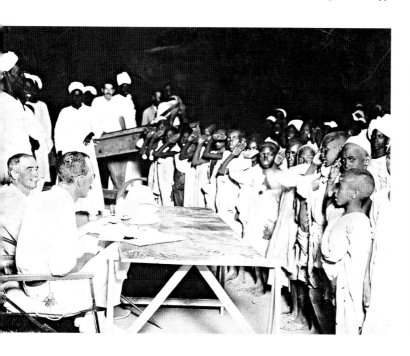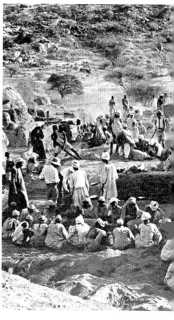

9 Wellcome and his
employees at Jebel Moya.
WL, M13043

men and boys were employed – 500 at the site of Abu Geili, directed by
Crawford, and 3,500 at Jebel Moya itself (fig. 10). The scene on the site
must have been reminiscent of the excavation scenes from *The Raiders of
the Lost Ark*, and the numbers of workers put an intolerable burden on
the staff trying to record the excavations and finds, with the result that
the quality of the archaeology suffered. There was a strict hierarchy on

the site, with the controlling presence of Wellcome at the top, European staff to oversee archaeology, ethnology and physical anthropology, as well as organise the camp, and professional excavators from Egypt to supervise the diggers who were Sudanese locals. There were also local women employed to cook, wash and clean. The trenches were named after the villages from which the workers came (Segadi New Trench, Moya New Trench, the Egyptian Trench). After a chaotic first season when Wellcome himself directed the digging, professional archaeologists were brought in, like O.G.S. Crawford, fresh from Oxford, who, despite occasional difficulties with Wellcome, saw his work at Abu Geili as a life-changing (and life-enhancing) experience.

The policy of employing all who wished to work meant that not everyone could be accommodated on the digs and other projects were

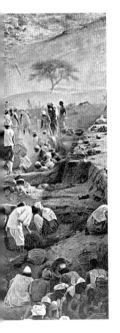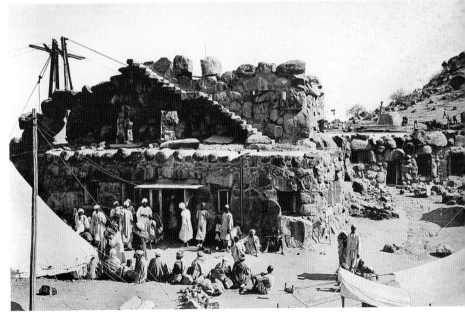

10 ABOVE LEFT Excavations in progress at Jebel Moya, 1913–14. WL, L14548

11 ABOVE RIGHT The House of Boulders at Jebel Moya. WL, M13041

devised lest their hands become idle. The most fantastical of these was the building of the House of Boulders, which was to be Wellcome's headquarters, but was only barely finished before he left for the last time (fig. 11). Work on this edifice was a multi-national affair. Italian granite workers trimmed the boulders and their erection was supervised by Greek stonemasons, but all the really hard work of dragging the huge stones into place was carried out by the Sudanese. Major Uribe, Wellcome's camp commandant, was to live in the House every winter for twenty-seven years when he returned to oversee some minor charitable work and to keep the camp and equipment ready for Wellcome's ever-delayed return. After this the site reverted to the

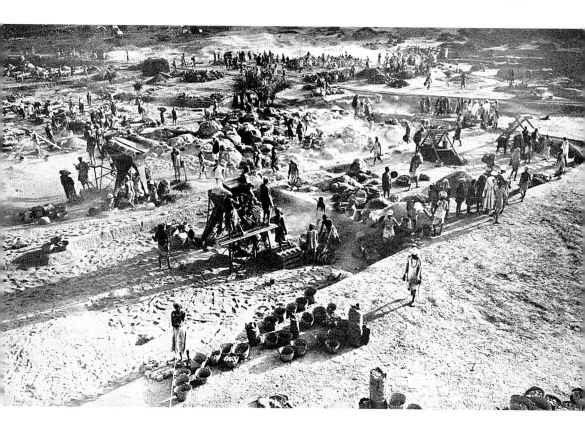

12 Jebel Moya – the sifting machines. WL, M13051

control of the Sudanese government and the area became open for others to excavate. The House of the Boulders still stands today.

Contributions which did last were some of the technical innovations employed (and developed) by Wellcome. Present good practice on archaeological sites is to sieve the soil removed to recover artefacts hard to find in the process of excavation, but sieving has only been regularly employed since the 1960s and then not by all. Wellcome's teams used 'sifting machines' (fig. 12) through which all soil was passed, with large teams of people employed for this purpose and the sieved soil removed by light railway. Crawford, himself a careful fieldworker, was unsure about the usefulness of this huge labour: 'But it must nevertheless be admitted that the results were not by any means valueless, for it was from the siftings that some of the best small finds, including two coins, were found'.[7] But he was openly sceptical about another policy of Wellcome's which is now also common (although not universal) practice, that everything should be kept: 'Every fragment of pottery, brick and stone had to be kept; we were obliged to make a special compound and pile in it classified and labelled heaps of this useless rubbish'.[8] Wellcome's view that the smallest and least significant things can be informative, in aggregate if not individually, accords with the present spirit of our times.

One innovation of Wellcome's own which had a huge influence on Crawford, and through him on archaeology more broadly, was aerial photography: 'I must pay tribute to Wellcome's initiative in this matter of box-kite photography, which was his own invention. It was the first time that air-photography had been used in archaeology, and it is one of the things that led me ultimately to develop this technique'.[9] Wellcome developed a huge box-kite to hold a camera aloft, the shutter activated by remote control from a wire attached to the camera. Barrett, his site photographer, must have spent hours with this contraption (which sometimes fell to the ground) as well as up ladders and hoisting the camera using pulley systems (fig. 13). The results, whether of Wellcome's camp (fig. 14), the nature of the features (fig. 15), or the workings of the excavation (fig. 16), are both beautiful and informative. More conventional photography was used to make detailed records of finds *in situ* (fig. 17). In his use of the best techniques of the day, Wellcome demonstrates his desire that his investigations be scientific, which indeed they were in a technical sense. Cutting across good science was the drive to save the natives from drink, which led to huge amounts being dug at a speed not consonant with control or detailed recording.

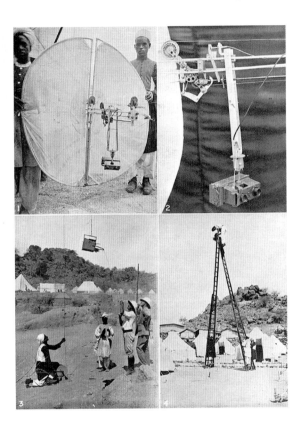

13 Aerial photography at Jebel Moya. Plate XVII from *Jebel Moya, the Wellcome Excavations in Sudan*, vol. 2, by Frank Addison, London, 1949. WL, ZCl.12

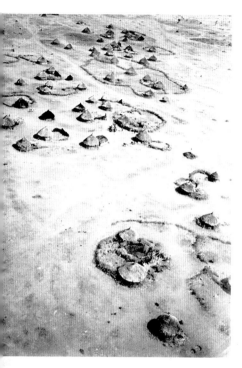

14 Aerial
photography of
the camps at
Jebel Moya. WL,
M13049a (above),
M13049b (below)

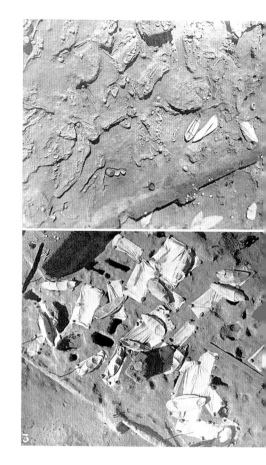

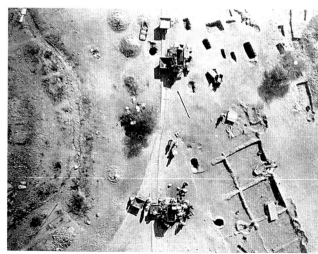

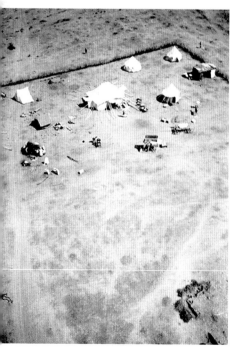

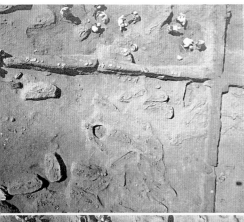

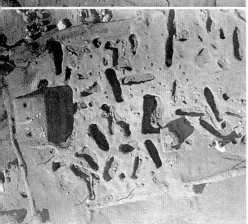

15 The nature of the features
at Jebel Moya. Plate XVIII from
Addison's *Jebel Moya*.
WL, ZCI.12

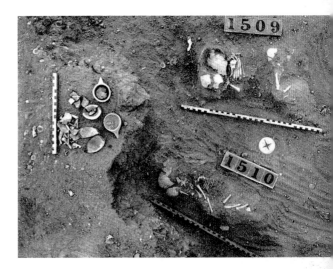

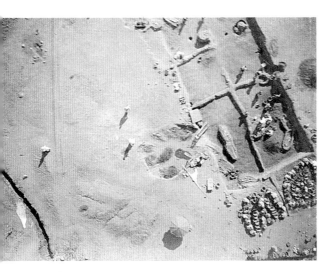

16 LEFT The
workings of the
excavation at
Jebel Moya.
WL, M13048c (left),
M13048d (right)

17 Jebel Moya – burial
1509 under excavation.
Plate XXXIV from
Addison's *Jebel Moya*.
WL, ZCI.12

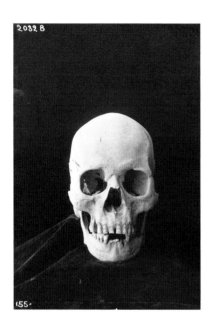

18 and 19 Photographic
records of human remains.
WL, Jebel Moya album, 1913–14,
photographs 155 (above) and
91 (below)

In all at Jebel Moya, 2,838 graves were recorded together with their grave goods, making this one of the largest ever excavations of a cemetery. The bones were recorded in the field in a manner again according to the dictates of science (figs 18 and 19). Many of the artefacts were stored in London warehouses, moved and then moved again, some being discarded after Wellcome's death. Wellcome's secretive nature is partly to blame for lack of publication, which led the archaeological community to fear that he had something to hide: 'We were both [Crawford and Reisner, a well-known archaeologist of Egypt who advised Wellcome on field techniques] aware of the fact that Mr. Wellcome's mania – I do not think the word is too strong – for secrecy had given rise to much unfavourable criticism in archaeological circles';[10] '. . . and in the Gezira strange legends of gold and temples grew up and established themselves around the name of Jebel Moya'.[11]

Eventually Wellcome's trustees employed Addison to write up Jebel Moya[12] and Crawford helped with the publication of the site of Abu Geili that he had excavated so long before.[13] Towards the end of his life, Crawford returned to the Sudan as a guest of the Sudanese government: 'Being here at all was the realization of a dream, for I had been living here in imagination for years past'.[14] It is not hard to believe that Wellcome may well have felt the same. As usual we lack Wellcome's own words and must use proxy evidence to reconstruct his feelings, just as the prehistorian works.

The area of the southern Sudan became the province of anthropologists and little archaeological work followed Wellcome's own. This was partly due to his own permission from the Sudanese government which limited the scope of others' work and partly because northern Sudan, with its proximity to Egypt, was more obviously attractive. This hiatus in work gave Wellcome's results little surrounding context and their

20 Necklaces of faience
beads and pendants.
Canaanite, from Lachish
(modern Tell ed-Duweir),
Israel, c. 1500–1200 BC.
BM, ANE 132125-6

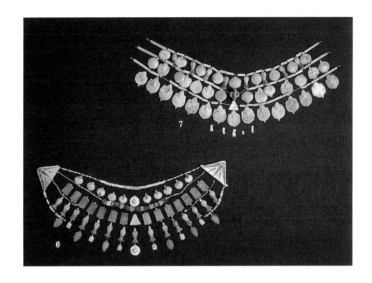

impact was decreased enormously by lack of publication. These were
important excavations in terms of scale and for the technical innovations they produced, but if you look in the best histories of archaeology Wellcome's name will be absent.

Wellcome's only other contact with archaeology was indirect, through
his funding of the Wellcome-Marston research expedition to excavate at
the late Bronze Age site of Lachish, today in Israel. Under the direction of
J.L. Starkey, the team excavated within Lachish, with striking discoveries
in the so-called Fosse Temple, including artefacts showing strong
Egyptian influence on this part of the south Levant (figs 20–22).

21 Ivory hand. Canaanite,
from Lachish, c. 1400–1200 BC.
BM, ANE 1980-12-14, 12036

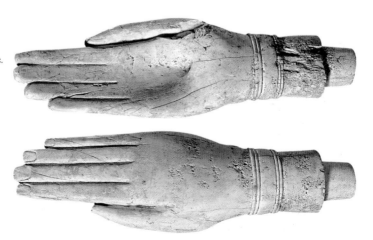

Wellcome's social being survives beyond the grave in many ways, not the least of which are through his collections and excavations. A very private man, he set up a mass of relationships with others, mostly through objects he collected or had dug up. We can reconstruct his persona to a degree by examining his objects and his practical activities, complemented with other people's words.

I am privileged to work at one of the most extraordinary museums in the world, the Pitt Rivers Museum (fig. 23). Lieutenant-General Pitt Rivers, after whom the museum is named, is seen as one the great

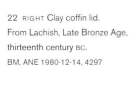

22 RIGHT Clay coffin lid.
From Lachish, Late Bronze Age,
thirteenth century BC.
BM, ANE 1980-12-14, 4297

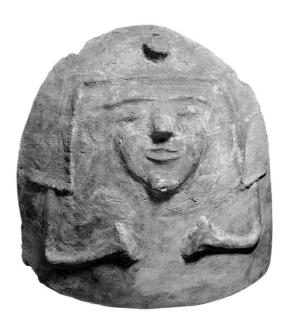

Victorian collectors and was a role model for Wellcome in his own collecting practice. Pitt Rivers stressed the importance of the everyday object in understanding human history and Wellcome followed him in this. Pitt Rivers tried to build up series of objects, showing the changes in form from the simple to the complex in (for instance) the movement from digging sticks to ploughs, or sticks to clubs. Again, this inspired Wellcome to attempt some form of completeness in his collections and his excavations, where he made his workers keep even the most mundane bits of brick and tile. A critical view of Wellcome was that he acquired Pitt Rivers' habits of mind – a belief in evolution and progress, the need for completeness, the desire for order – in the

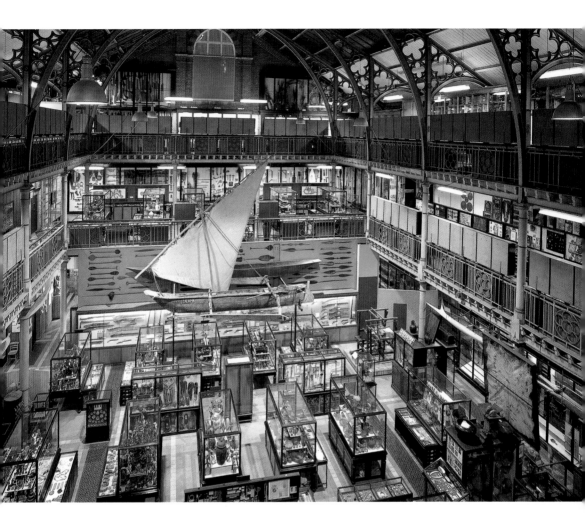

23 The Pitt Rivers Museum,
Oxford. PRM

Edwardian era when many of these intellectual habits were being questioned, making him seem behind the intellectual times.

The nineteenth-century Darwinian revolution (or was it evolution?) re-immersed human beings in nature by showing that our long-term history is shaped by the same sets of pressures as other species. In the last couple of decades social science has tried to reconnect people to the object world, showing that the animate human subject is not opposed by inanimate, brute objects, but rather that our sense of self as individuals and as groups is built up through objects which connect us to others, or isolate us as individuals. Wellcome was certainly a Darwinian in his belief, and evolution was a central theme of his medical, anthropological and archaeological interests. But I think he also doubted the subject/object distinction, even if he did not have the language to express those doubts. Such doubts may have derived from his own connections to objects. Wellcome was a very private man (he ate in his own tent on the excavations, where other whites dined communally) and this increased with age. His connections to people were through the medium of objects, making apparent the social role of things. His collections and his deep involvement with technology were not just an echo of a bygone age, but an attempt to express something of his own about the nature of the social world and its complex histories, which in the end was inexpressible.

In *The Order of Things* Foucault starts with a quote from Borges who in turn quotes from 'a certain Chinese encyclopedia' where 'animals are divided into: (a) belonging to the Emperor, (b) embalmed, (c) tame, (d) suckling pigs, (e) sirens, (f) fabulous, (g) stray dogs, (h) included in the present classification, (i) frenzied, (j) innumerable, (k) drawn with a very fine camelhair brush, (l) *et cetera*, (m) having just broken the water pitcher, (n) that from a long way off look like flies'.[15] Wellcome's collection takes us into a similarly puzzling world, where familiar logics fall away. Strangeness can seem exotic, quaint, diverting or merely misguided. But in reflective mood we realise that the things and values we hold dear and take for granted might seem odd to others. I think Wellcome realised this. Hence the range of things that he bought, many of which are confronting and odd at first sight. He also knew that any one scheme he came up with to display his collection would be too unidimensional to do justice to the material as a whole. His excavated material also made no immediate sense. Wellcome was on an intellectual journey which involved much travel, but held no real possibility of a final destination. There are many things that can be done with a great collection, such as that of Pitt Rivers or Wellcome. Not the least of these is to encourage habits of mental travel. A canopic jar, a three-thousand-year-old pot sherd, a bronze pendant which is part-woman, part-horse, part-phallus, a clay leg or ear – all of these can make us wonder about ways of life foreign to our own and how much our lives might be foreign to others. There are universals in human life, in that we all build our social lives through objects, we all speak, think, dance and die. But we are also different as individuals and as groups, which is something, as Wellcome realised, to be cherished and not merely classified, dismissed or reviled.

NOTES

1 James, R.R. 1994. *Henry Wellcome*. London:
Hodder and Stoughton, p. 14.

2 Meskell, L. 2002. *Private Life in New Kingdom Egypt*. Princeton:
Princeton University Press, p. 182.

3 Accession no. A97578.

4 Addison, F. 1949. *Jebel Moya*. Vols I and II. Oxford:
Oxford University Press, p. 1.

5 Crawford, O.G.S. 1955. *Said and Done. The Autobiography
of an Archaeologist*. London: Weidenfeld and Nicolson, p. 97.

6 Crawford 1955, p. 98.

7 Ibid., p. 102.

8 Ibid.

9 Ibid.

10 Crawford, O.G.S. and Addison, F. 1951. *Abu Geili*. Oxford:
Oxford University Press, p. 5.

11 Addison 1949, p. 9.

12 Addison 1949.

13 Crawford and Addison 1951.

14 Crawford 1955, p. 280.

15 Foucault, M. 1970. *The Order of Things*. New York:
Vintage Books, p. xv.

ACKNOWLEDGEMENTS

We sometimes lose sight of the fact that scholarly activity should be enjoyable, but my work with the 'Wellcome team' has been a great pleasure. I am extremely grateful to Ken Arnold for initially involving me with work on Wellcome, to Christine Bradley who has helped greatly with images and text, and to Danielle Olsen who has always been full of ideas and inspiration and has also helped with images and words for this piece.

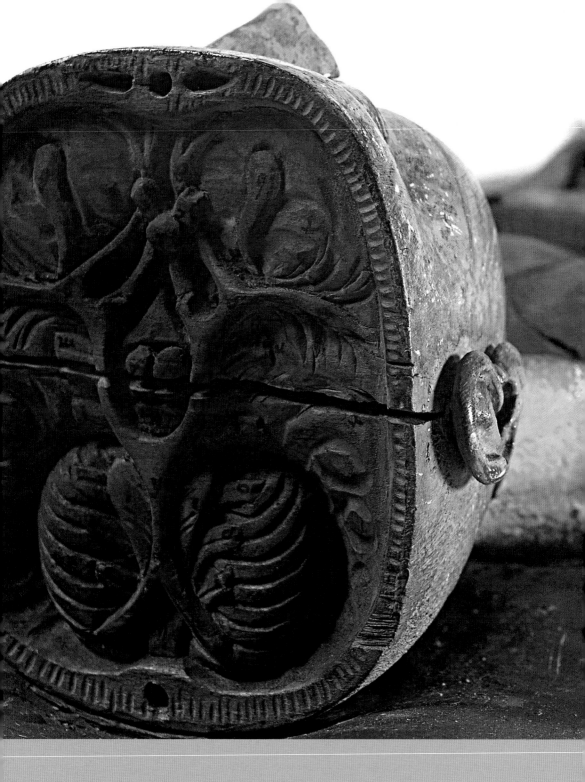

Wooden anatomical figure with
removable parts. German, c. 1700.
SM, A118272

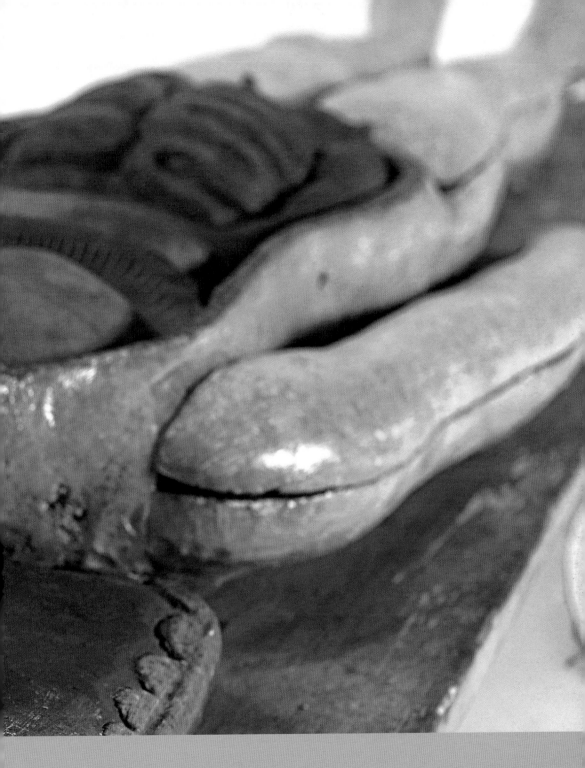

Understanding the body

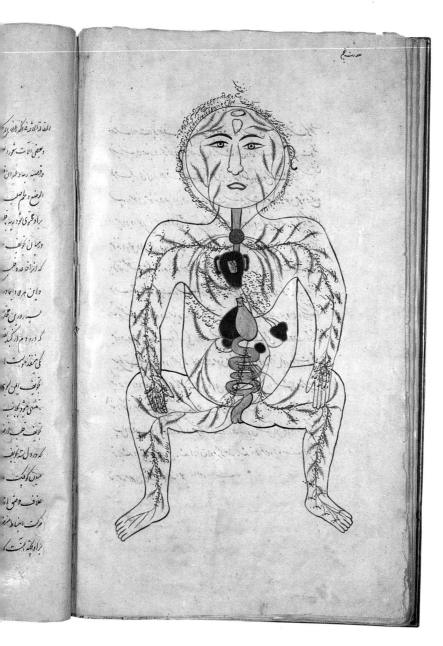

Arterial figure from *Tashrīḥ-i Manṣūrī* (*Mansur's Anatomy*). This treatise contains chapters on the five 'systems' of the body: bones, nerves, muscles, veins and arteries. Mansur came from a Persian family of scholars and physicians, and composed this work in the late fourteenth century. This copy was made in the eighteenth century.
WL, Persian MS 449

BELOW Votive male torso, dissected to show viscera. Such offerings were made to the gods either in the hope that they would cure the part of the body depicted, or to thank them for a cure already obtained. Roman, 200 BC–AD 200. SM/SSPL, A634998

OVERLEAF (LEFT) A Persian broadside copied on Western paper depicting the 'zodiac man' in which different parts of the body are shown to be influenced by various planetary conjunctions. The appropriate times and places for different treatments are indicated by the signs of the zodiac. Acquired in 1933. WL, icon. accession number 65620.7

OVERLEAF (RIGHT) Anatomical figure showing muscles. Plate IV from A.E. Gautier d'Agoty's *Cours complet d'anatomie, peint et gravé en couleurs naturelles*, Nancy, 1773. WL, EPB F.432

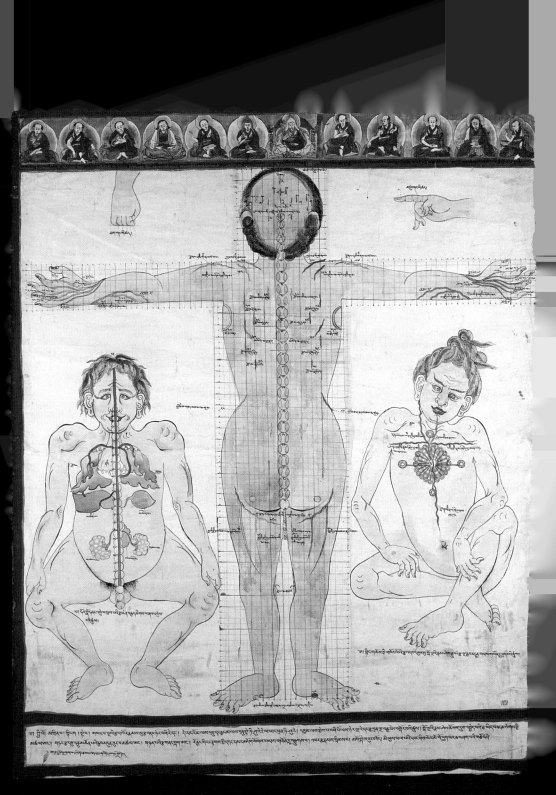

Tibetan anatomical chart showing different organs, the vertebral column, the solar plexus and the system of channels connected with the five senses and with consciousness. Twelve great medicine teachers are depicted at the top. Acquired in 1920. WL, Tibetan catalogue no. 53

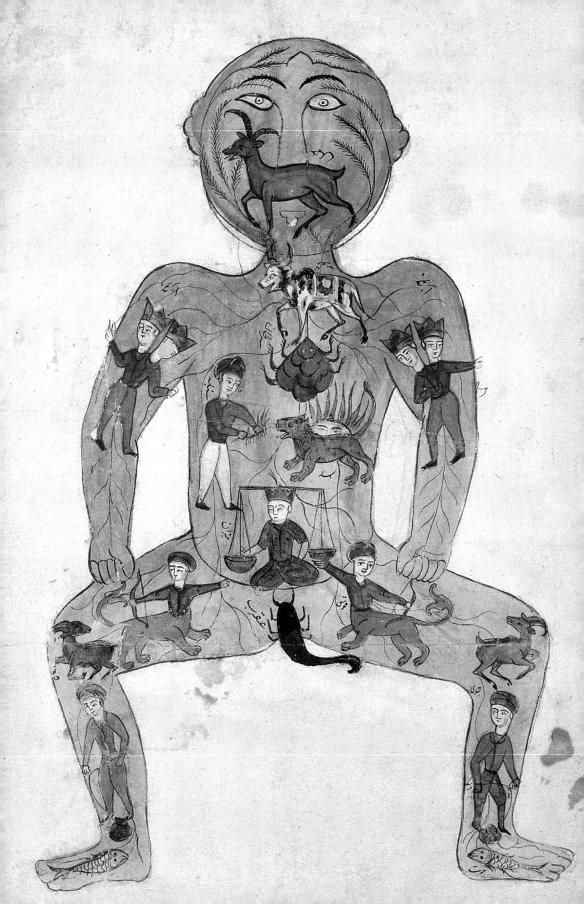

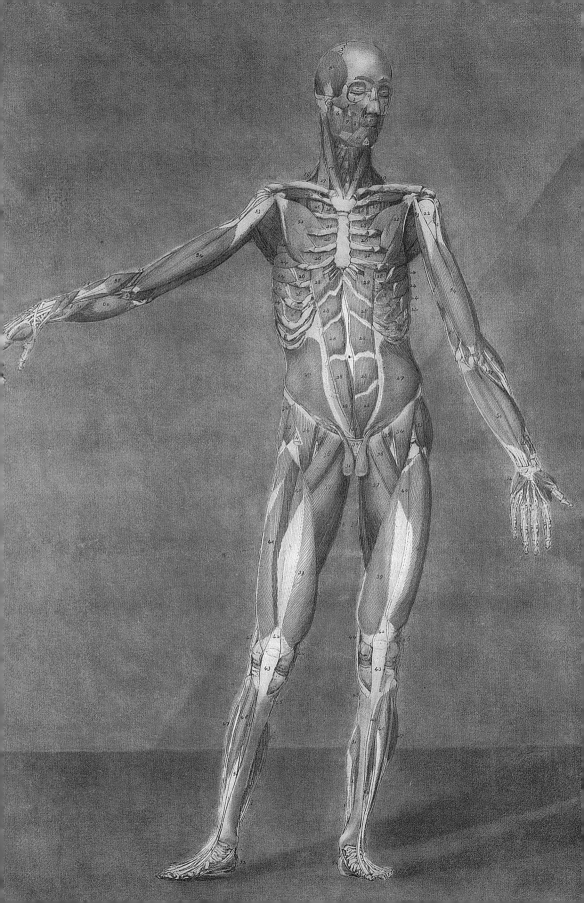

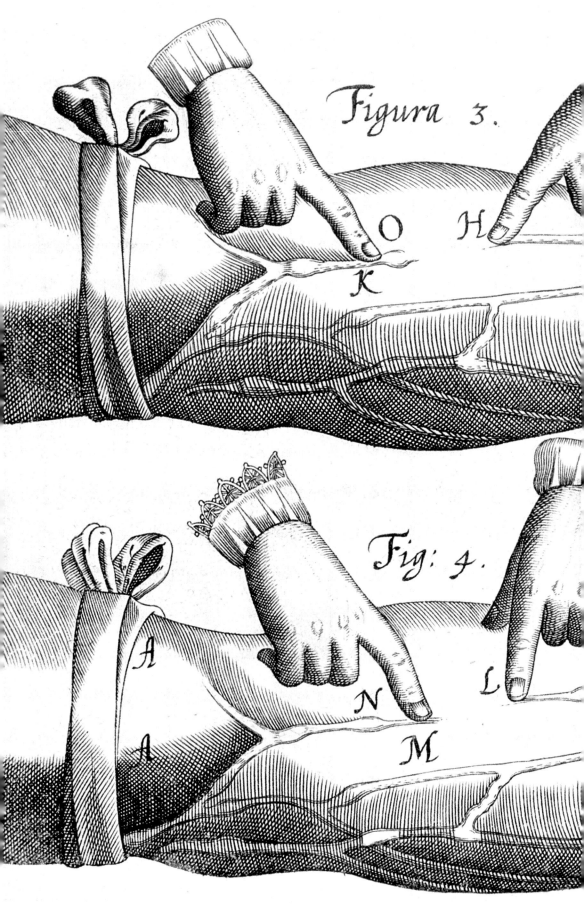

Figura 3.

O   H
K

Fig: 4.

A
A
N   L
M

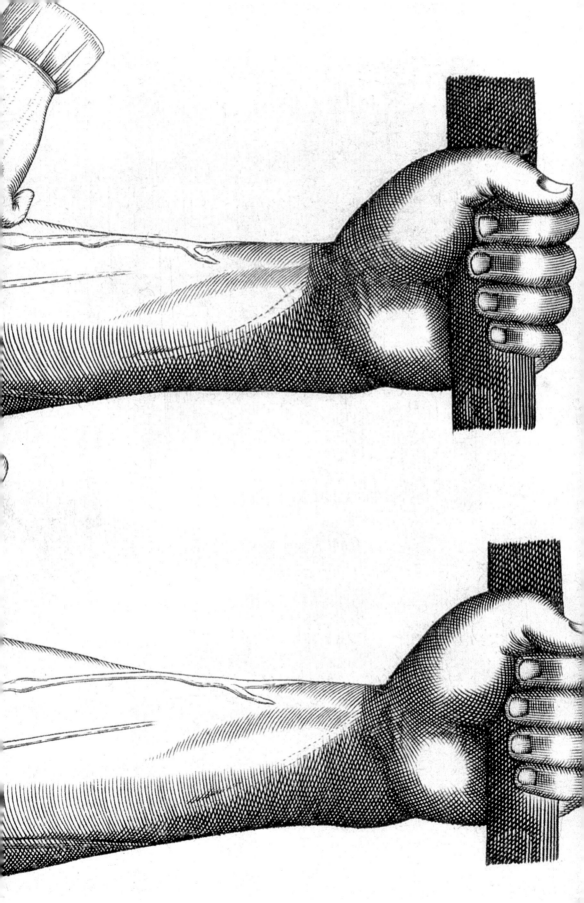

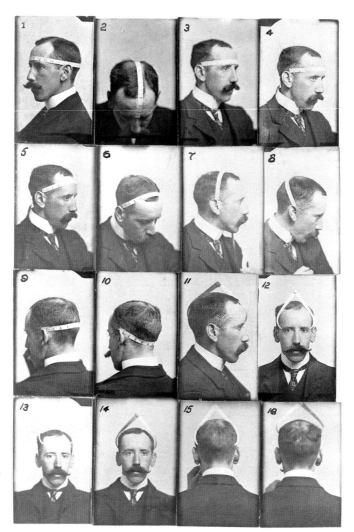

The British phrenologist Bernard Hollander illustrating with his own head his system of cranial measurements. A panel of sixteen photographs, c. 1902. WL, 27949i

PREVIOUS PAGES Illustration from William Harvey's *Exercitatio anatomica de motu cordis et sanguinis in animalibus* (*An Anatomical Study of the Motion of the Heart and of Blood in Animals*), Frankfurt, 1628. Harvey undertook groundbreaking research into the movement of the blood and the function of the heart. This picture is designed to show that valves in the veins make blood flow in one direction only. WL, EPB 3069/B

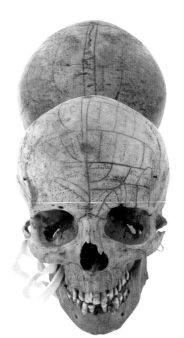

LEFT Skull inscribed in French with phrenological markings. One half shows the head according to the system of Gall, the other according to that of his colleague, Spurzheim. Nineteenth century. SM, A25407

RIGHT Chart of a head containing over thirty images symbolising the phrenological faculties. Coloured wood engraving by Henri Bushea after Orson Squire Fowler, c. 1845. Imprint: London. WL, 27923i

SYMBOLICAL HEAD.

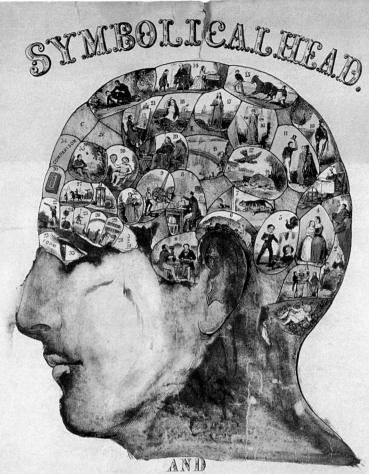

AND
PHRENOLOGICAL CHART,
BY DR BUSHEA, L.L.D.

EXPLANATION of the CUT. The design of this Cut is, to show the natural language of the mental organs situated in the various parts of the brain. For example—Veneration is represented by a devotional attitude; Benevolence, by the good Samaritan; Secretiveness, by the Cat catching the Rat; Destructiveness, by the Tiger destroying his Prey; Sublimity, by the Niagara Falls; Acquisitiveness by the Miser, weighing and counting his money; Causality, Newton philosophising upon the falling of the apple; Alimentiveness, by two persons eating and drinking; Firmness, by the Donkey, &c.

ARRANGEMENT; NUMBERING AND DEFINITION OF THE FACULTIES.

Animal Propensities.

1. AMATIVENESS.—The passion of love and attraction between the sexes as such; desire to caress and fondle.

A. MATRIMONY.—Desire to pair; to unite for life; and to be constantly in the society of, and to share with, the loved one.

2. PHILOPROGENITIVENESS—Parentallove, regard for children, pets, and animals, and attention to their wants.

3. INHABITIVENESS.—Love of home; attachment to the place where one lives, or has lived; desire to locate and remain in one place.

3*. CONCENTRATIVENESS.—Unity and continuity of thought and feeling; disposition to dwell upon one subject until it is completed.

4. ADHESIVENESS.—Friendship; attachment; affection; desire for society; to congregate; to associate; and to entertain friends.

5. COMBATIVENESS. — Self protection ; defence, personal courage ; resistance; boldness; resolution; the let-me-alone disposition.

6. DESTRUCTIVENESS.—Executiveness ; energy; indignation; hatred; retribution; and a destroying exterminating disposition.

*ALIMENTIVENESS.—Appetite; hunger and thirst; desire for nutrition; and enjoyment of food and drink.

7. SECRETIVENESS.—Secrecy ; concealment; cunning; evasion; policy; management; ability and disposition to disguise, and to play oppossum.

8. ACQUISITIVENESS.—Desire to acquire and possess; to trade; save; and take care of property, the mine-and-thine feeling.

9. CONSTRUCTIVENESS.—Contrivance; skill; ingenuity; desire and ability to use tools, and understand machinery; manual dexterity.

Religious and Moral Sentiments.

10. SELF-ESTEEM.—Self-respect; dignity; independence; love of liberty and power; self-reliance, and desire to command respect.

11. APPROBATIVENESS.—Regard for character and reputation; ambition; affability; desire for popularity, fame and distinction.

12. CAUTIOUSNESS.—Sense of danger; precaution; solicitude; fear; apprehension; regard for present and future safety; dread of results.

13. BENEVOLENCE.—Kindness; humanity; sympathy; pity; disinterestedness; munificence; desire to make others happy.

14. VENERATION.—Worship of God; feeling of devotion and respect; regard for superiority, things sacred, authority, and antiquity.

15. FIRMNESS.—Will; decision; stability; perseverance; determination; fixedness of purpose, and unwillingness to change; fortitude.

16. CONSCIENTIOUSNESS.—Sense of moral obligation; regard for duty, justice, integrity, and right; penitence for sin; and desire to reform.

E. CIRCUMSPECTION.—Discretion; consistency; uniformity; balancing; regulating power, and desire to harmonise the character.

17. HOPE.—Sense of immortality; of a future state; anticipation of success and happiness; looking forward to future results.

18. MARVELLOUSNESS.—Faith; belief in Divine Providence; sense of the omnipresence of God; of spiritual existence; wonder; surprise.

19. IDEALITY.—Refinement; delicacy of feeling; taste; love of perfection and beauty in nature, art, and composition; ecstacy.

B. SUBLIMITY.—Sense of the vast; grand; sublime; terrific; extravagant; endless; wild and romantic in nature, art, or composition.

20. MIRTHFULNESS.—Wit; sense of the absurd and ridiculous; ability to joke, make fun, ridicule; gaiety; levity; playfulness; humor.

21. IMITATION.—Power of imitating; copying, and representing; versatility of action; doing as others do; describe and act another's part.

Perceptive Faculties.

22. INDIVIDUALITY.—Observation of things, and power to examine; to identify individual objects; to be an eye-witness; curiosity.

23. FORM.—Recognition of shape; likeness, or outline; memory of countenance and configuration; and ability to commit to memory.

24. SIZE.—Perception of bulk; magnitude, and proportion; ability to judge of length; breadth; height; angles; perpendiculars and distances.

25. WEIGHT.—Sense of gravity, and power to apply its principles to machinery and muscular motion; shooting; balancing; walking on ice, &c.

26. COLOR.—Sense of colors, their different shades, and harmony in their arrangement in nature and painting; delight in seeing them.

27. LOCALITY.—Memory of place; location; direction; where we have seen persons and things; the geographical faculty.

28. CALCULATION.—Perception of numbers, and their relations; numerical computation; ability to reckon figures in the head.

29. ORDER.—Arrangement; system; neatness; method; desire for convenience and method; and economy in business operations.

30. EVENTUALITY.—Sense of active events; love of experiments; desire for knowledge and information; fondness for narrations of occurrences.

31. TIME.—Knowledge of chronology; of the duration and lapse of time; memory of when, and how long; equality in step, and the beat in music.

32. TUNE.—Perception of sound, melody and proper emphasis in reading, speaking, or singing; ability to compose music.

33. LANGUAGE.—Ability to talk; to communicate ideas; to use appropriate language; versatility of expression; memory of words.

Reflective Faculties.

34. COMPARISON.—Sense of resemblance; ability to analyze; classify; compare; infer; critical acumen; inductive reason.

35. CAUSALITY.—Perception of the causes of things; the why? and wherefore? power of abstract thought; penetration; planning; originality.

C. Capacity to judge of the true motives, characters, and intentions of others, aside from their actions; perception of thoughts and desires unexpressed; the faculty of like and dislike.

D. Adaptation of causes to their effects; intuitive perception of results; power to perfect and apply an argument; ability to act and speak as to accomplish a desired end.

TEMPERAMENT.

There are Four kinds of Temperament.

THE LYMPHATIC, or PHLEGMATIC, in which the secreting glands are the most active portion of the system, producing both corporeal and mental languor, inactivity, and dulness; an aversion to exercise the corporeal and intellectual functions.

The SANGUINE, in which the arterial portion of the system is the most active, indicated by a strong and rapid pulse, strong feelings and passions, and more of ardour, zeal, enthusiasm, and activity, than of strength and powers.

The BILIOUS, in which the muscular portion of the system predominates in activity, producing strength and power of body, with great force and energy of mind and character.

The NERVOUS, in which the Brain and the nervous system are most active, gives the highest degree of excitability and activity; vividness of emotion, intensity, rapidity, and clearness of thought, perception, and conception; sprightliness of mind and body, but less endurance.

EXPLANATION

The written figures refer to the Developement and Strength of the Faculty, thus, when marked 2, Idiocy; 4, very small; 6, small; 8, rather small; 10, moderate; 12, rather full; 14, full; 15, rather large; 18, large; 20, very large; 22, extra large; 24, ultra extra large.

Entered at Stationers' Hall.

Second Edition, Improved.   LONDON:—PRINTED FOR THE AUTHOR, BY S. STRAKER, 80, BISHOPSGATE STREET.   Price 2s. Plain; 2s. 6d. Coloured.

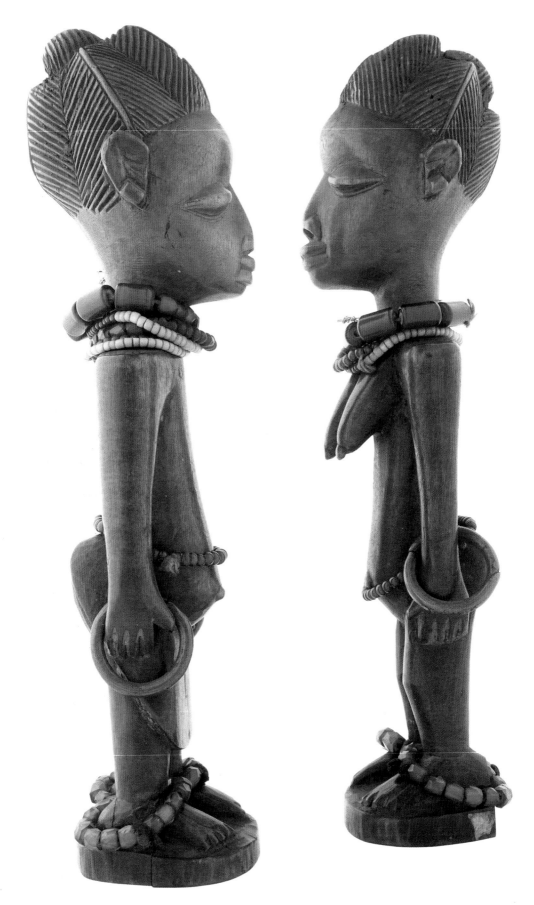

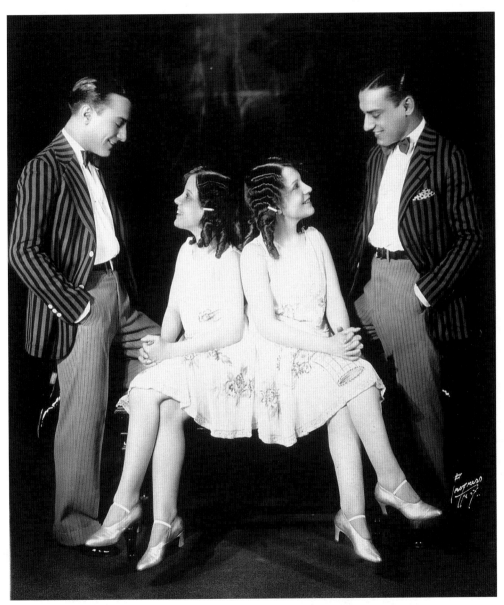

LEFT Yoruba Ibeji figures, representing twins. When images such as these are first carved, they are soaked in an infusion of medicinal plants, and adorned with amulets to ensure the twins' good fortune. The Yoruba have one of the highest twinning rates in the world. Nigerian, 1871–1910.
SM, A655924, A655927

Daisy and Violet Hilton, conjoined twins, being wooed by two young men, c. 1927. Daisy and Violet were born in Brighton, England, to a poor unmarried barmaid called Kate Skinner. Skinner sold the twins to her employer, Mary Hilton, who trained them to sing, dance and play music, and exhibited them all over the United States and Europe. This photograph was taken at Progress Studios, New York.
WL, 33703i

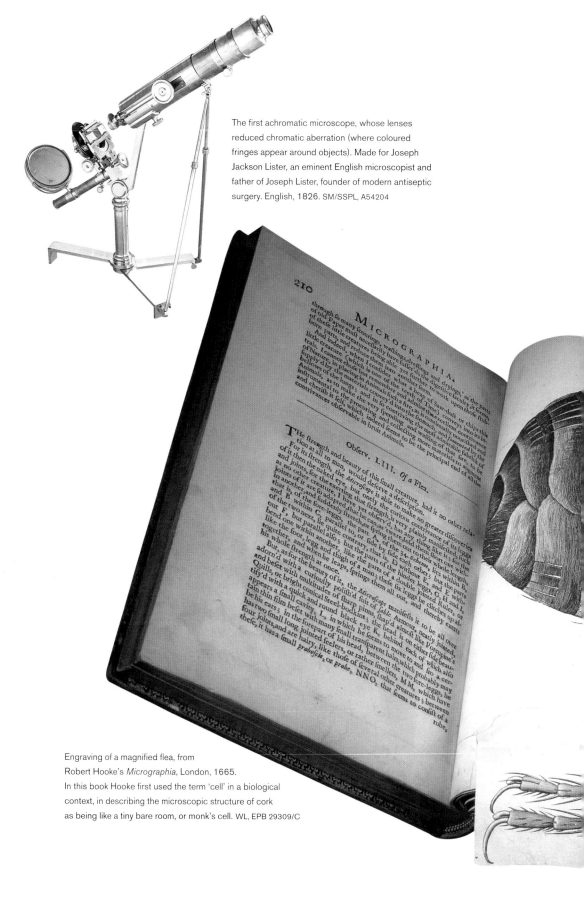

The first achromatic microscope, whose lenses reduced chromatic aberration (where coloured fringes appear around objects). Made for Joseph Jackson Lister, an eminent English microscopist and father of Joseph Lister, founder of modern antiseptic surgery. English, 1826. SM/SSPL, A54204

Engraving of a magnified flea, from Robert Hooke's *Micrographia*, London, 1665. In this book Hooke first used the term 'cell' in a biological context, in describing the microscopic structure of cork as being like a tiny bare room, or monk's cell. WL, EPB 29309/C

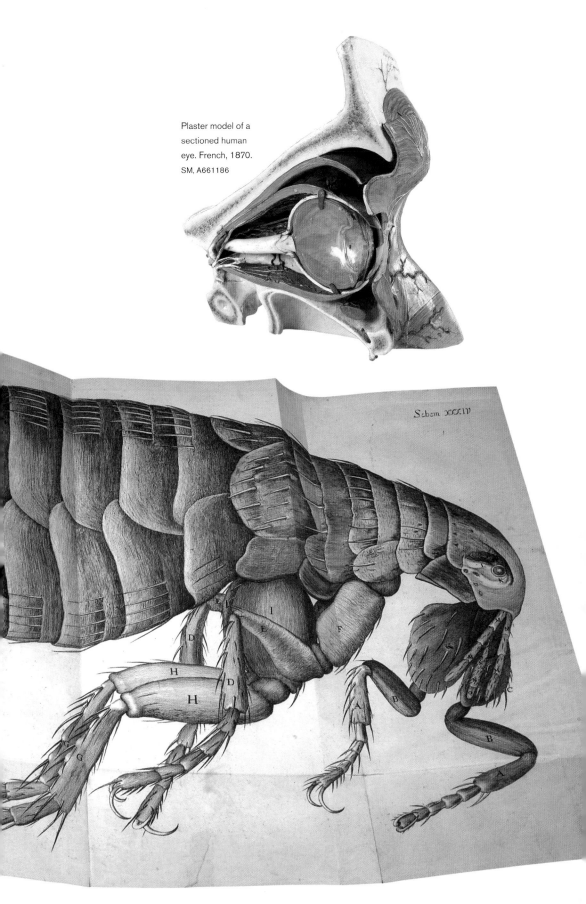

Plaster model of a
sectioned human
eye. French, 1870.
SM, A661186

Schem XXXIV

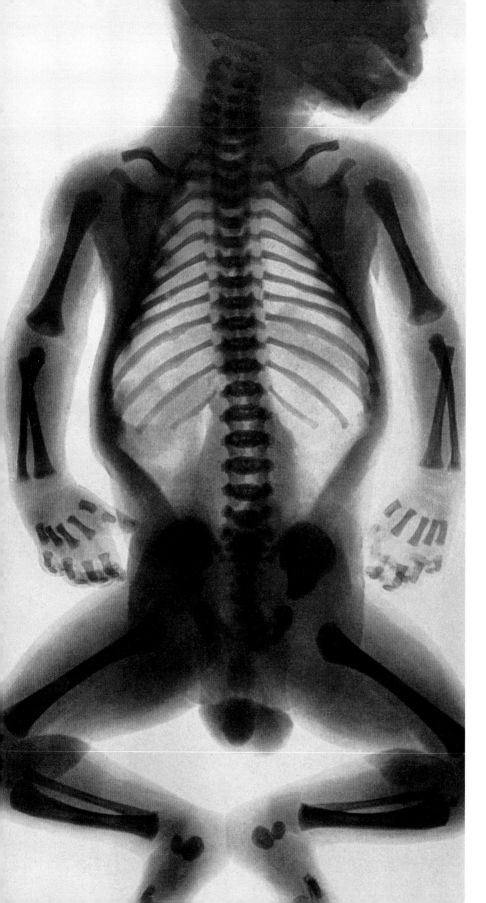

Radiographic images by G. Leopold and T. Leisewitz, Dresden, 1908. On the left, the skeleton of a mature child, and on the right, the injected arterial vessel system of a nine-month-old foetus. WL, 17137i (left), 17141i (right)

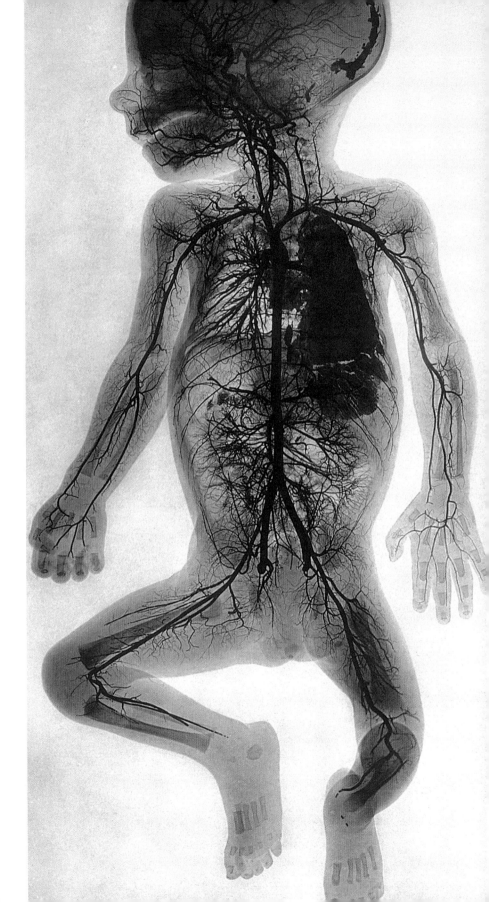

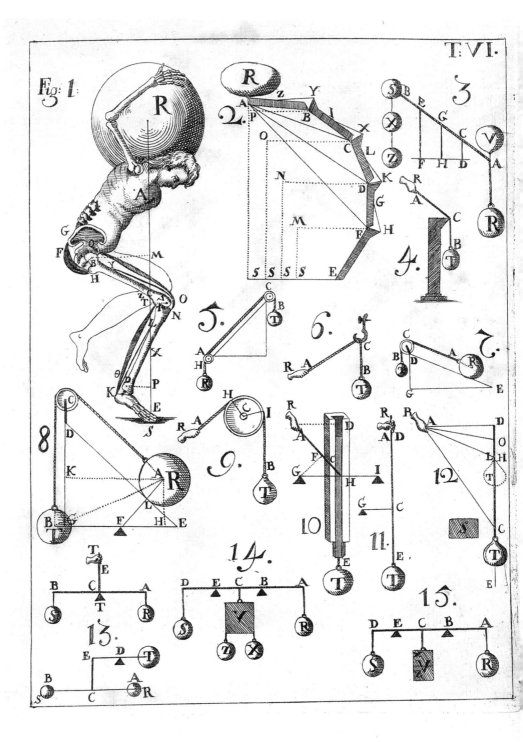

T: VI.

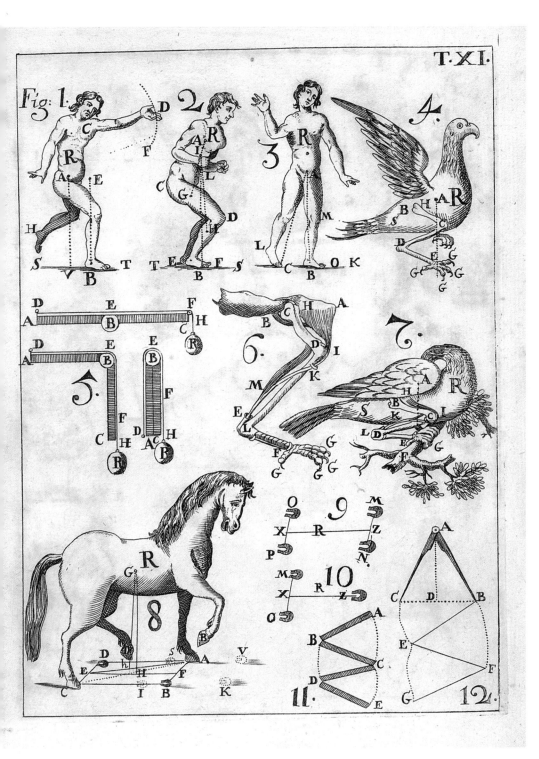

Illustrations from Giovanni Alfonso Borelli's *De motu animalium*,
Naples, 1734. Borelli (1608–79) was the first to systematically
apply the new mechanics of Galileo to physiology. WL, EPB 14628/B

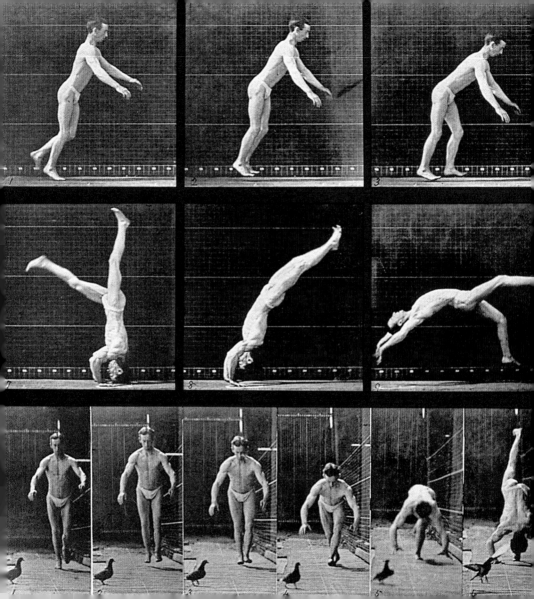

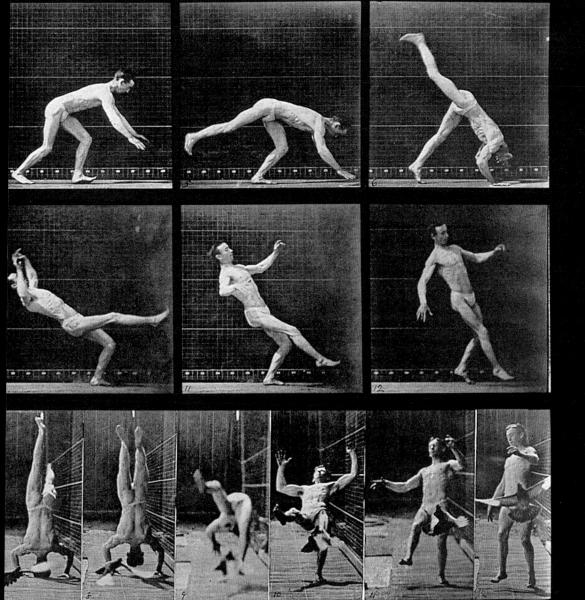

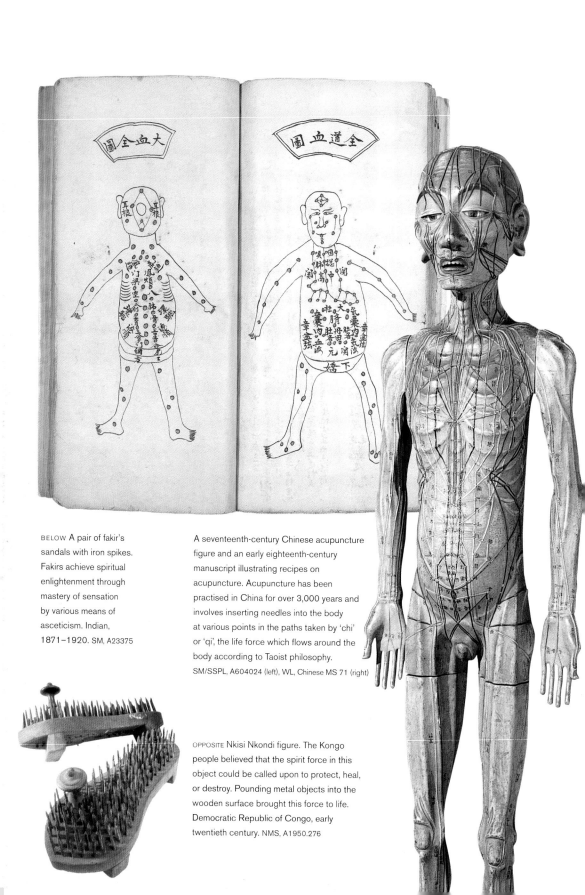

大血全圖

全道血圖

BELOW A pair of fakir's sandals with iron spikes. Fakirs achieve spiritual enlightenment through mastery of sensation by various means of asceticism. Indian, 1871–1920. SM, A23375

A seventeenth-century Chinese acupuncture figure and an early eighteenth-century manuscript illustrating recipes on acupuncture. Acupuncture has been practised in China for over 3,000 years and involves inserting needles into the body at various points in the paths taken by 'chi' or 'qi', the life force which flows around the body according to Taoist philosophy. SM/SSPL, A604024 (left), WL, Chinese MS 71 (right)

OPPOSITE Nkisi Nkondi figure. The Kongo people believed that the spirit force in this object could be called upon to protect, heal, or destroy. Pounding metal objects into the wooden surface brought this force to life. Democratic Republic of Congo, early twentieth century. NMS, A1950.276

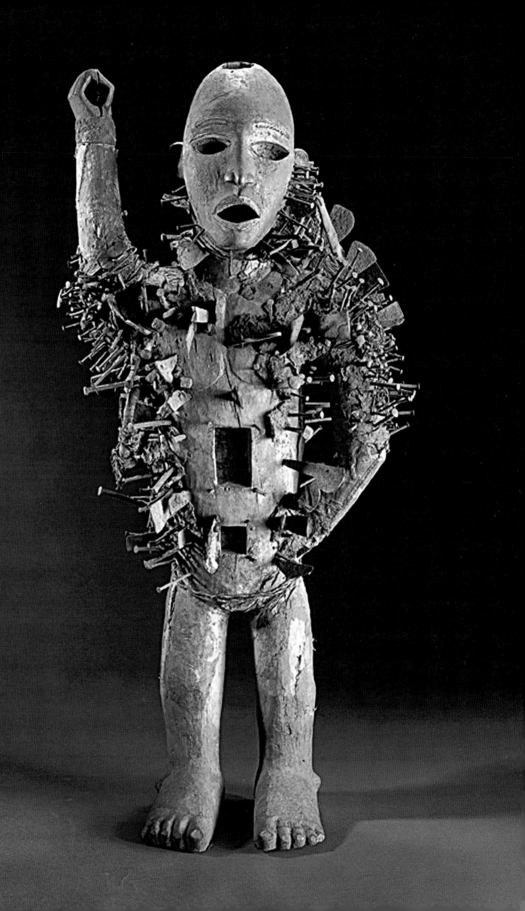

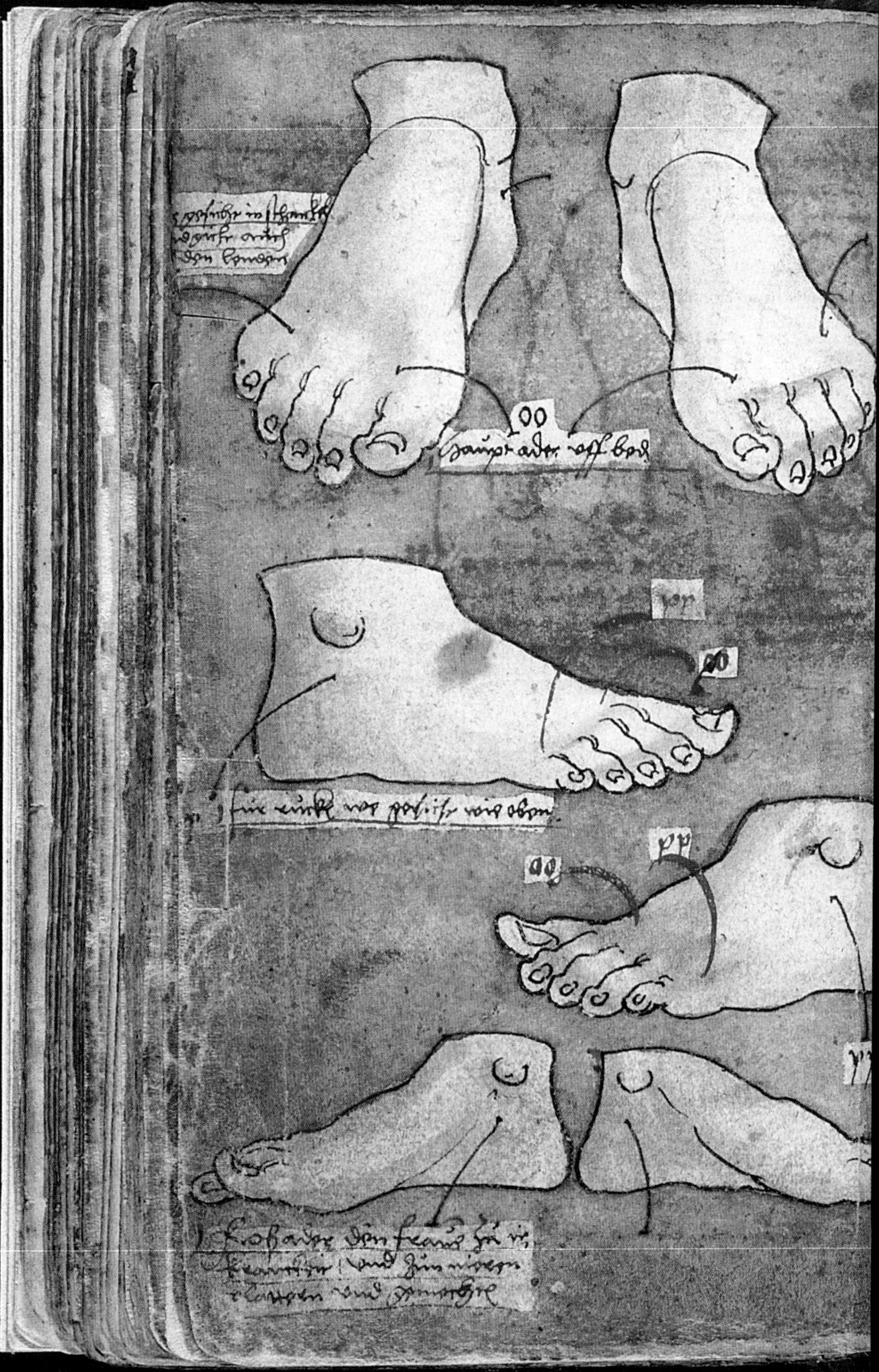

gefucht in ffrancke
wurd ortis
den lunzen

gainot aider offbord

fur einke wer geluse wer obom

pp

00

qq

Kohader den frans zu v.
kraucher und zu widern
clappen und zunwhe

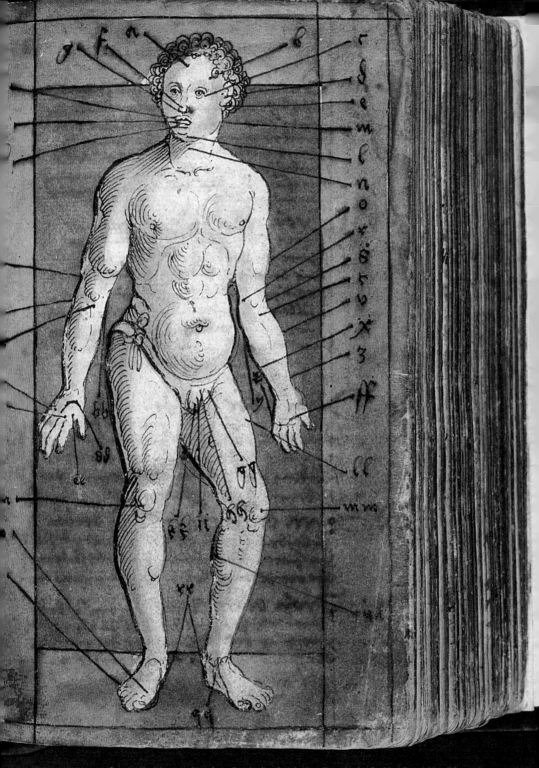

Illustrations from a German health manual, or *Arzneibuch*, showing the location of veins for bleeding. 1524–50. WL, Western MS 93

Et si 12 dicte quarta sexta in abecedario gelando quod signum lune ad
istum diem sit signum questionis Ergo signum questionis una sittab
gradum ad arbitrium cuius est tradita hec sitta loco 4 sunt 2 2 quos
quos gradus adde ii gradibus et faciunt 36 gradus in
signis lune iam mutetur adde numerum ... transitorum et faciunt
22 signa Et quia faciunt 36 gradus dico quod anno domini 143x
9 hora ... in festo mathie luna ... medium
motum eius erat et fuit in 17o gradu cancri ...

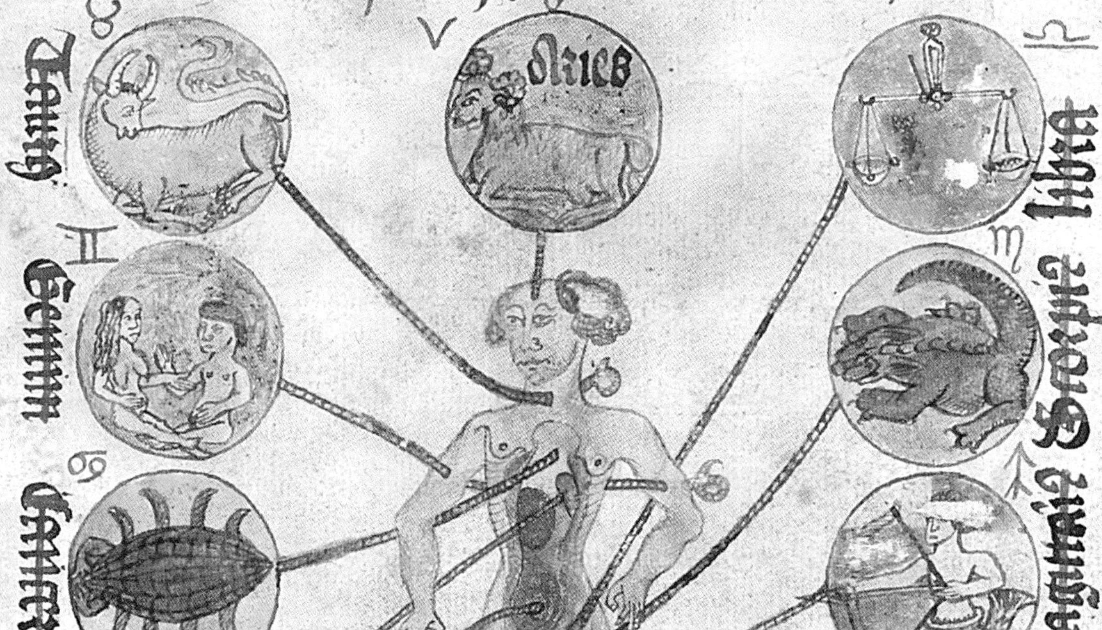

Item Aries ist hoeft. Thaurus in die hals. Gemini in die arme. Cancer
in die borst. Leo in dz hartz. Virgo in de buwick. Libra in den nauel. Scorpio in de
macht. Sagittarius in de diech. Capricornus in de knie. Aquarius in de scheen. Piscis in de voet.

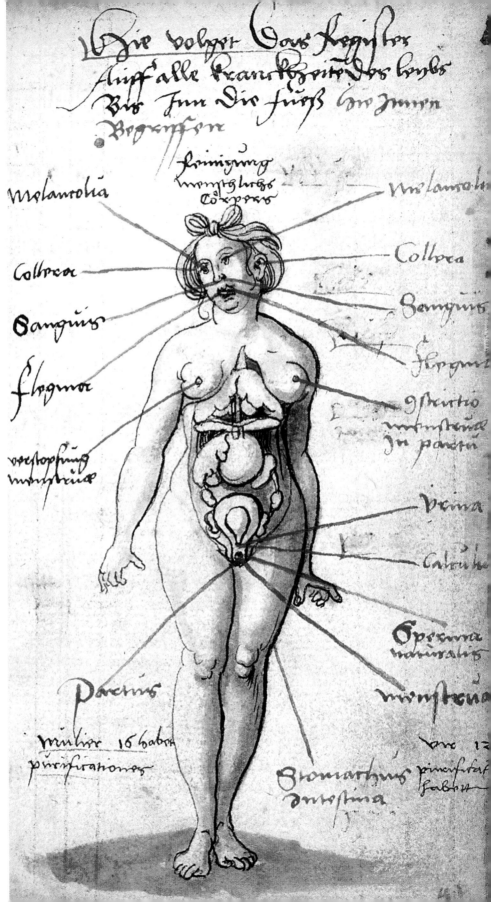

LEFT 'Astrological Man' linking parts of the body to the corresponding signs of the Zodiac. Taken from Heymandus de Veteri Busco's *Ars Computistica*. This manuscript includes notes on the calendar, medical astrology and fortune-telling. Dutch, 1488. WL, Western MS 349

RIGHT Illustration from a German health manual, or *Arzneibuch*. This figure introduces a section on diseases based on the humoral model of the body. 1524–50. WL, Western MS 93

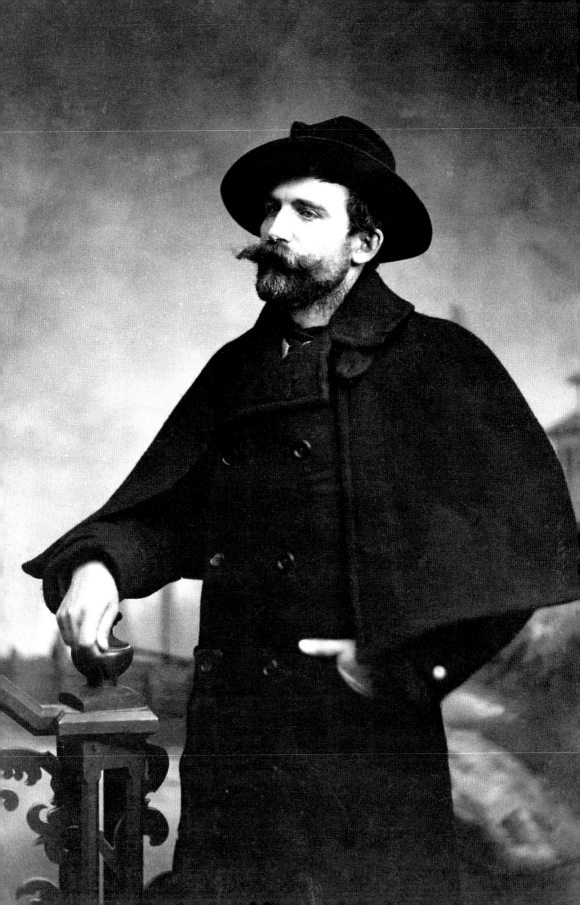

Henry Wellcome, 1887.

'All my life I have been a keen

student in the field of anthropology

and have made extensive

collections of ethnological objects

from various parts of the world.

These collections form a

predominant part in my Historical

Museum in London, although

at the present time, for want

of adequate housing space,

The Historical Medical Section

is the most prominent.'

LETTER FROM HENRY WELLCOME TO COLONEL HAY, 22 JUNE 1929.

Medicine and Anthropology in Wellcome's Collection

John Mack

'Actually my interest in anthropology came before the medical, but still they have both continued on parallel lines or have merged. My collections of anthropological material, considered as such, are vastly greater than the strictly medical, while most of the anthropological material possesses strong medical significance, for in all the ages the preservation of health and life has been uppermost in the minds of living beings, hence the omnipresent medical man and the *religio medico*, or priest physician.'

(Henry Wellcome in *Great Britain, Royal Commission on national museums and galleries*, London, HMSO, 1929)[1]

The Hall of Primitive Medicine, which started life as a temporary exhibition and became a significant part of the Wellcome Historical Medical Museum established in Wigmore Street, London, from 1914, was the most substantive physical expression of Wellcome's vision of the links between medicine and anthropology. It was hard to avoid the Hall: it was on a major artery through the Museum such that visitors were obliged to pass through it, a situation echoed by the new Wellcome Gallery on the main through-route of the British Museum (although, in that case, without the implication that it is 'primitive'). The gallery, and its earlier predecessor – the initial exhibition put up in 1913 to coincide with the Seventeenth International Congress of Medicine held in London that year – contained what to modern expectations would seem a somewhat bewildering range of displays. Included were methods of food preparation, examples of edible substances, culinary equipment, shields, spears and other weaponry, implements used in theft and in the punishment of miscreants, masks, figures, divination implements, amulets and other magical devices, and so on. The objects displayed would not be out of place in the scheme of a general ethnography gallery (figs 1–2). Furthermore they were a microcosm of the eclectic collecting habits of Wellcome himself. The question of whether his displays of objects were just a *melange* of

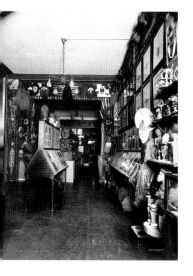

things which happened to have interested him across a long life is addressed above (see Ghislaine Lawrence essay). Wellcome's curators helped to shape the Museum's displays as they evolved, and his writings and instructions to the Museum staff suggest that he had a wider vision that was not fully realised in his galleries. But the question to be addressed here remains: do Wellcome's collecting habits and the displays in his Museum have any meaningful rationale which we can recover and which is significant today?

The central questions raised by the Commissioners taking Wellcome's evidence concerned the utility of anthropological museums and the possibility of creating a central museum for the display and study of ethnographic collections. Wellcome's responses could be somewhat impenetrable; but he was clear about one aspect of the value of such collections: they would benefit native races by enhancing better government and more humane colonial administration. After all, he argued, if you were to ask a Sudanese who was the greatest person who had ever lived, the unvarying reply would be 'Mahommet'. Yet if you were to ask who was the greatest living person, the answer would be 'Kitchener', the victor over the Khalifa's forces at the Battle of Omdurman but also, Wellcome argued, its benign, anthropologically informed Governor General through to the restoration of peace. The Sudanese had been unable to fight for Kitchener in the Great War but instead, Wellcome remarked, had contributed generously to funding the British Red Cross.

1 Hall of Primitive Medicine, Wellcome Historical Medical Museum, 13 Wigmore Street, London, *c.* 1914.

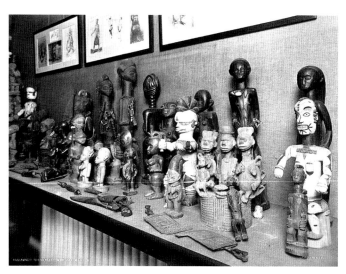

2 Figurines of West and Central African origin in the Hall of Primitive Medicine, *c.* 1914.

They recognised, it was asserted, just treatment and good government when they saw it. Wellcome supported other apologists for enlightened colonial rule such as the collector and ethnographer whom he provided with medical support in the Equatorial Forests of Central Africa, Emil Torday.[2] Both saw acquaintance with ethnographic collections as the essence of a sound grounding in administrative nouse overseas, 'for the man who understands native peoples and their habits, customs, superstitions, their beliefs, and fears, has an enormous advantage over the man who does not'.[3]

But when it came to his views on the relations between anthropological or ethnographic collections and his medical interests, Wellcome had struggled to make the members of the Royal Commission understand. He had run through a number of scenarios which would lead his examiners to think of them together. Most of his examples, however, seemed to stress concurrence rather than convergence. In the person of the informed medical missionary (fig. 3), he found the closest point of intersection – people like the Cook family, doctors in Uganda inspired by the Christian faith, whose example encouraged Wellcome to open the 'Lady Stanley Women's Hospital' in 1931 to support maternity and child welfare.[4] Important as this hospital was to become (and when Wellcome gave his evidence he was yet to fund the initiative), it must have seemed to the Commissioners somewhat vague because, rightly or wrongly, the most compelling reason he seemed to be giving for merging his ethnographical and medical interests was expressed as autobiographical rather than conceptual. It is worth following him down these unconventional, and to an extent unfashionable, byways to see what modern thinking might make of this. In the two sentences with which we start, Wellcome sought to come up with a definitive statement of where and how anthropology and medicine relate. What follows in this chapter is a reflection on their intent and significance.

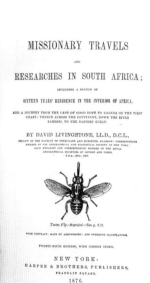

3 Title page of David Livingstone's *Missionary Travels and Researches in South Africa*, New York, 1876. Wellcome was much attracted to the larger-then-life figures of African exploration, becoming close to Henry Morton Stanley, the 'finder' of Livingstone, in the 1880s. WL, BZP (Livingstone)

'My collections of anthropological material . . . are vastly greater than the strictly medical'

Wellcome famously bought huge quantities of objects offered for sale at auction and elsewhere in the opening decades of the twentieth century – and then failed to unpack them systematically. Much remained boxed up in storage until redistributed after his death to Museums with more rigorous approaches to registration and curatorial housekeeping (fig. 4). The diversity of his collection, his apparent lack of honed discrimination and his tolerance of copies where originals were otherwise unavailable to him are regarded by some as an embarrassment. The suspicion is that Wellcome did not know, or was sufficiently wealthy not to bother about a distinction treasured by the tyros of the market in ethnography and antiquities. Fakes or transgressive images of one sort or another were apparently as acceptable as the 'authentic'. The spirit of the collecting, as demonstrated elsewhere in this volume, however, was one of urgency: as is still to an extent the case today, the pace of change led to a heightened sense of the need to document what was still extant by acquiring it before it disappeared. There are reasons why Wellcome, and by extension his employees, sometimes bought first and inspected their haul of objects later, sometimes rejecting objects, sometimes too pressed to examine them closely. In any case, Wellcome himself told the Royal Commission, collecting in duplicate was a good thing for it meant you could have one example for exhibition and another to be studied and handled by those wishing to learn from the collections. The spirit was that it would, if not now, potentially one day all be useful – and, of course, 'handling collections' are now much in vogue.

Museums have different methods of registering and recording their objects. The arrival of electronic options and digitalised imagery have transformed this

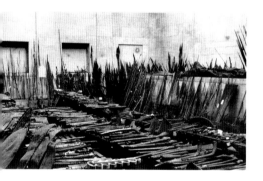

4 Weapons originally belonging to the Wellcome Historical Medical Museum laid out in the Duveen Gallery at the British Museum, 1955. The photograph shows one section of the gallery only, probably about one twelfth of the whole.

process. In the British Museum a different approach was in place until quite recently. Indeed my first job, which was so large that ultimately it was overtaken by electronic advances, was to identify, describe, research and draw the African objects donated by the Trustees of the Wellcome Historical Medical Museum in a major distribution of the original collection in 1954. This was done in large brown leather volumes. Many young curators have learnt their trade from being obliged to undertake these tasks, of which the now-abandoned duty to draw was the most time-consuming and controversial (fig. 5). Some were better at it than others. It did, however, teach initiates like myself how to look systematically at objects and how to interpret them.

In a stimulating essay, the art historian and critic John Berger has described the technique used by the pre-war German photographer August Sander.[5] His method was to invite each of his sitters to stare at the camera with the same expression. Whether priest or paper-hanger, their approach in front of the camera was the same, allowing

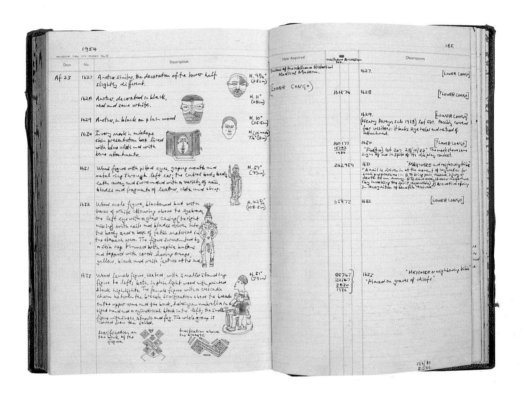

5 Page from the accession register of part of the Congolese objects donated to the British Museum in 1954 by the Trustees of the Wellcome Historical Medical Museum. The descriptions and drawings are those of the author. BM

the differences arising from experience and character to emerge when photographs of different subjects are placed side-by-side. Similarly curators developed an 'eye' from systematically scanning each object, always on the look-out for difference among otherwise similar things. The purpose in drawing was not necessarily to represent the thing as it was, but to highlight the features that made it distinctive from other objects with which it might later be confused. It helped develop a strong sense of objects as part of a series of creations, whilst focusing attention on distinguishing detail. Like the colonial administrators whom Wellcome imagined picking up an understanding of native culture from the process of handling and studying indigenous artefacts, curators learnt their trade from these intense sessions of looking and drawing.

The methods of registration adopted by Wellcome's curators were somewhat less rigorous than this: their labels still attached to the objects donated to other institutions and the original registers which support them from the 1950s provided little guidance to those of us who undertook the task afresh in later years. This is not necessarily a criticism: they were not unique in this. Most museum curators of the same period similarly worked with artefactual categories of little analytical subtlety. Orientalism was rife, but was not regarded as the problematic approach it is seen as being today. As in the Registers, there was a rough classifactory system at work in the storerooms: weaponry, furniture, masks, figures and so forth. The strictly medical, it will be noted, was at best a subsidiary category subsumed beneath the broad umbrella of anthropology.

'The *religio medico*, or priest physician'

Many of the issues that arise in an attempt to understand Wellcome are about the difficulties of cross-cultural classification. In the registers and the stores, a grand catch-all term, 'ritual object', applied to anything that defied the descriptive vocabulary; it signified something out of the ordinary, something eccentric. The term is likewise adopted as a flag of convenience by archaeologists and many ethnographers faced with aspects of activity that escape the existing categories. In front of the Royal Commission, Wellcome might well have used the term when talking of his interest in the overlaps between the fields of religion and medicine; but he preferred instead to run his categories together – to merge them.

In many parts of the world, 'eccentric' behaviour, disturbing dreams and associated physical affliction are diagnosed as the product of spirit or demonic possession. During anthropological fieldwork in Madagascar, I worked for a time with a young administrator in one of the southern towns of the island. He had been an impassioned man with a large appetite for life and an energetic, impatient nature; but when I got to know him he had started to be greatly impeded by debilitating bouts of uncertainty, outbreaks of sweating, and vivid, troubling dreams. He consulted a traditional healer and learnt that he was afflicted by a foreign spirit (*tromba*). At this time a wave of spirit possession, which would itself repay analysis as an historical phenomenon, was sweeping Madagascar.[6] Many of the most powerful possessing spirits were identified with exotic, external origins. Of these, some of the strongest here in a distant coastal region were linked to Andrianampoinimerina, the founder and ruler of the expansionist kingdom in the centre of the island in the late eighteenth century. In the case of my unfortunate colleague, the diagnosis was that the invasive entity was derived from a foreign sailor; it had disembarked from one of the ships visiting the local port, only to dock within his person.

The method of cure in such circumstances is to expel the invading spirit by inducing it to speak, which it did through the mouth and gestures of the administrator when in trance. The afflicted had to confront and ultimately overcome the possessing spirit by taking on its characteristics. The preparations were lengthy. Firstly, a white tunic reminiscent of a sailor's suit was sewn together for my colleague to wear during the expulsion process. A large model ship was made as a vessel for the voyaging spirit and this was placed on a table facing him when the ceremony began. Finally, a *zebu* (or humped cow) was bought which would be sacrificed at the end to seal the event.

The whole procedure was overseen by a spirit familiar – a female relative who had herself been possessed and who guided him through the lengthy and threatening process. The ceremony took several exhausting days as the afflicted moved in and out of a state of trance, convulsed periodically, stuttering and swaying to the accompaniment of music, the consumption of rum, and the inhalation of smoke from burning substances which were placed on the model ship in front of him. Throughout the process he was the centre of attention, his unpredictable swings of mood guided by his more experienced, solicitous assistants. At dawn on the second day the voice of the afflicted gained a new level of fluency and certainty, and the spirit finally began to speak, almost to sing, in a babble of language which mixed bits of Malagasy (the language of Madagascar) with what seemed to be snatches of French and Swahili. The resultant speech became a flood that needed translation, which the spirit familiar provided in a colourful but still relatively incoherent interpretation. As psychoanalysts in the West undergo psychoanalytic treatment themselves as part of their training, so here the administrator, having successfully expelled the unwelcome spirit guest, regained his former zest for life, and himself became a spirit medium.

Such processes of exorcism have an ironic aspect: to get rid of the possessing spirit you have to submit body and soul to the possessing spirit. The sailor's suit, the ship and the voice of the possessed are all expressive of the identity of the matelot, the unwanted intruder. As a spirit medium in his own right, my colleague might adopt other persona in order to advise other sufferers of appropriate strategies and effect cures. Like an actor performing different parts in different costumes, the varying identities of spirits implies varying presentations. One of the most remarkable exponents of spirit mediumship in the region was a young schoolgirl who, when I visited her, was doing her homework, studying a French primer with the evocative title *A Toi de Parler*. Her spirit identity was signalled by the simple expedient of loosening her hair (something female relatives otherwise only do as a mark of mourning) and putting on a hat. Nonetheless the identification of illness and disorder with invasive spirits which

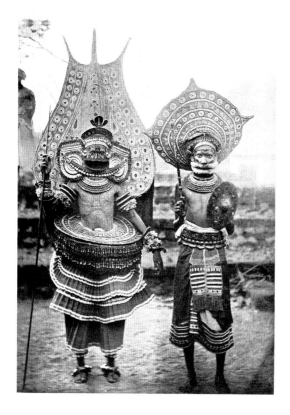

6 Image said to be of 'two Malayan exorcists' wearing appropriate ritual costume. From a photograph by Wiele & Klein, *c.* 1900. WL, 21487i

need to be expurgated establishes a link between expertise in the spirit realm and the practice of healing. So Wellcome was right to insist on the connectedness of medical and religious considerations in many cultural contexts. Indeed, one of the leading British anthropologists of the opening decades of the twentieth century, W.H.R. Rivers, himself a physiologist, psychologist and anthropologist, had defined the complex as the cluster of conception, diagnosis and treatment which links medicine, magic and religion.[7] And it is worth noting that L.G.W. Malcolm, who from 1926 was the Wellcome Museum's Conservator, was himself a Cambridge graduate trained in anthropology by A.C. Haddon and by Rivers. Haddon was to offer his services to the Museum, as he did also to the Horniman Museum in south London and to the Museum of Archaeology and Anthropology in Cambridge.

Wellcome's photographic collections are replete with images of 'ritual specialists' from around the world. Some are copies of original photographs; others have been re-photographed from travel writings, biographies and early twentieth-century ethnographic monographs. The archival prints range from Malayan exorcists 'clad in the appropriate disguises for carrying out their professional avocation' (fig. 6) to 'A Zulu medicine-man fighting a coming hailstorm' (fig. 7) and a Nigerian 'shaman' who 'has to wear numerous charms not only to make certain that he possesses magical powers, but also to advertise the fact he depends upon them, some of which he sells for a high price'. 'The clothes of the man,' the inscription continues, 'are almost concealed by the number of amulets, while a leopard-skin does duty as a hat' (fig. 8). The terms 'medicine-man' and 'shaman' in this vocabulary are generous categories dealing with the sources of all manner of conditions: physical discomfort, psychic or psychological disorder, and even adverse weather forecasts.

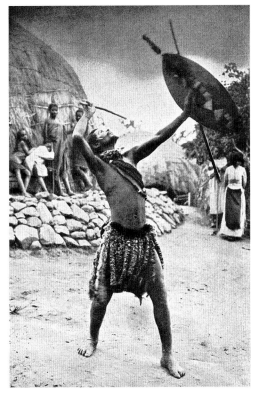

7 Zulu ritual specialist said to be combating a threatening hailstorm. From a photograph by the Trappist Mission at Mariann Hill, Natal, South Africa. WL, 21325i

It seems likely that the selection of images for the archive was implemented with direct instruction from Wellcome himself. However, as an indication of what was considered worth preserving in support of the collections and displays, it is a good indication of how the wind was blowing that Wellcome's employees conducted their trawl of the potential sources against a classificatory system that happily merged the medical and the ritual.

In the Hall of Primitive Medicine, the display of masks was similarly focused on the convergence of these categories. Some masks certainly do function in ways comparable to the garb of the possessed

9 OPPOSITE Sinhalese mask used in exorcism and showing the heads of the eighteen disease-spreading demons on either side of the central figure. Sri Lanka. Acquired before 1900. SM, A51293

in Madagascar. They assert a separate persona; they alter the state of mind of the individual such that, in the flow of ritual performance, they not only represent spirits, but the masker is himself also entranced, suffused with spirit. The human agent within the concealing frame of the mask becomes the vessel of the spirit, a wholly owned subsidiary (to borrow from the vocabulary of the other side of Wellcome's life), rather than simply an external mechanism. They thereby obtain the potential to cure and to be cured. But there are clearly gradations within this. Subsuming all masking within a single category risks confusion. The Sinhalese masks in Wellcome's original collections are a good example of some of the modalities.

In Sri Lanka there are two cycles of masked performance which are common to many parts of the island. Of these, one, *Kolam*, is essentially a form of mythic drama in which stories of origin are presented by masked performers. The origins of masking practice are traced to Vesamuni, the god of good fortune whose name translates as 'disguised face', suggesting that the 'artifice' of masquerade is well understood to be a contributory element in the drama.[8] There is little explicit connection to illness and healing in the conception of this masking complex. However, a second sequence of masking gets much closer to our theme. *Sanni* refers to masking that is a part of exorcism rituals, the term itself being associated with disease-spreading demons, which number eighteen in the Sinhalese cosmos (fig. 9). *Sanni* exorcism is concerned with redressing imbalances which have arisen through demonic intrusion into the person of the individual. Health and wellbeing are seen as being dependent on a proper balance of the humours: wind, blood and bile, and phlegm. Demonic intervention disrupts a healthy humoral balance.

8 Medical specialist photographed at Maiduguri, north-eastern Nigeria, wearing amuletic devices. From a photograph by Mrs C.L. Temple. WL, 21326i

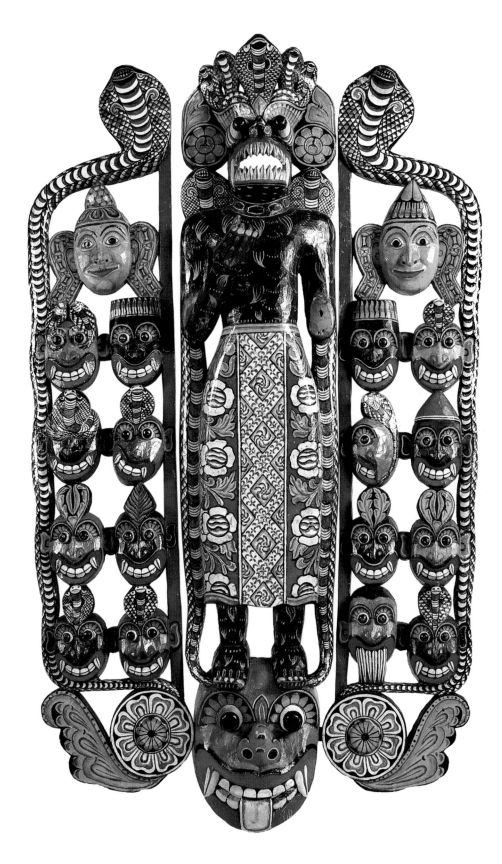

Its restoration is achieved by returning the possessing demon to its own appropriate place in the demonic order through exorcism from the body of the patient.

Exorcism follows a sequence of more or less complex actions depending on the seriousness of the demonic possession to be confronted. One of the most feared of all is *Mahasona*, the Great Cemetery Demon, whose name is given to exorcism itself. As the power of *Mahasona* comes from its drawing of lesser demons into itself (including the *Sanni* demonic order), so its exorcism subsumes the features of other rites that are appropriate to lesser demons in Sinhalese conception.[9] The process of exorcism thus requires the successive presentation of the demonic elements which contribute to the state of disorder and illness to be resolved; these are confronted by invoking the overarching power of the divine and ultimately their effectiveness is thereby sublimated. In the case of the *Sanni* demons, they are first invited into the arena that has been constructed for the

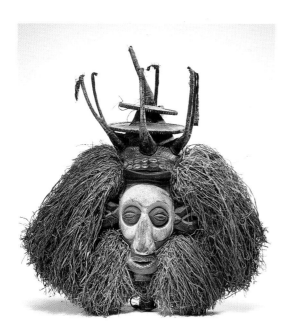

10 Mask used in male initiation into adulthood. Yaka people, Democratic Republic of Congo. Acquired before 1936. FMCH, X65-5447

exorcism rites. Their entrance is presented through dance performance, offerings are made and they enter the 'palace' which has been constructed for them. During these proceedings the patient falls in and out of trance. Finally, the performance ground is purified, the divine presence of Shiva is invoked and with the singing of appropriate songs the shadow of illness is lifted. In the context of *Mahasona* exorcism, this is but one episode as the *Sanni* demons subsumed within the greater demonic order are in effect returned to their subordinate place within the cosmic hierarchy. Other demons have different methods of expurgation and realignment. Similarly less fearful cases of demonic possession may be addressed through the performance of the individual elements of episodes brought together in the exorcism of the Great Cemetery Demon.

Within Sinhalese practice, then, there are two distinct uses of masks, the one theatrical, the other curative. In the Hall of Primitive Medicine, and even more so in the wider Wellcome collection, all these were mixed together. Many of the masks from Africa that were included are associated with initiation procedures, often connected with circumcision and, until recently, with the withdrawal of initiates to enclosed initiation camps where they remained in isolation for lengthy periods during which they were instructed into adulthood (fig. 10). One of the secrets learnt by initiates is that the masked figures which police their retreat are articulated from within the concealing envelope of the costume by their fathers and older brothers. This knowledge of the mechanics of masking, of course, does not necessarily make masquerade fraudulent, as one of its meanings in English asserts. The masks may be held to represent ancestral spirits, spirits of the bush and so forth (fig. 11). These entities are no less powerful a point of reference for initiates because, unlike women and children, they are now 'in' on the intelligence that masking is orchestrated by human agency. The masks are still expressions of jeopardy: dangerous, powerful and threatening.

Yet where masking challenges the presence of spirits in the cultural contexts we have considered, other traditions have a more placatory character. The Elema of the Papuan Gulf live on long sandy beaches bordered on one side by the depths of the sea and on the other by the extensive forests. Both are conceived as the dwellings of potentially dangerous spirit-monsters. Up until the 1930s, the period when Wellcome died, a vigorous tradition of entertaining these various spirits in a series of festivals was observed. The sequence of ritual performance lasted over periods of up to twenty-five years and followed a series of developing episodes. As different communities along the coast were at varying stages in the cycle, a regular pattern of events was followed. Wellcome acquired a number of the masks associated with these ritual performances, including a tall-necked form worn on the top of the dancer's head, conveying great height (fig. 12). The masks and other ritual objects produced for these events

11 Headpiece of an 'egungun' mask depicting an ancestral hunter. Yoruba people, Nigeria. Acquired before 1936. FMCH, X65-9051

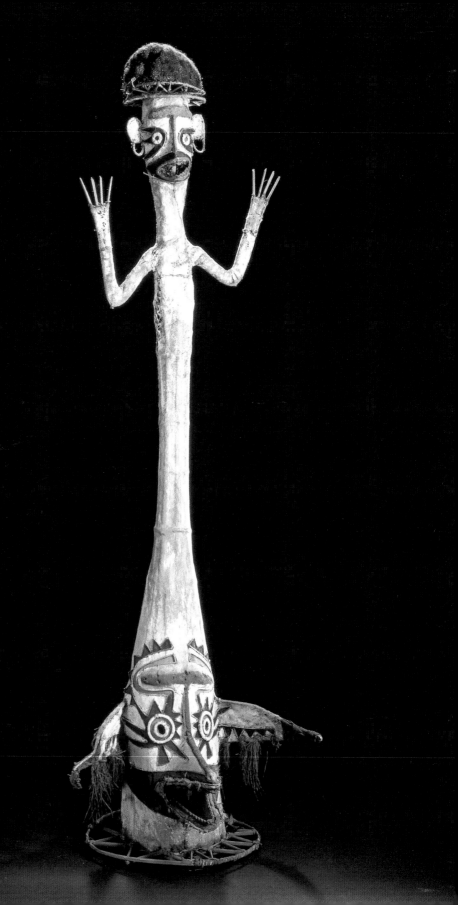

are conceived as temporary dwellings for the spirits of the depths of land and sea. And the rituals themselves, rather than invoking the threatening or healing powers of the spirit world, are focused on inviting in and entertaining spirits. They have a deliberately comic aspect. Where exorcism is a palliative, enacted after illness has occurred, Elema ritual is more like preventive practice.

'The preservation of health and life has been uppermost in the minds of living beings'

12 Tall headpiece from a masquerade designed to entertain potentially malign spirits as part of a cycle of masquerade performances. Elema people, Papuan Gulf. Acquired before 1936. FMCH, X65-4344

Even if we leave to one side the uses of masks in antiquity, they are familiar devices employed in the modern world in a wide variety of contexts, which appear to move us a significant distance from straightforward so-called 'medical' applications. They are worn variously by burglars, terrorists, wrestlers, welders, hunters, children at birthday parties, surgeons, executioners – *and* performers in rituals of healing. From a simplistic point of view, masks have in common the fact that they transform: the person donning the mask looks different with the mask on than without it. However, the extent to which that capacity is exploited varies considerably in human cultures. Assembling all the different types together and thinking of them as the same will not work (figs 13–16). Yet what this does point out is the need to take these categories of the material world one step back. Masking is not so much a type of object as a technique of transformation which can be exploited in various ways.

We have looked above at the wide range of material assembled in the original Wellcome museum to illustrate his theme of primitive medicine – everything from amulets to weapons, from enemas to food bowls. Like the elastic category 'mask', much of this may seem to stretch credibility. What, we may well ask, has the display of quantities of spears and shields got to do with medicine? Surely this is taking us beyond the bounds of reasonable association. Wellcome, in one of his promotional pamphlets, uses the image of a spear juxtaposed to a 'tabloid' (his word for one of his patented pills). The latter, in his astute marketing language, is described as a 'weapon'. Wellcome's products were a kind of protective shield. Where earlier generations had seen strength of will and character as an aid to seeing off tuberculosis or cancer – and the lack of such qualities as a cause of their development in the first place – Wellcome was patenting a cure which took the older image and made the unequal fight against illness more winnable.

In English, the language of possession and of exorcism is replete with ideas of uninvited intrusion, of guests who neither knock before coming in nor are willing to recognise a time to leave, and whose presence is only detected when things really start to go wrong. So too sorcerers are often said to have 'shot' malign substances into the victim, hence the dramatic sequences in which sorcerous material is apparently extracted from the body of the sufferer. This is the same

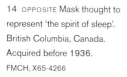

13 Ekpo society mask which represents an elephant. Ogoni people, Nigeria. Acquired before 1936. BM, Af23.877

14 OPPOSITE Mask thought to represent 'the spirit of sleep'. British Columbia, Canada. Acquired before 1936. FMCH, X65-4266

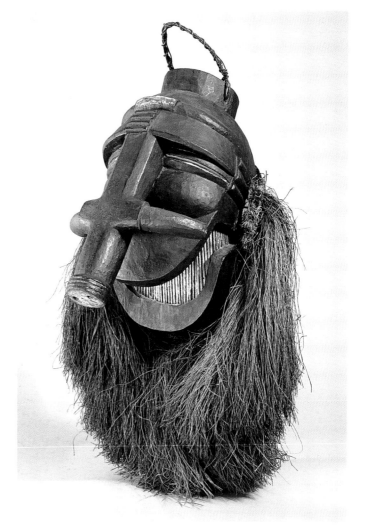

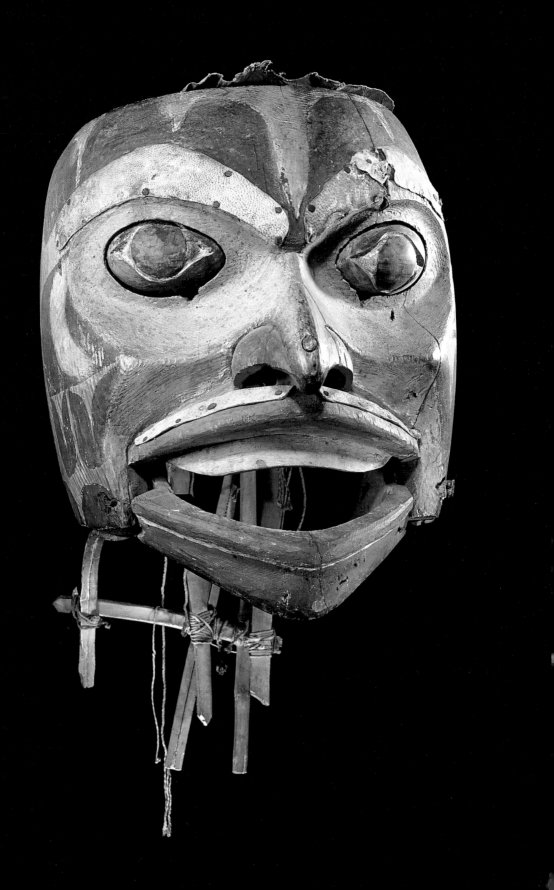

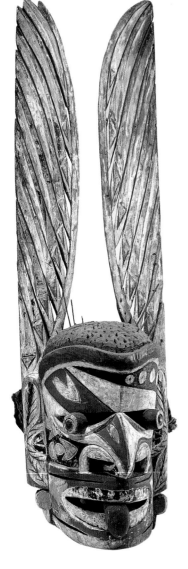

15 Mask used in complex mortuary ceremonies (*malangaan*). New Ireland, Papua New Guinea. Acquired before 1936. FMCH, X65-4360

vocabulary as that of bacteriology, where the imagery of warfare predominates. Bacteria are likewise invasive: sufferers 'battle' against their symptoms and their treatments seek to 'kill off' the unseen microbes.[10] The physical drama of the entranced 'fighting' the possessing spirit, wrestling to 'overcome' and 'expel' the intruder, suggests the metaphoric connection is a well-established cross-cultural form of understanding of illness and disorder. In other languages two basic forms of vocabulary prevail: one talks of restoring balance, the other of fighting off and protecting against intrusive illness. In Swahili, for instance, there is a range of terms describing illness and disease. The common understanding of the aetiology of disease is the belief that it is evil people who send you illness or wish it upon you. The term *kujikinga* is the commonest for describing protection against the onset of malaise. It refers to charms and devices which 'shield' individuals and households from illness. There is much theatre and much word-play in this – apart from Wellcome as publicist and showman, Sinhalese exorcists, Swahili ritual specialists and Shakespeare, amongst others, have all been here. These are at root ways of thinking about and understanding fundamental human experience. As Roy Porter has eloquently shown,[11] to see illness as injury is deeply embedded in our conception of its causes, and to see all injury as preventable – given the right protective shields (whether of weapon, amulet or tabloid) – expresses a common convergence of apprehension in the minds of living beings. This convergence is therefore not diminished or replaced by the advent of modern medicine.

'My interest in anthropology came before the medical'

Autobiographical reflection provides us with a metaphor for a rationale Wellcome took into a wider understanding of the human condition. He introduces us, as he did the Commissioners in 1929, to the sequence of his own interests: from anthropology to modern medical science. Anthropology – those palaeolithic arrowheads and artefacts of native American life which initially interested him – was of his own childhood. So, too, in the evolutionary scheme he advocated, anthropology was the route to an understanding of the childhood of man, earlier conditions brought forward as memory to modern times. His

Museum, after all, was an educational museum of the *history* and *context* of medicine, not of the *practice* of medicine – that was dealt with elsewhere in his Museum of Medical Science. As a visitor, you had to pass through the Hall of Primitive Medicine to get anywhere else in the building, as humanity had been obliged to pass through a condition where all things were subsumed together before medical science became separated out. The Hall of Primitive Medicine is also a glimpse into the hall of Wellcome's own mind and intellectual orientation. A visit to the Museum was a trip through the evolution of man and his cultural creations. What had been merged together was the sequence of Wellcome's own interests with that of human history – and this in its turn became an ordering device designed into a museum.

16 Wood mask in a style associated with the Ngunie River area of Gabon. Such masks are often worn by men mounted on stilts enhancing the effect of other-worldliness. Acquired before 1936. FMCH, X65-5270

Of course, as has been well documented,[12] all this was about Wellcome's adoption of the anthropology of the later nineteenth century. With present-day suspicions of master narratives of human history, of applying rooted Western-centred categories of analysis across cultures, this is easily dismissed as old-fashioned – indeed, even at the time when Wellcome was applying such ideas, they were already becoming out of date. In his evidence to the Royal Commission and elsewhere Wellcome mentioned his gratitude to the leading figures of museum anthropology of his day: Charles Hercules Read at the British Museum or Henry Balfour at the Pitt Rivers in Oxford. But he was not talking of intellectual debts or the sources of his own inspirations. If there was anyone who filled that role it was probably Pitt Rivers himself, though what we know of Wellcome's self-contained self-motivated character suggests he would have seen Pitt Rivers as a fellow traveller rather than a guiding light. Pitt Rivers' approach was similar to Wellcome's. He took in a broad sweep of human history and sought in his displays to reveal the progress of man from his infancy through to technological and intellectual advancement. The display of the Pitt Rivers collection disregarded cultural context and put objects together as technological categories, showing thereby successive phases of technological advancement within single object types. Cultural variation was comprehended and subjected to a discipline of evolutionary principles.

This worked best for displays of weapons or tools; and when it worked well in display terms, an emergent visually coherent structure of development was evident in the arrangement of the objects on the walls and in the cases. When it did not, the gaps and 'missing links' were evident. It is reminiscent of the obsessive ordering of things by someone like Samuel Pepys. Pepys, of course, collected books. He reportedly arranged and rearranged his library, and finally classified his books according to size. This he did in double rows on the shelves of his study with the larger volumes placed behind the smaller so that the titles of all could be seen; and in order that the tops were aligned with each other, wooden blocks were placed under the shorter books to give a uniformity of height. These were then gilded to match the bindings.[13] As in evolutionist displays, the individuality of each item in the collection was subsumed within their formal presentation in series. They could only be rescued by being taken out of their allotted place – though once done, the gap would become obvious by breaking up the sequence. It is hard to imagine Pepys putting the books he had been working on in a pile for the night rather than replacing them in their proper places on the library shelves. No more can we imagine a Pitt Rivers being happy with a gap in the sequence of his evolutionary displays.

This was the spirit of the Wellcome exhibitions in his museum – a visual sequence coherent with an evolutionary sequence, and ultimately coherent with an autobiography. In 1925 Wellcome closed the Museum for six months to allow his new appointee, Malcolm, to make changes. As Skinner has described,[14] the result put weapons together in an overall sequence which started with animal tusks and ended with the repeat firing musket, whilst more directly medical sequences dealt with the surgical knife, the toothbrush, the enema and the gas mask. For evolution of a common design to be visually coherent required closer proximity of form than any of these sequences could possibly achieve. In 1928, when a new tranche of training staff were recruited, they included four anthropologists. They would have been entirely conversant with the new theoretical stance that was emerging: an emphasis on functional categories and inter-relationships. The Hall of Primitive Medicine, within which all of this was subsumed, would have made some sort of sense to them. What the sequence is actually about is displaying a series of functionally related objects arranged in a broadly chronological sequence, in which medical science is allocated a part, but is not an imposing measure of the rest. It does for medicine and its contexts what the British Museum does for British history and culture: it locates it in its wider field, the better to apprehend it for what it is. And perhaps in the end the underlying contemporary message to be drawn from Wellcome's perception is that institutions of this kind need an anthropological perspective to comprehend them as wholes.

NOTES

General reference: James, R.R. 1994. *Henry Wellcome*. London: Hodder and Stoughton.

1 'Oral Evidence, Memoranda and Appendices to the final report'. London: HMSO, pp. 103–9.

2 Mack, J. n.d. (1990). *Emil Torday and the Art of the Congo, 1900–1909*. London: British Museum Publications.

3 Wellcome 1929, p. 103; see also Torday, E. 1925. *Causeries Congolaises*. Brussels: Vromant.

4 Wellcome 1929, p. 106; Turner, H. 1980. *Henry Wellcome, The Man, His Collection And His Legacy*. London: The Wellcome Trust and Heinemann, p. 27.

5 Berger, J. 1980. *About Looking*. New York: Vintage International, pp. 31–40.

6 Estrade, J.-M. 1985. *Un Culte de Possession a Madagascar: le tromba*. Paris: L'Harmattan.

7 Rivers, W.H.R. 1924. 'Medicine, Magic and Religion.' The FitzPatrick Lectures delivered before The Royal College of Physicians of London in 1915 and 1916. London: Kegan Paul, Trench, Trubner and Co.

8 Goonatilleka, M.H. 1978. *Masks and Mask Systems of Sri Lanka*. Colombo: Colombo University Press.

9 Kapferer, B. 1991 (1983). *A celebration of Demons, Exorcism and Healing in Sri Lanka*. Oxford and Washington DC: Berg with Smithsonian Institution Press, esp. Chapter 6.

10 Sontag, S. 1979. *Illness as Metaphor*. New York: Vintage Books.

11 Porter, R. 1997. *The Greatest Benefit to Mankind, A Medical History of Humanity from Antiquity to the Present*. London: Fontana Press, Chapter 2.

12 Skinner, G.M. 1986. 'Sir Henry Wellcome's Museum for the Science of History' in *Medical History* 30, pp. 401–18.

13 Rigby, D.L. 1944. *Lock, Stock and Barrel: The Story of Collecting*. Philadelphia: J.B. Lippincott, p. 79.

14 Skinner 1986, p. 398.

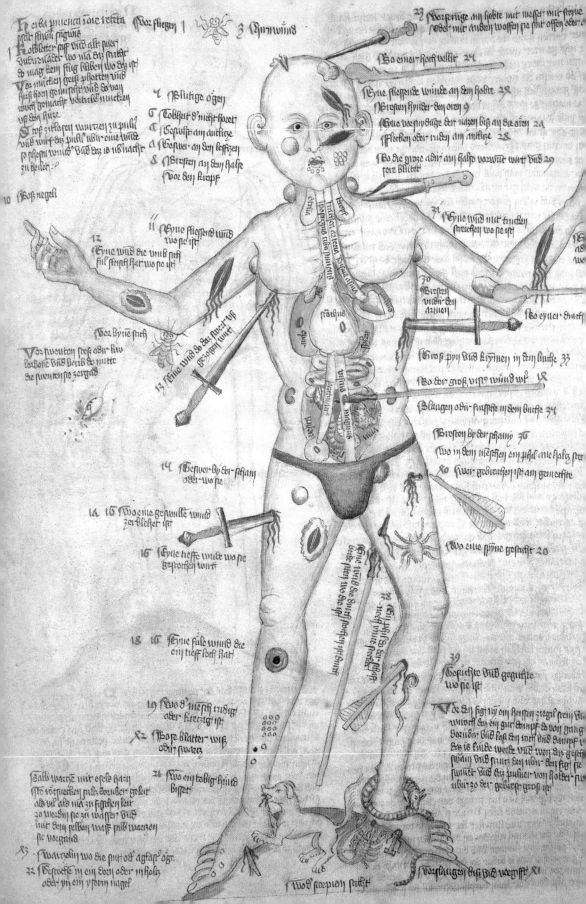

The body
under attack

'Wound man' illustration from a
German manuscript which depicts
a whole range of wounds that a
medieval surgical might be called
upon to treat. c. 1420.
WL, Western MS 49

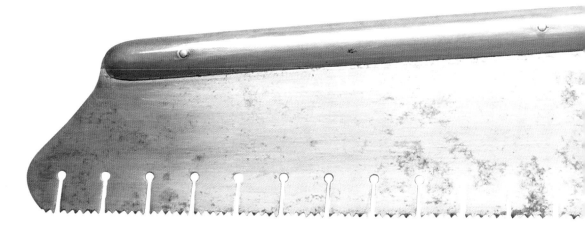

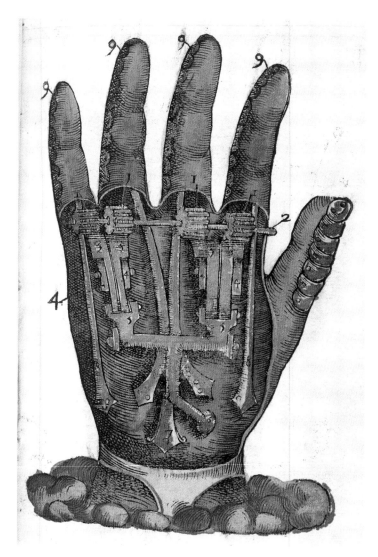

These two woodcuts are from Ambroise Paré's *Instrumenta chyrurgiae et icones anathomicae*, 1564. As a French army surgeon, Paré made significant contributions to amputation surgery and prosthetics. WL, EPB 4818/B

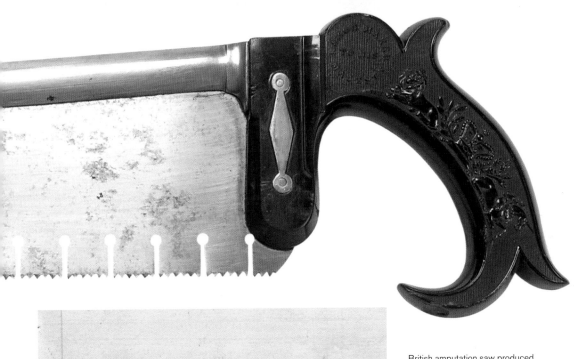

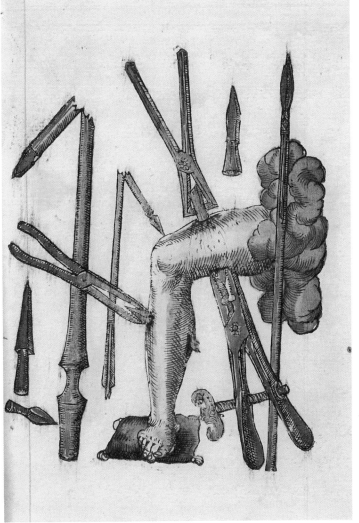

British amputation saw produced by John Weiss. The deep notches on this saw were designed to prevent bone and tissue clogging the blade. Nineteenth century.
SM, A600563

Augenmaß zuschieß-
sens, vund zurichtens, ains
Ins annder zaigt onne die linien
daran das augen steett, ꝛc

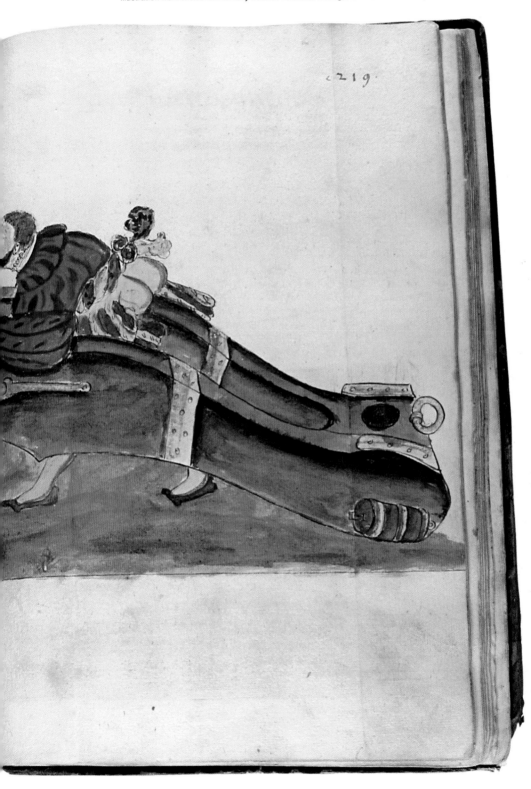

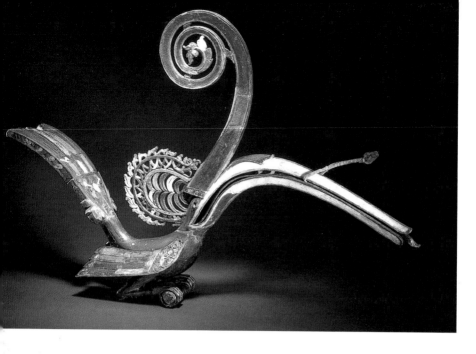

Ancestor bird figure (*Tenyalang*) of the Iban Dayak people of Borneo. Displayed in festivals honouring the God of War and at celebrations of successful head hunting. Acquired before 1936. FMCH, X65-5653

BELOW Photograph showing Major General Horatio Gordon Robley with his collection of tattooed Maori heads. 1895. WL, Icv 31763

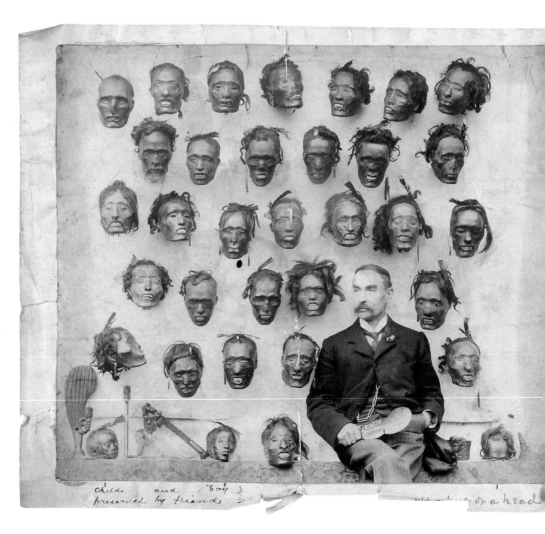

child and boy preserved by friends

RIGHT War shield. The deep indent in the top edge allowed an archer freedom of movement to fire his arrows whilst standing side-on to his adversary. Papua New Guinea. Acquired before 1936. FMCH, X65-4325

FAR RIGHT Shield of woven fibre decorated with a pattern of pearl shell inlaid on black resin. Probably carried for dancing and display by a wealthy and powerful community leader. Central Solomon Islands. Acquired before 1860. BM, 1954.Oc6.197

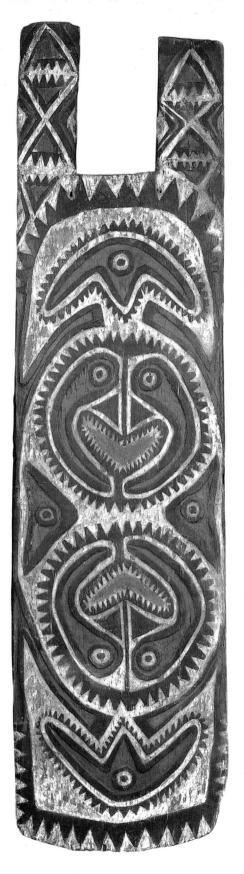

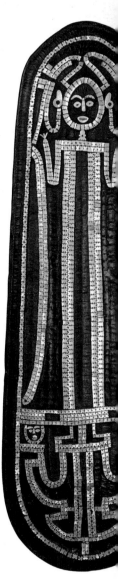

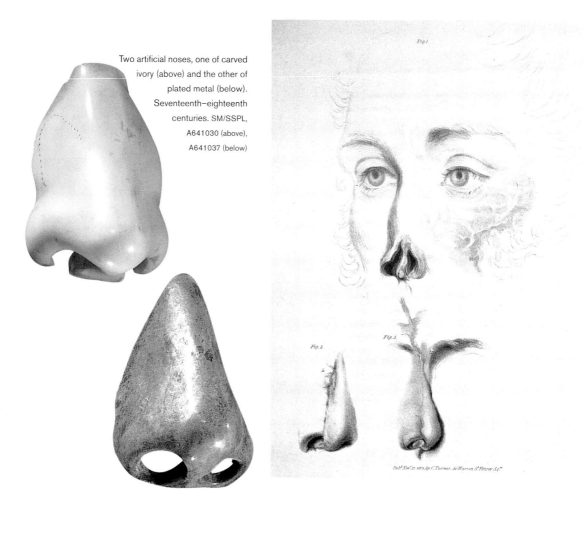

Two artificial noses, one of carved ivory (above) and the other of plated metal (below). Seventeenth–eighteenth centuries. SM/SSPL, A641030 (above), A641037 (below)

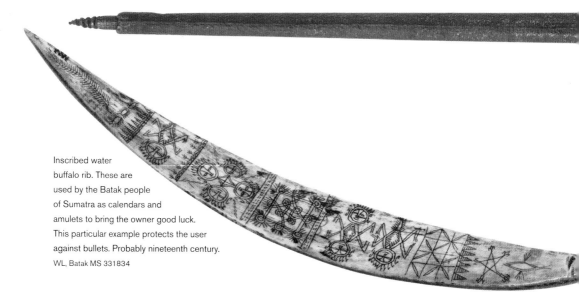

Inscribed water buffalo rib. These are used by the Batak people of Sumatra as calendars and amulets to bring the owner good luck. This particular example protects the user against bullets. Probably nineteenth century. WL, Batak MS 331834

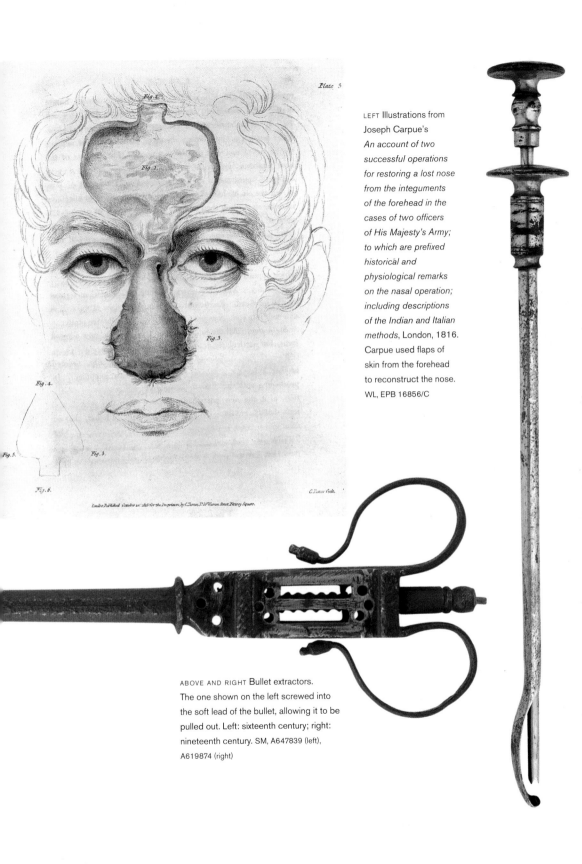

LEFT Illustrations from Joseph Carpue's *An account of two successful operations for restoring a lost nose from the integuments of the forehead in the cases of two officers of His Majesty's Army; to which are prefixed historical and physiological remarks on the nasal operation; including descriptions of the Indian and Italian methods*, London, 1816. Carpue used flaps of skin from the forehead to reconstruct the nose. WL, EPB 16856/C

ABOVE AND RIGHT Bullet extractors. The one shown on the left screwed into the soft lead of the bullet, allowing it to be pulled out. Left: sixteenth century; right: nineteenth century. SM, A647839 (left), A619874 (right)

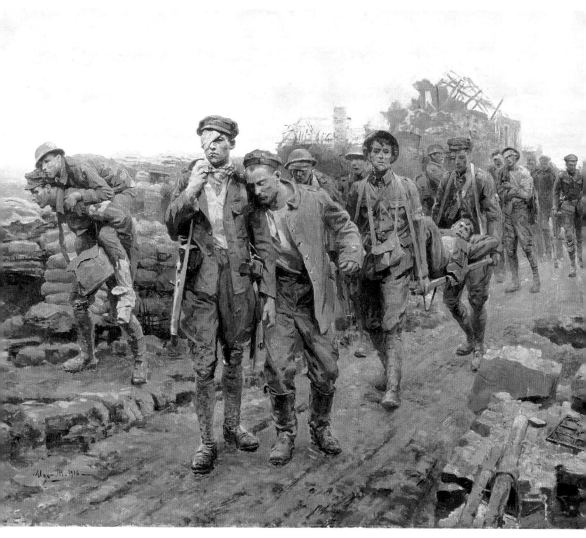

Oil painting by Ugo Matania
depicting wounded First World War
soldiers. 1916. WL, 45949i

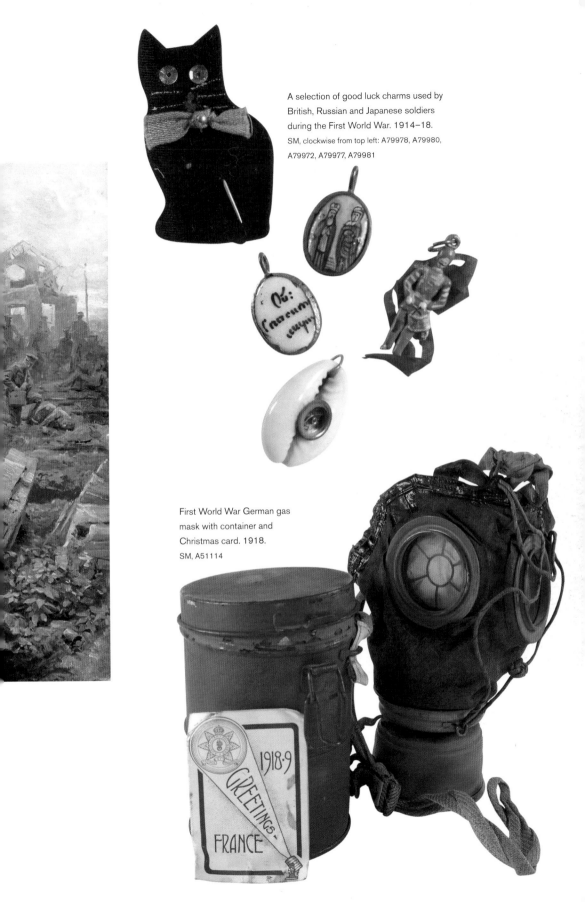

A selection of good luck charms used by
British, Russian and Japanese soldiers
during the First World War. 1914–18.
SM, clockwise from top left: A79978, A79980,
A79972, A79977, A79981

First World War German gas
mask with container and
Christmas card. 1918.
SM, A51114

Edward Jenner's *An inquiry into the causes and effects of the variolae vaccinae* in which he announces his discovery of smallpox vaccination. The illustration is of the cowpox-infected hand of a dairy maid, Sarah Nelmes. London, 1798.
WL, EPB 30385C

BELOW Row of ancestor figures (*adu zatua*) from Nias Island, Indonesia. These figures represent supernatural helpers against disease and other calamities. Collected before 1907.
FMCH, X65-5679

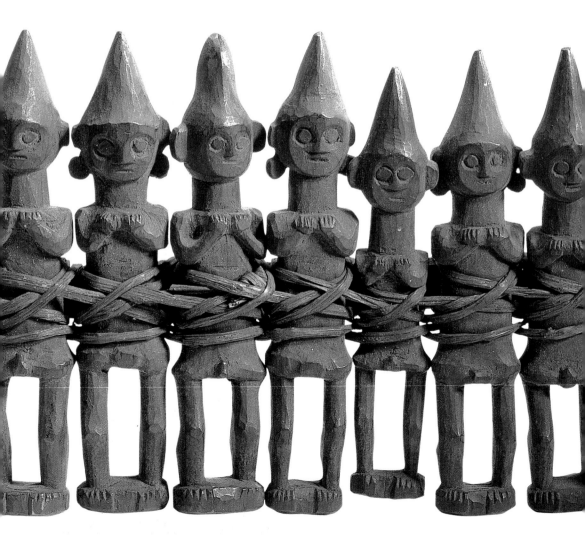

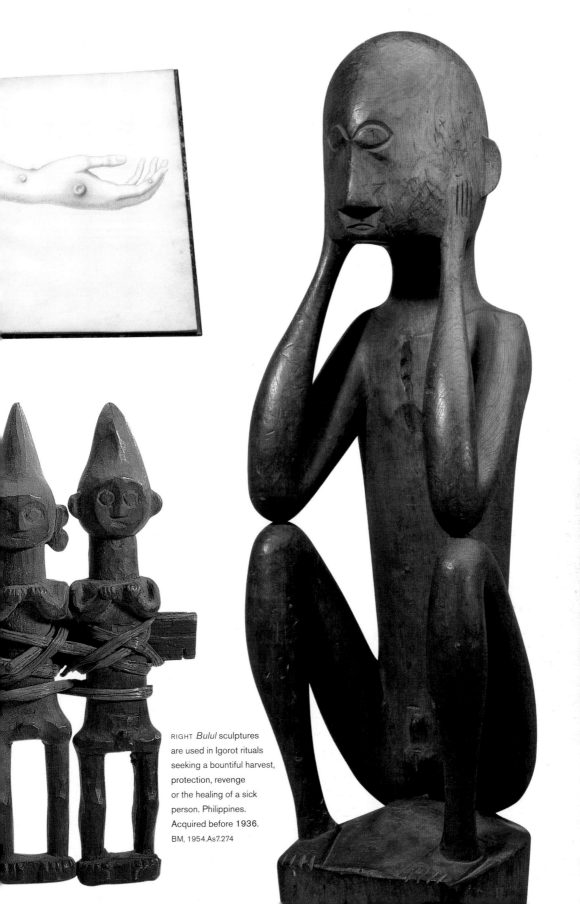

RIGHT *Bulul* sculptures
are used in Igorot rituals
seeking a bountiful harvest,
protection, revenge
or the healing of a sick
person. Philippines.
Acquired before 1936.
BM, 1954.As7.274

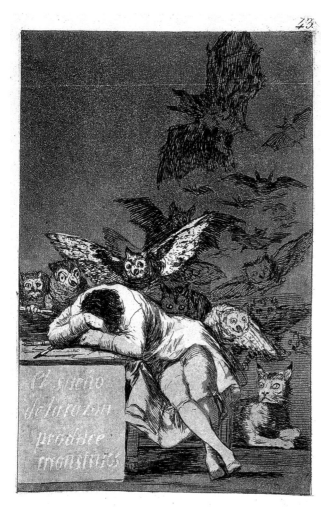

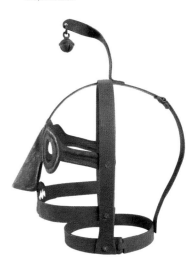

BELOW Iron 'scolds bridle' mask, used to publicly humiliate and punish people, mainly women. Probably German, 1550–1800. SM, A138325

ABOVE A man asleep dreaming of monsters. Etching by Francisco Goya (1746–1828) from his *Los Caprichos* series. Goya made these prints after a serious illness that rendered him deaf. This image represents monsters of the imagination, created by the dreams of sick and delirious men. Spanish, 1796–8. WL, 36752i

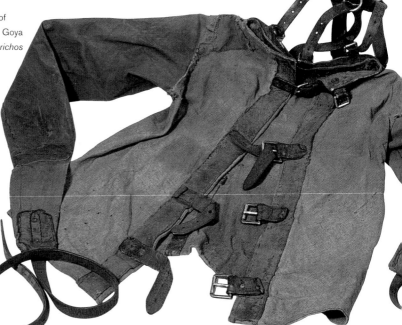

Copy of a canvas and leather strait-jacket. English, *c.* 1930. Acquired at a London auction, 1933. SM/SSPL, A130344

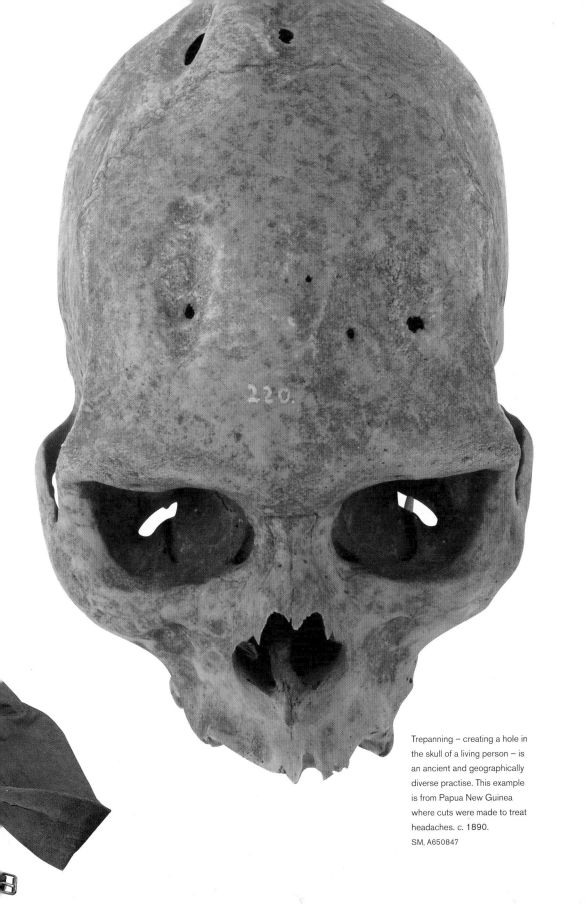

Trepanning – creating a hole in the skull of a living person – is an ancient and geographically diverse practise. This example is from Papua New Guinea where cuts were made to treat headaches. *c.* 1890.

SM, A650847

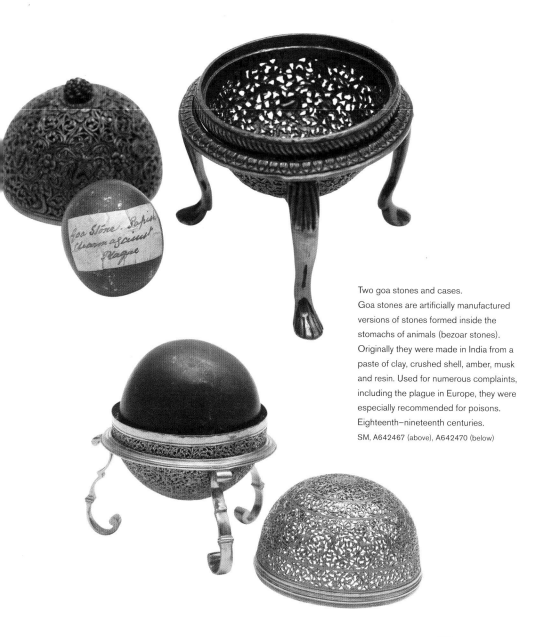

Two goa stones and cases.
Goa stones are artificially manufactured versions of stones formed inside the stomachs of animals (bezoar stones). Originally they were made in India from a paste of clay, crushed shell, amber, musk and resin. Used for numerous complaints, including the plague in Europe, they were especially recommended for poisons. Eighteenth–nineteenth centuries.
SM, A642467 (above), A642470 (below)

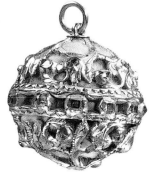

Gold pomander set with diamonds, designed to hold perfumed wax as protection against foul smells or infection. Sixteenth century.
SM/SSPL, A629434

Ethiopian scroll containing charms against the evil eye and various diseases including rheumatism. Nineteenth century.
WL, Ethiopian MS 9

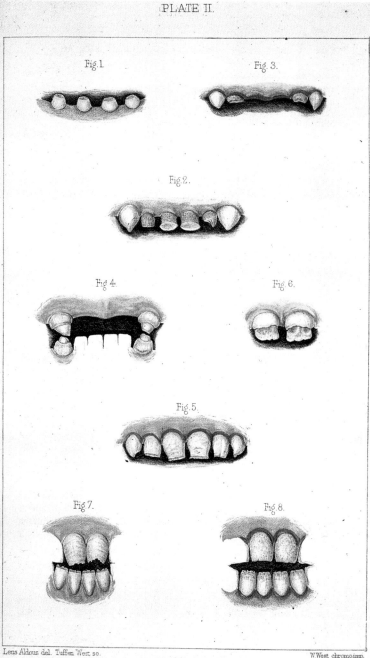

PLATE II.

Fig. 1.

Fig. 3.

Fig. 2.

Fig 4.

Fig. 6.

Fig. 5.

Fig 7.

Fig. 8.

Lens Aldous del. Tuffen West sc.

W. West chromo.imp.

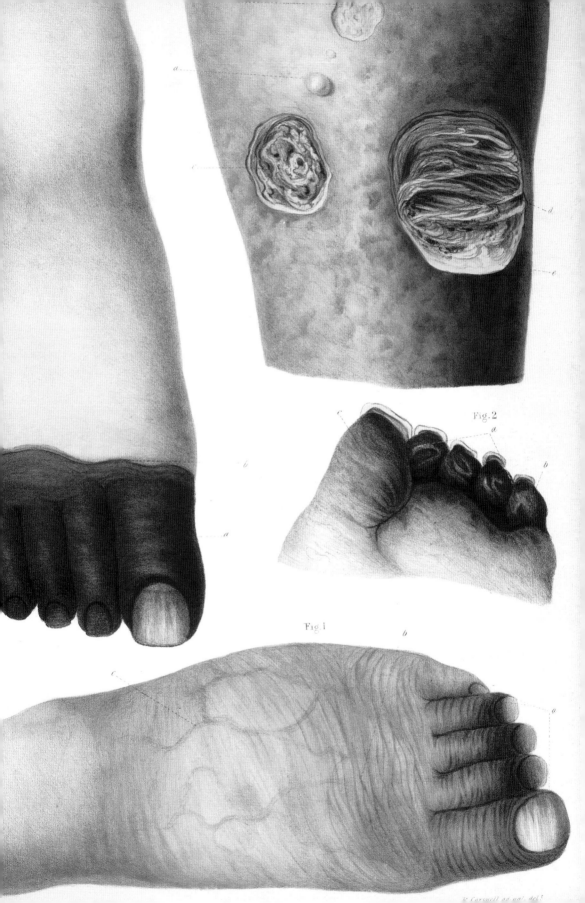

Fig. 2

Fig. 1

E. Carswell ad nat. del.

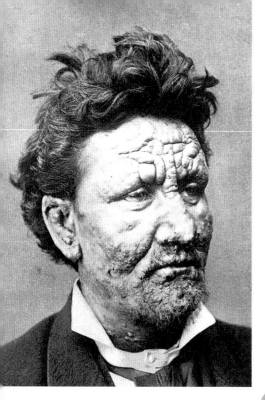

Illustration showing tuberous leprosy of the face from *Leprosy in its clinical and pathological aspects*, by G.A. Hansen and C. Looft. Bristol, 1895. WL, Med.2 8973

BELOW Reproductions of seventeenth-century clappers used at the leper hospital of Saint Nicholas in Kent. Lepers would sometimes use clappers like these to make a noise that would warn others of their approach. SM/SSPL, A635022 (left), A635021 (right)

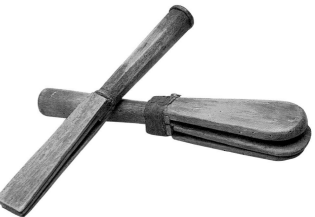

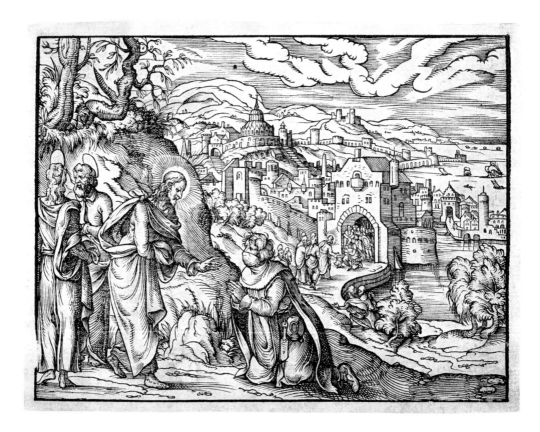

BELOW A Portuguese watercolour drawing of a woman with scales on her upper body and grossly enlarged lower limbs, perhaps representing elephantiasis. 1695. WL, 87i

Illustration of a diseased kidney from Richard Bright's *Reports of Medical Cases*, vol. 1, London, 1827–31. WL, EPB 15395/D

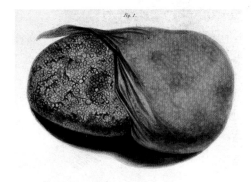

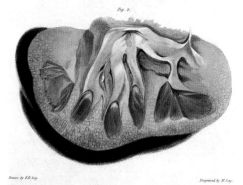

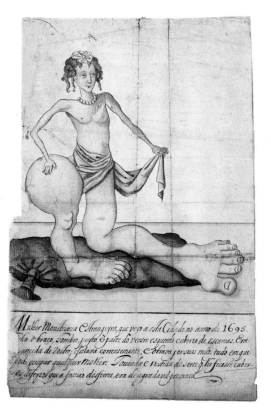

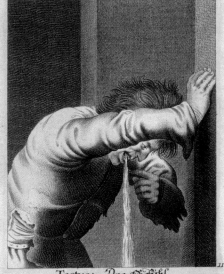

LEFT Christ healing a leper. Woodcut by an unidentified artist, after Jost Amman. Frankfurt am Main, c. 1571. Note the clapper tied to the leper's belt. WL, 6i

A man vomiting after overeating and drinking. Engraving by J.J. Kleinschmidt after Jan van de Velde the younger. Augsburg, Germany, eighteenth century. WL, 27165i

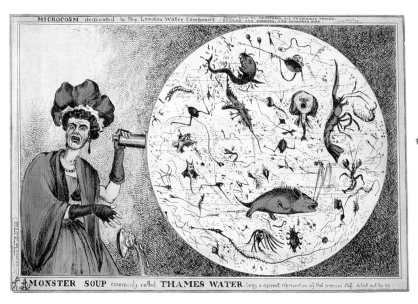

Monster soup. Etching by William Heath. In the nineteenth century, sewage and waste contaminated the River Thames in London making it a prime source of water-borne diseases. 1828. WL, 12079i

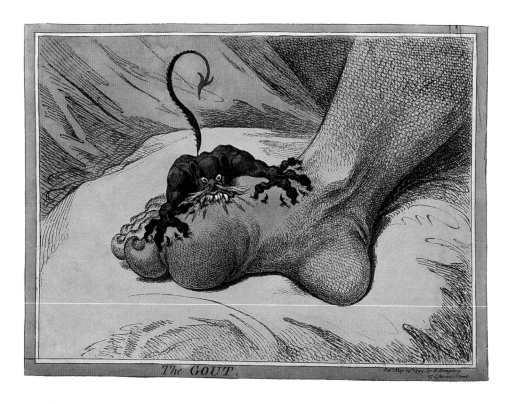

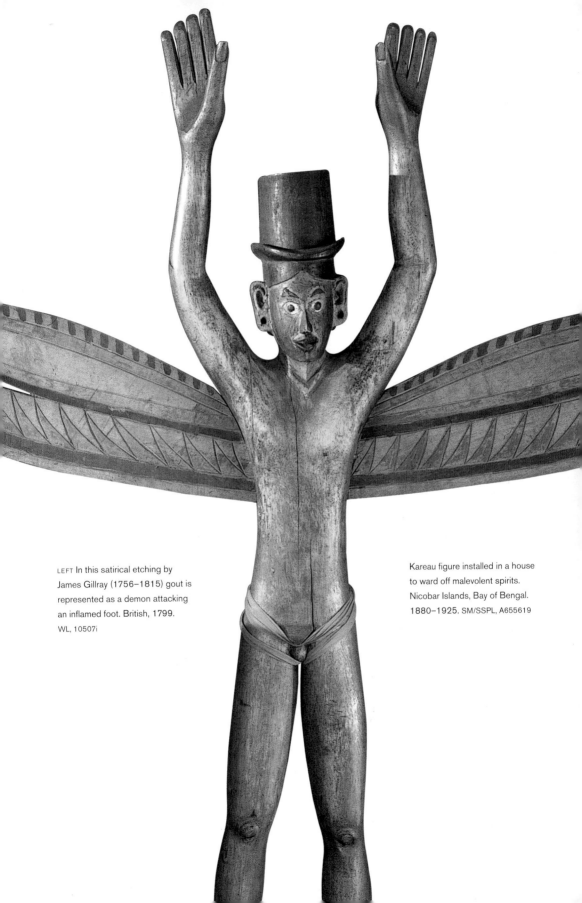

LEFT In this satirical etching by
James Gillray (1756–1815) gout is
represented as a demon attacking
an inflamed foot. British, 1799.
WL, 10507i

Kareau figure installed in a house
to ward off malevolent spirits.
Nicobar Islands, Bay of Bengal.
1880–1925. SM/SSPL, A655619

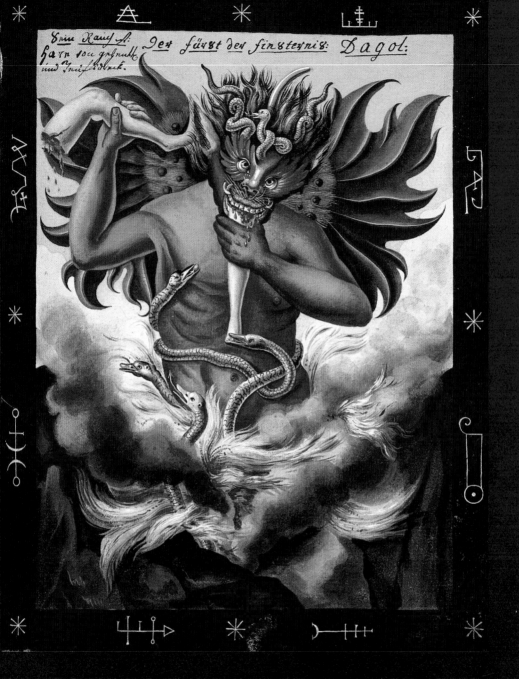

Illustration of 'The Prince of Darkness: Dagol' devouring human limbs, from *Compendium rarissimum totius Artis Magicae sistematisatae per celeberrimos Artis hujus Magistros*. This general work on magical arts contains drawings of various demons. Possibly German, *c.* 1775. WL, MS 1766

RIGHT Detail from Georg Bartisch's *Ophthalmodouleia*, Dresden, 1583, a treatise on various eye conditions and treatments. WL, EPB 697/D

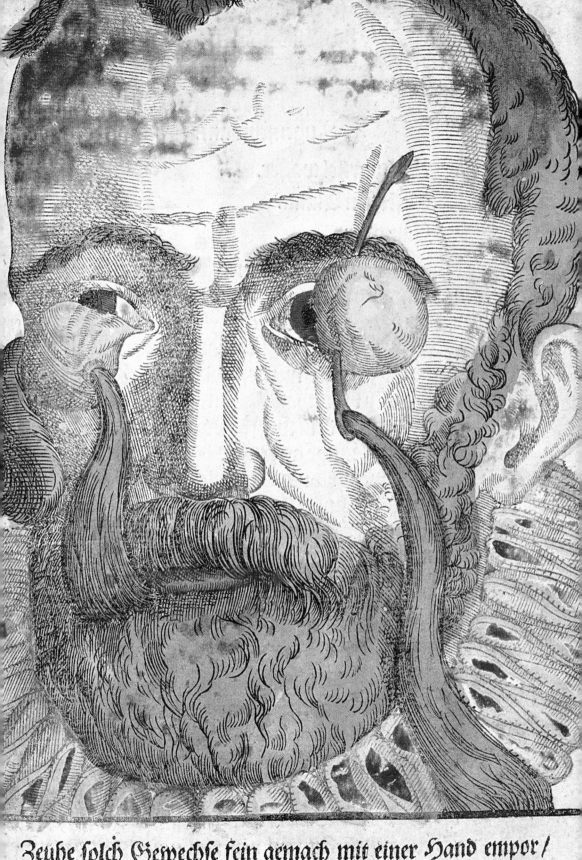

Zeuhe solch Gewechse fein gemach mit einer Hand empor /
s genaweste als du kanst / wol heraus / Darnach nim ein fein

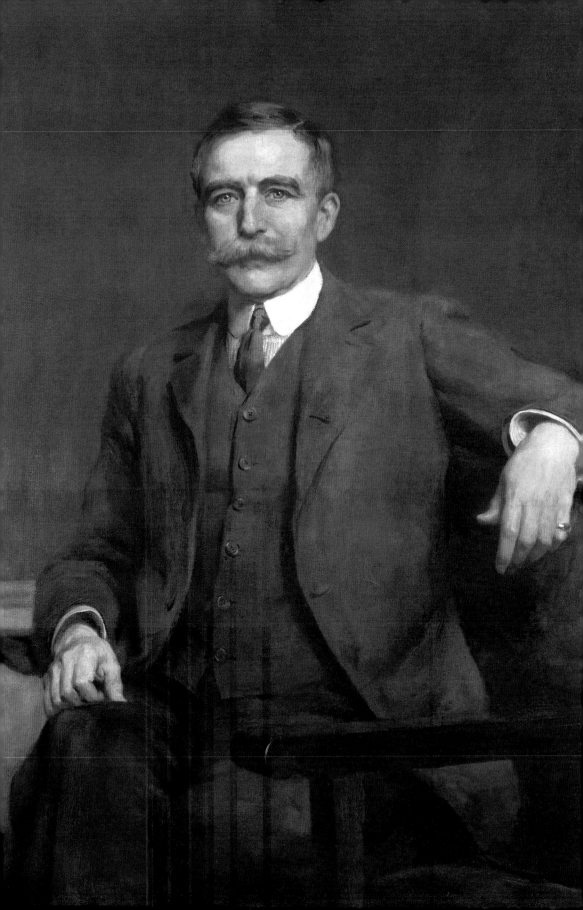

Henry Solomon Wellcome.
Oil painting by
Hugh Goldwin Riviere, 1906.

'I shall try to drown my sorrow

in work. Work is a great comforter,

and my life work is one that

contributes to the welfare of others,

as well as myself, and this thought

helps to brighten one's life.'

LETTER FROM HENRY WELLCOME TO SENATOR ROBERT LANSING,

AUGUST 1910, FOLLOWING HIS SEPARATION FROM SYRIE.

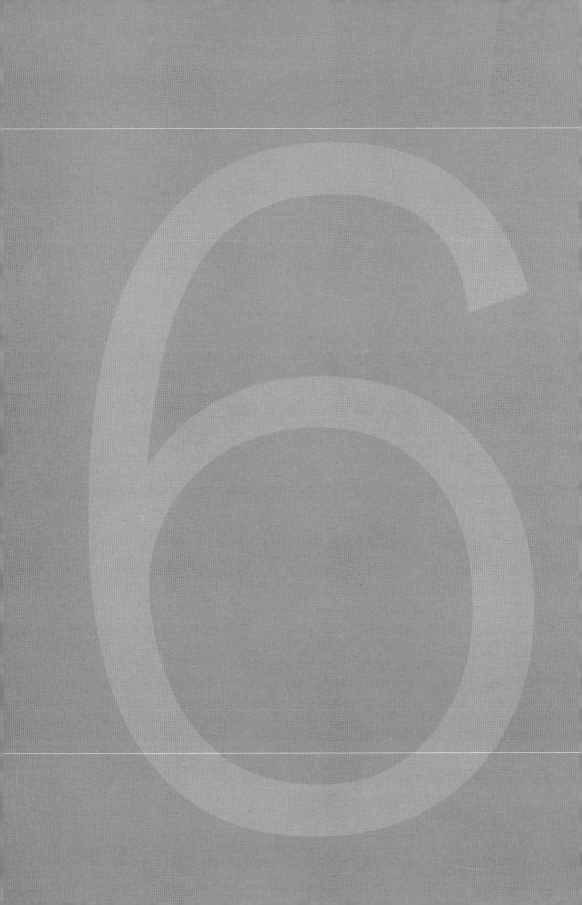

Objects of Modern Medicine

John Pickstone

The exhibition at the British Museum that this book accompanies represents but a fraction of the mind-boggling collection assembled for Henry Wellcome. There can be no single way to understand this richness. Each object, picture or grouping will suggest many ideas; and any of these ideas could be developed through new objects, pictures and groupings. Our age relishes the prolix babble of such collections. Indeed, we may be more comfortable with this miscellany than was the age in which Wellcome himself collected – when tidy minds might have seen his endeavours as a Bohemian fringe of good order.

But we resonate to his collection now – at a time when many museums no longer feel bound by the taxonomic disciplines and can mount displays which turn artefacts into art objects, to be savoured more than studied. Because museum arrangements are now less tied to type or date, we do not miss the ordering for which Wellcome's aides never found the time. And because we celebrate the varieties of culture more than the progress of Western civilisation, we can feel at home with Wellcome's eclectic, non-hierarchical view of non-Western and early modern medical cultures.

For though Henry Wellcome was a major user and an early sponsor of biomedical science, and his firm well known for its advanced research, 'scientific medicine' was not central to his collecting policy. Though he acquired artefacts of some 'medical greats', notably Louis Pasteur (figs 1 and 2), his collections generally reflected the global variety he had himself experienced while travelling the world as a pharmaceutical salesman. They also reflected the variety of cultures in any given place – as in the Minnesota of his youth where American-Indian medicine co-existed with the domestic medicine of European 'pioneers' and with the beginnings of the very modern Mayo clinic (fig. 3).[1]

But as we relish the variety, richness and disorder, we may also wonder how it sits with our more 'progressive' representations of medicine – with the story of scientific 'take-off' from the later nine-

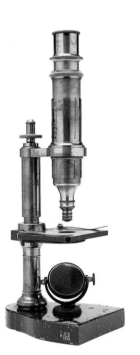

1 Objects used by Louis Pasteur and collected for Henry Wellcome include this brass compound monocular microscope made by Nachet et Fils of Paris. 1861–70.
SM/SSPL, A55114

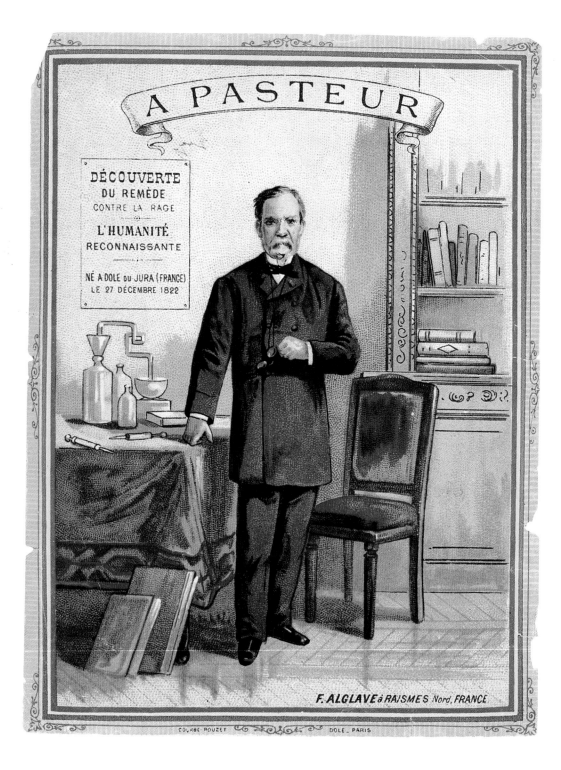

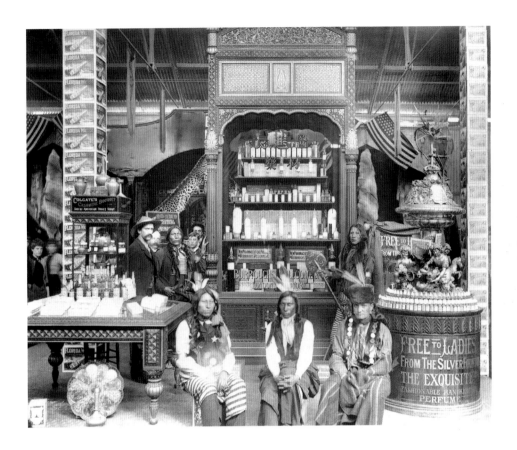

3 Burroughs Wellcome exhibit at the Chicago Exhibition of 1893. Wellcome is on the left, wearing a hat. WL, M7870

2 LEFT Chromo Lithograph label of Pasteur as discoverer of vaccination against rabies. Produced c. 1890 and evidence of his status as a French hero in humanity's fight against disease. WL, 38595i

teenth century, a story in which Wellcome himself played an important part. By the 1930s and the end of Wellcome's career, anaesthetics, antisepsis, bacteriology, vaccination, and the proliferation of analytical methods from autopsy to antibodies had already come to constitute a new medicine. And for us now, a lifetime later, that story is twice the length and so much richer – including antibiotics, new types of drugs and surgery, intensive care, scanners, aided reproduction and the new genetics. But this modern story is about a series of technical accomplishments rather than cultural variety. How, then, might these two accounts be related? How can we understand the variety which Wellcome collected, alongside the more technical stories which were established by his time and which have been extended and underlined since his death?

For us now, scientific medicine from the later nineteenth century has become a part of history – a stage of an ongoing drama that has come to seem problematic as well as promising. We can see its instruments and equipment as period pieces from another age, as well as aspects of a scientific present. But do we need to choose between history and science? Perhaps instead we can bring them into focus together. Perhaps, like some microscopes, we can be 'binocular'; we can get a rounded view of instruments and other artefacts as devised and used for projects that made sense to their makers and users, and which remain alive for us now (fig. 4). We can see instruments as historically particular ways of locating diseases, say, or of analysing bodies, or focusing healing thoughts, removing dangers, or trying out remedies. And, in helping answer our questions about these various long-term projects of medicine, the objects can help us trace the continuities and the changes over time, or measure the similarities and differences between geographically separated medical cultures.

So when we look at an object in a museum we should be asking how and why was the object made? Was it handcrafted or mass-produced, and by whom? When, where, by whom and to what effect was the object used? What did it mean to the doctor and the patient; how did it fit into their views of the body and of disease? And then come other sets of questions about how the object or picture came to be on display or in a museum. Why was it kept? What other objects might have been used by different people, and perhaps not kept? What does that selection tell us about the impact of the techniques in question and the values of succeeding times? By trying to answer such questions, we can take these survivals of medical pasts and reconstruct the medical projects of which they were a part. And then we can ask how the projects of past medicine relate to those we live with now.

Illuminating such issues has been the central task of the university discipline from which I now write – the social history of science, technology and medicine – though it has found it easier to engage with texts than objects! In its present form, that enquiry dates from the 1930s, when a number of European scholars sought to see medicine

4 Satires can be useful ways of reconstructing public understandings. This etching by G.M. Woodward, from 1802, depicts a quack doctor beginning business. Note that the 'Physic for Man and Horse' includes twenty potions for specific types of people.
WL, 10932i

and technology as part of cultural history or the history of ideas. After the Second World War, and especially from the late 1960s, the enterprise broadened and deepened, in the USA and later in the UK where Wellcome Trust support for historical studies of medicine became crucial. Historians of science and medicine have interacted profitably with philosophy, anthropology and sociology, social and cultural history, and with 'science studies'. Intellectual fashions have come and gone, and groups of scholars differ – of course – in their preferred methods; but all have access to a set of useful tools which can help us bring medical history to (our) life.

Tools for history

5 A nineteenth-century English scarificator, used as a blood-letting instrument. SM, A216750

The key is to see the processes of science or medicine as truly part of history – not just to allow that a bleeding apparatus now seems repulsive (fig. 5), but to unearth the understandings and practices which made bleeding desirable in the medicine of that period. Why, for example, was it common in the eighteenth century for patients to 'spring clean' their bodies by shedding a pint or so of blood? How did some people appear dominated by 'blood' or by 'bile'; and how did understandings of bodily qualities relate to temperament and to character? We can try through such questions to reconstruct a world of ideas and practices; and we must maintain the same sympathetic, enquiring stance whether the period in question be the Middle Ages or the Cold War. As historians, we try to get inside the heads of the past, thinking their thoughts after them, whilst also concerned with our own times.[2]

The complementary knack, often, is to focus on the 'local', and on practices and skills as well as understandings – on the particular circumstances and surroundings of the actions or the artefacts in question. Who was doing the medical work – with what, where and to whom? And who was taking notice? And then we can ask how the results travelled from that place and time, and how localities were linked into regional, national or global nets. What were the key communities to which practitioners,

researchers or patients related, and how did these communities
change over time? How was a new instrument invented, who took it
up, and how was it then marketed? How might artefacts or pictures
reveal the ways in which local stories became part of a bigger phenomenon, extending widely in both space and time (fig. 6)?

And a third prescription, for some cases, is to try looking 'from the
bottom up'. Think what medicine felt like from the patient's point of
view. Try to work out the common, vernacular understandings of the
body and its surroundings – not just to understand the reception of
expert knowledges, but to see how expert views were constituted from

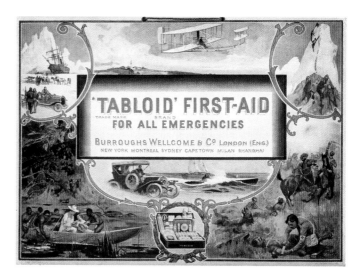

6 Tabloids packed in a
medical chest and advertised
by Burroughs Wellcome and
Company. Tabloids were a
new and convenient way of
taking (and trading) medicines.
By promoting them when most
medicines were sold 'loose',
Wellcome built a business
which spanned the world,
gradually drawing the colonies
and economic dependencies
into the Western system of
pharmaceutical manufacture.
WL, 16398i

or against more widespread perspectives. See, for example, how
medical instruments were related to other technologies – how the
stomach pump (fig. 7) that was high-tech around 1830 was manufactured and sold alongside pumps for watering the gardens of gentle-
men, or novel first-aid devices for passing stimulating smoke up the
backsides of the nearly-drowned (fig. 8).[3]

From these prescriptions come three tensions which energise and
guide the best of medical history (and the history of science and
technology more generally) – the tension of past and present, of local
and global, of expert and vernacular.

And to them we can add a further consideration – about the complexity of all human understandings, wherever and whenever, and

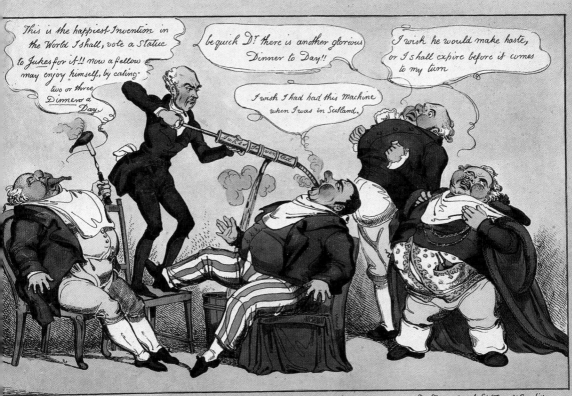

7 ABOVE Satirical coloured etching by W. Heath, 1824, showing the newly invented stomach pump of Dr Jukes, here being used to extract 'superfluities, excuses and poisons' from 'Aldermen, corporations and gourmandizers in general'. Such pumps were rare and especially associated with emergency treatment for opium poisoning. WL, 12220i

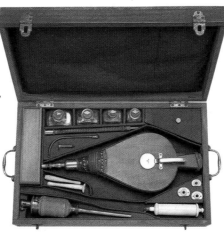

8 English Tobacco Resuscitator Kit from 1774, used in the 'Humane Society' movement which promoted the rescue and revivification of the apparently dead, especially the drowned. SM/SSPL, A640992

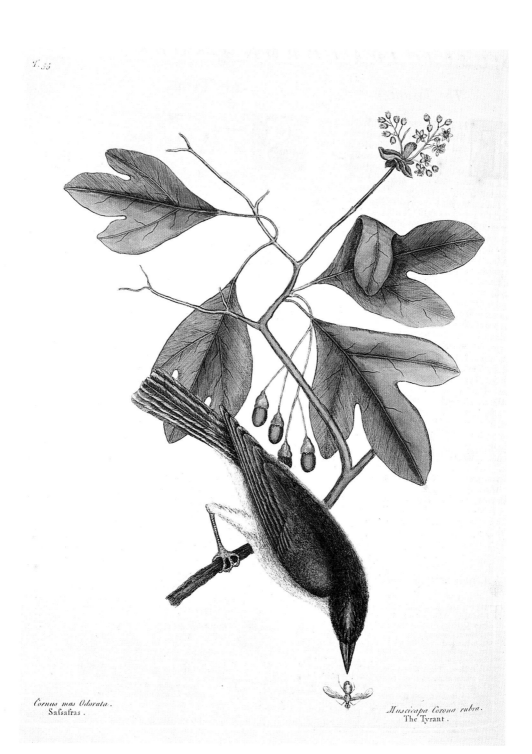

T. 55

Cornus mas Odorata.
Safsafras.

Muscicapa Corona rubra.
The Tyrant.

9 LEFT 'The tyrant bird on a sprig of sassafras': from Mark Catesby, *The Natural History of Carolina, Florida and the Bahama Islands*, vol. 1, London, 1731–43. WL, EPB F.963-4

10 Analysing disease as organic lesion. A colour-stipple engraving by W. Say in Richard Bright's *Reports of Medical Cases*, vol. 1, London, 1827–31. Bright was a London physician remembered for the exploration of kidney diseases. WL, EPB 15395/D

hence the need to go beyond the simple contrasts and oppositions that dog our discussions of medicine, science and arts. Oppositions such as scientific versus non-scientific, or rational versus magical, are not very helpful – especially if we restrict the title 'science' to the 'natural sciences' and assume it is all done in laboratories, and in much the same way; or if we simply contrast the scientific method claimed by some modern medicine with the variety of practices attached to medicine in other cultures.

We might better recognise that there are *many* ways of gaining knowledge that is more or less secure, systematic and useful; and that voyages, museums, hospitals, factories and armchairs can be places of 'research', as much as laboratories. 'Medical science' has much in common with linguistics, say, and medical practice with horticulture. But our terms often mislead us; and the word 'science' cuts out so much of what we ought to value – from the natural history of daffodils, dolphins or diabetics, to the systematic analysis of politics, patients' groups or poems. So I am here suggesting that we might gain by thinking of medicine (and science and technology more generally) not as monolithic, but as compounded of several projects or *ways of knowing*, some of which are shared with many other forms of scholarship, and none of which are entirely restricted to the 'natural sciences'.[4]

I am suggesting that we think of four such projects which we might see as the elements of medicine (and of other subjects), compounded in various ways over time and space. *Natural history*, in a general sense, will serve as a name for the practices of describing, collecting, classifying and displaying, which are used in medicine as

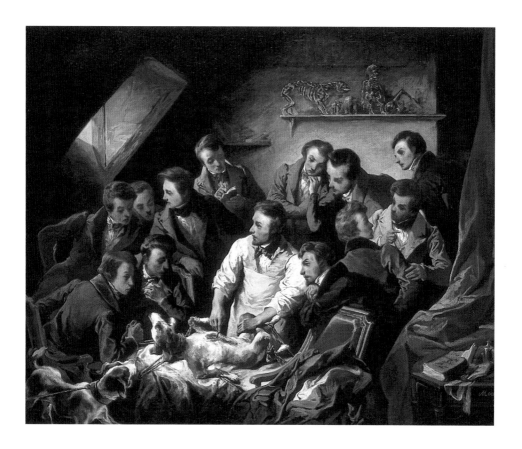

11 Oil painting by Emile-Edouard Mouchy, 1832, of animal vivisection in Paris. To its proponents, especially in France and Germany, experimentation on live animals was the new road to technical effectiveness in medicine; to its opponents, especially in England, it was immoral cruelty. WL, 44579i

much they are as for birds and buttercups (fig. 9). *Analysis* refers to the dissection, in theory or practice, of complex entities into their elements – whether the entities be planetary motions, chemical compounds, geological formations or human bodies (fig. 10). *Experimentation*, in medicine or in physics, is the practice of trying out novel ideas and combinations – of systematically going beyond analysis to find ways of changing the world (fig. 11). But we must recognise too the role of *human meanings* in all medicine. Diseases, for example, may threaten or humiliate; they are parts of culture and politics, as well as of our natural history; with or without doctors, we work out what our diseases may signify.[5] And that remains true, even in the most modern of medical encounters, even in the world where scientific occupations, industry and government have converged into a project which is sometimes called techno-science or techno-medicine – the systematic mobilisation of all these ways

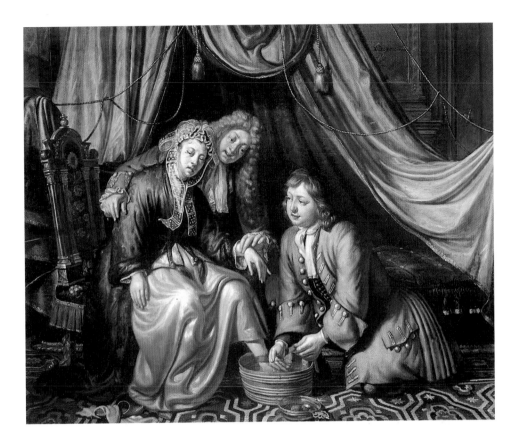

12 A physician and a surgeon attending to a high-status patient. Oil painting by Mathijs Naiveu (1647–1721).

WL, 44718i

of knowing into the production of scientific commodities such as advanced pharmaceuticals.

And whether separately or variously compounded, these ways of knowing all generated and used artefacts, pictures and texts, some of which have come down to us.

Modes of medicine

To get a taste of the natural historical in medicine, we can imagine the gentleman-physician in conversation with a rich patient and patron – assessing the patient's reports, fears and aspirations, and seeing disease as disturbances of a life, probably produced by environmental changes, and remediable perhaps by medicines, bleeding, diet or by regimens to rebalance the body. This form of medicine we can describe as biographical or bedside medicine. It was developed in classical

Greece but is known to us best from eighteenth-century Europe. It has much in common with other great medical traditions in the Middle East, China and India (fig. 12).[6]

We might also note that this kind of biographical medicine comprises both the natural history of patients or diseases, and the symbolic, human meanings which diseases hold for patients (and for doctors). So the diagnosis of arthritis, say, is both a statement about likely 'natural' outcomes (as might also apply to an arthritic horse), and a label with a certain symbolic resonance and social significance for the doctor, the patient and the social group. The patient comes to terms with both these aspects, and may rethink them for his or her own case.

At any period, there is lots of *natural history* involved in medicine. The accumulation of careful 'case histories' is an example, or the collections and museums of medicine – whether of herbs and minerals, bones or pickled brains, or of the many types of human blood proteins to be found across the world.

To see a medicine dominated by *analysis*, we can move from aristocratic patients to the vast 'poor-houses' of France after the French Revolution. We picture the French clinical professor, around 1820, walking the wards of a Parisian state hospital full of sick paupers. He speaks to students more than to patients, and listens more to the patients' chests than to patients' tales. For him, diseases are anatomical lesions, not disturbances of the body's equilibrium; and anatomical clarity can only be obtained through dissection of bodies after death. But disease as lesions could be searched for in life, and this was the significance of the stethoscope which was invented there and then. A simple tube placed to an ear allowed the doctor to 'see' into the patient's chest, where murmurs might reveal the irregularities of heart and lungs (fig. 13).[7]

From about this time, Western medicine became marked by the sustained attempt to analyse sick (and well) bodies in terms of their minute structures and chemical composition. The model was the new chemistry associated with Antoine Lavoisier in Paris, which replaced the classical elements with new substances, defined in a new way. And from autopsy and simple chemistry there developed a

13 Stethoscope which once belonged to Laënnec, the Parisian physician who invented the instrument. Initially the stethoscope was a simple wooden tube, or even a roll of paper – hardly a product of technical ingenuity, more a symptom of a new view of disease in which 'peering into the body' made sense. SM/SSPL, A106078

whole range of analytical techniques and instruments that multiplied over two centuries, populating laboratories in hospitals and clinics, universities and industrial companies.

For scene three, from about 1840 and especially in Germany, we switch to a University biomedical laboratory with microscopes and

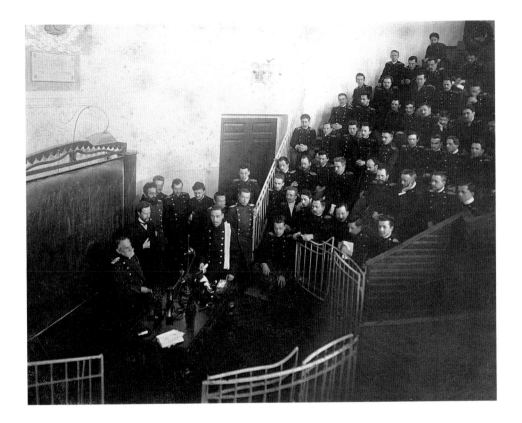

14 Photograph of I.P. Pavlov demonstrating an experiment on a dog at the Imperial Military Medical Academy, St Petersburg, 1904. By 1900, experimental physiology was a standard part of medical education. Pavlov became world-famous for his work on gastro-intestinal physiology, especially on 'conditioned reflexes'. WL, 11935i

measuring apparatus. This kind of laboratory extended analysis, but it also added the possibility of animal experimentation, through which mastery of living processes could be achieved and demonstrated. Biomedical *experimentation* became common in the later nineteenth century, as university teachers analysed and displayed the workings of living animals (fig. 14).[8]

Such academic experimentation was echoed in the new workrooms of professional inventors, especially in America; and whenever experiments had commercial potential, or inventions could aid systematic investigation, then the academy might converge with the institutions

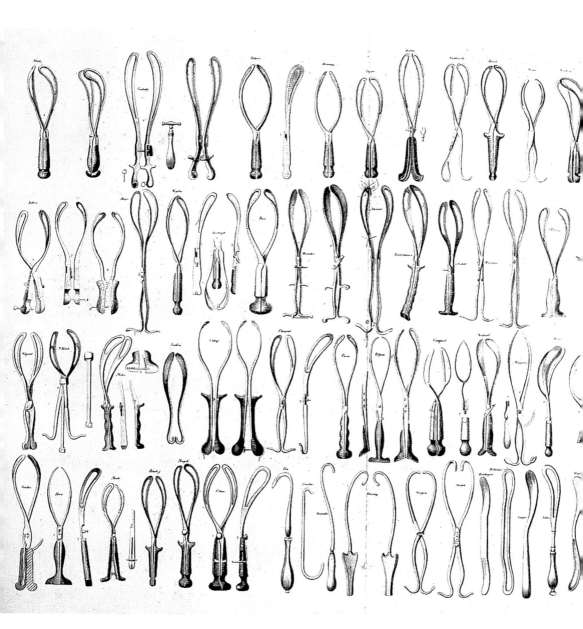

15 The will to be different? An illustration of the
astonishing variety of obstetrical forceps, from a
German *Geburtshülficher Atlas*, by H.F. Kilian,
Düsseldorf, 1835–44. WL, EPB F.442

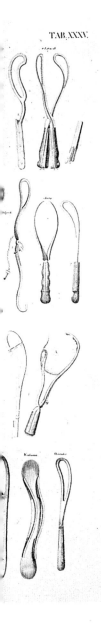

T.AB.XXXV.

of industry. And from these *techno-scientific* complexes came the scientific commodities sold by industrial companies which in the twentieth century became increasingly central both to medical practice and to bio-medical investigation.[9]

But if we reflect a little on what we all know of present medicine, if only as patients, then we soon realise that this sequence of ways of knowing, however refined or extended, can be no simple series. All the types of medicine are still more or less in play in our time, as can be seen if we go from a GP to a hospital. We can discuss the disruption of our lives in terms of natural history and meanings, and we may be prodded and poked in clinical examinations meant to uncover the lesions within us. The GP or a consultant may send for lab tests, and then prescribe pills developed by industry from experiments on animals, and sold perhaps by advertisers who know more than we do about our systems of symbolic meanings!

So better not to envisage a simple series, but rather a set of different medical ways of knowing – of human meanings, natural history, analysis, and experiments – variously mixed and structured in different times and places. But how, then, might that perspective help elaborate the questions we can put to our medical objects – for example, to a pair of obstetric forceps from the Victorian period? How might we 'read' them at the various levels just sketched?

We may know that there were many kinds of forceps – Victorian obstetricians liked to design their own and have them manufactured. So in some museums we can see many 'species' of forceps laid out like natural history specimens, each speaking of its maker and of craft, and of the will to be different (fig. 15). Or we might trace the use of forceps through the records of doctors, and so compile another kind of history. We might see them as expressive of a mechanical analysis of childbirth, and a correspondingly mechanical practice. We might look for evidence that forceps were celebrated for their use in emergencies, or feared as representing an 'unnatural', impersonal approach, perhaps a form of assault; and we might reflect how Victorian attitudes to forceps were related to later attitudes. And by so seeing meanings in objects, we may come to recognise and contrast different styles of medicine and the variety of approaches to the body.[10]

But medicine, of course, is not just sets of understandings – it is also sets of actions, by doctors or patients, in the hope of cure, alleviation, or prevention. Doctors are usually expected to produce results, not just diagnoses or narratives about causes and likely outcomes. Maybe, however, we can see such interventions as in some ways paralleling the ways of knowing that we have just outlined. To each aspect of understanding, there may correspond characteristic modes of action or technique. So let's now work through the list just given, beginning with the practices, pictures and artefacts which were based on human meanings.

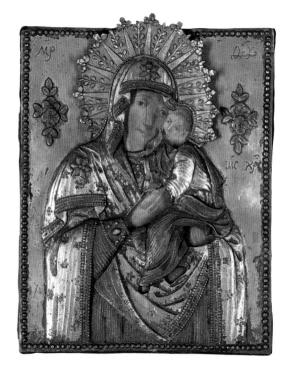

16 Icon of Virgin and Child, carried by a Russian soldier in the Crimean War. The Russian text on the reverse of this piece indicates that its owner was 'Staff Captain Constantine Meshcheriakoff. Died in the Marine Hospital Sevastopol of Disease in the month of May 1855'.
WL, 44966i

Techniques of morale

Prayer, exortations and ritual might thus appear as 'techniques of morale' – meant to alter our relation to the world, or of the world to us. Icons, for example, might assure of the presence and protection of a God, even through great dangers (fig. 16). And even materialists may prepare spiritually when they are about to suffer a serious operation (or to perform a very tricky experiment). One way or another, we all orient ourselves to the meanings of our worlds – perhaps by Sunday walks in the hills, or trips to historical museums, or by reading primers on Darwinian psychology that make monkeys of us all.

Votive offerings, representing our defective organs, were objects meant to focus attention, whether of the Gods or of people, in the hope that 'attitude' would make a difference. Call it 'magic' if you wish, but that is profitable only if we then ask about the roles of 'magic' in our own lives. Here I follow the philosopher R.G. Collingwood who maintained in the 1930s that magic was the technology of morale and that anyone who neglected morale – their own, their colleagues' or their enemies' – was doomed. The propagandists of our generation – whether advertising agents or spin-doctors – may not have read Collingwood, but one suspects they would agree.[11]

A century ago, Western doctors took great pride in their own magical effects – in their 'presence' and the faith it engendered in their patients (fig. 17). Of course, that would hardly pass muster in a world of 'evidence-based' medicine – except that in many clinical trials the placebo effect of dummy pills is greater than the extra benefit from

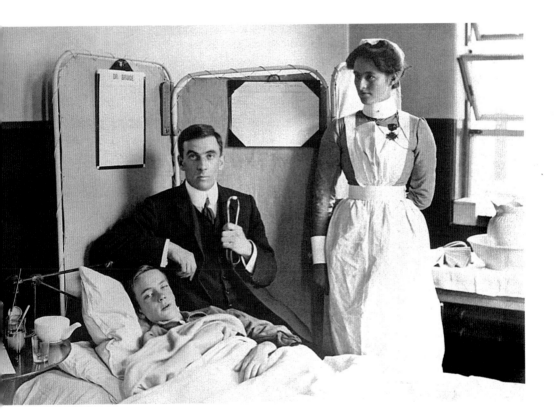

17 Photograph of Dr Basil Hood with a patient and nurse at Charing Cross Hospital, London, 1906. That doctors were now pictured 'at work', respectfully rather than satirically, suggests the increase in status of the profession. Medical consultants combined science and social authority; they expected to inspire confidence. WL, 28952i

pharmaceutically active medicine! Across all cultures past and present, faith, mutual support and the ability to come to terms with disease may be central to the maintenance and restoration of health; and modern Western cultures often fail to ensure those attitudes.

Objects of natural history

But, as another class of medical artefacts and illustrations can remind us, interwoven with the symbolic significance of health and disease is the lay and professional knowledge of our 'natural history' – the ways in which we blossom and perish like leaves on a tree, changing with the seasons and with age, according to our environments and the ways in which we choose (or are forced) to live. This is the medicine of diet and exercise, of massage instruments (fig. 18) and baths, and maybe of soporifics or stimulants. The classical traditions of East and West all have ways of relating bodies to their natural environments, and of discriminating between different kinds of bodies and environments. This natural history of bodies linked them with plants, animals and minerals, not least as medicines.

If rituals are technologies of meaning, then traditional medicines might be seen as practical extensions of our 'natural history' – using natural products to restore balance or combat specific disorders. That

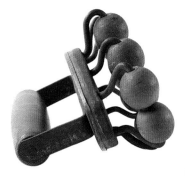

18 ABOVE Timeless technologies in timely forms? A German massage instrument, with rollers, in the shape of a flat iron. 1880–1920. SM, A602750

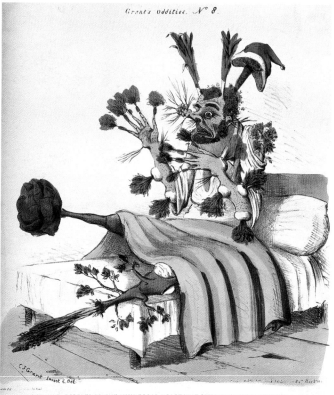

19 We are what we eat? The 'Singular effects of the universal vegetable pills on a green grocer'; a satire on J. Morison's Vegetable Pills. Coloured lithograph by C.J. Grant. 1831. WL, 11852i

Grant's oddities. N.º 8.

SINGULAR EFFECTS OF THE UNIVERSAL *VEGETABLE* PILLS ON A GREEN GROCER! *A FACT!*

Who *Green'un like* was order'd to live for the space of one Month upon *Vegetable Diet* & to Take during that time 132 Boxes of *Vegetable Pills* for the Cure of a *Gangreen*, & being caught in a Shower of Rain in the *Green Fields* in the evening of the 1.ˢᵗ of April last, was put to Bed 'midst *Shooting pains* & in the Morning presented the above Phenomenon of a *Moving Kitchen Garden* !!!

Query –   Is he not one of the *Productive Classes*.

kind of medicine is as old or as new as sleeping draughts or herbal drinks, as the gymnasia of classical Athens or the isometric machines of our health clubs. Whether as 'self-help', or professionalised or commercialised, this natural medicine resembles the crafts of horticulture or husbandry, and it remains very important – both at its own level, and as the basis for more elaborate and esoteric activities (fig. 19).[12]

It is also the basis for an environmentalist tradition in Western medicine which was alive in its classical form through the nineteenth century, and which we may need to reclaim in new ways. The environmentalism which is so prominent in the politics of our present offers new ways of seeing our diseases and our wellbeings as linked with global 'surroundings' in which the natural and the social are increasingly entangled.

But what lies behind the 'natural' in our health or our diseases? Is it spirits or quasi-human agencies – which takes us back to symbols and rituals? Or could medical and surgical interventions be based on the 'analysis' of underlying structures or functions, for the rectification of disturbances envisaged at the level of bodily elements – such as its organs, energy lines, humours, fibres, cells or chemistry? Such forms of analytical medicine have often been the provinces of 'experts' who claimed privileged access and judgement about the elements in question. What kinds of apparatus or pictures will reveal, or illustrate, those hidden causes?

Analytical devices

In the classical view, the fluids of the body were variously combined from the four elements and the four qualities: so blood (like air) was relatively hot and wet, and yellow bile (like fire) was relatively hot and dry; these humours corresponded to different kinds of food and drink, and to the seasons and the climates of particular places. People notable for their blood were sanguine or optimistic, others were bilious (hot and dry) in temper. In such ways the grid of qualities mapped a whole series of possible relations between the constitutions and temperaments of people and of places. In such medicine, diagnostic instruments had little place: forms of health or sickness were judged by direct observation of the pulse, or by the colour and consistency of blood or urine; but especially by the patient's account.[13]

20 BELOW LEFT The body as machine. An illustration from one of the key seventeenth-century texts on mechanical medicine: Giovanni Alfonso Borelli's *De motu animalium*, Naples, 1734. Borelli (1608–79) was taught mathematics by Benedetto Castelli, a student of Galileo. WL, EPB 14628/B

From the seventeenth century, new fashions in doctor-talk mostly followed the dominant modes of natural philosophy. So mechanical medicine thrived on the success of seventeenth-century 'mechanics' in explaining the motions of physical bodies, projectiles, levers and so on (fig. 20); and later, in the world of Jane Austen, the sensibility of the body parts came to the fore. But whatever the presumed elements of the body, the logic was much the same – the chosen properties linked wholes with parts, bodies with minds, and individuals with their environments.

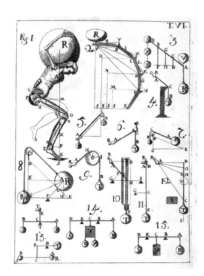

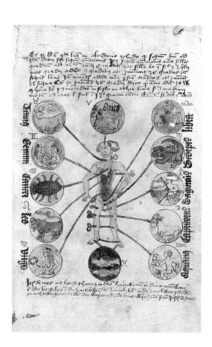

21 ABOVE RIGHT Cosmological analysis. An astrological chart showing the correspondences between organs in the body and the constellations in the heavens. Taken from Heymandus de Veteri Busco's *Ars Computistica*. Dutch, 1488. WL, Western MS 349

Indeed, the analysis of bodies was linked to the whole cosmos. Astrological medicine had high status in early modern Europe, and much modern astronomy was worked out in the service of astrological diagnosis and prediction (fig. 21). Eastern classical traditions had their own forms of analysis, for example the energy lines of acupuncture in Chinese medicine (fig. 22) – and here, too, the 'elements' of the body were linked with the body's surroundings and the world at large.[14]

Therapy, in many of the systems, was a matter of rebalancing – the removal of excess blood, fluid or energy, the tensing or slackening of fibres or nerves, or the addition of energy via stimulants or heat. The 'simple scales' of learned medical therapeutics were not very

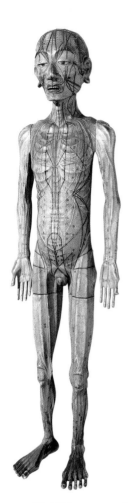

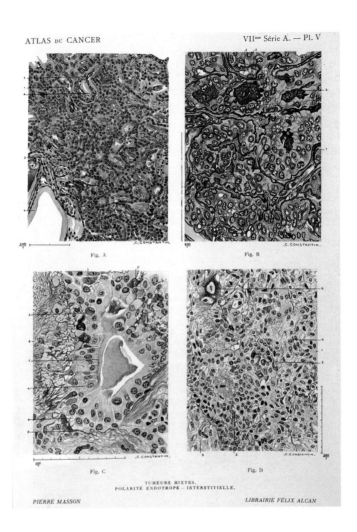

ATLAS du CANCER

VIIme Série A. — Pl. V

Fig. A

Fig. B

Fig. C

Fig. D

TUMEURS MIXTES,
POLARITÉ ENDOTROPE – INTERSTITIELLE.

PIERRE MASSON

LIBRAIRIE FÉLIX ALCAN

22 A Chinese acupuncture figure from the seventeenth century, made of wood. SM/SSPL, A604024

23 ABOVE RIGHT Mapping the microscopical elements of the body. J. Darier, *Atlas du Cancer*, Paris, 1922. WL, L23112

different from the regulation of inflation in present-day economies – the raising or lowering of interest rates according to whether the economic body seems to require stimulation or depletion. As in macro-economics, there was little reason to search for local causes.

But in the new medicine which developed from around the time of the French Revolution, disease became local – primarily a matter of tissue lesions, for tissues were the new elements of the body. Here was a new understanding of disease, and a new geography – one that was later redefined in terms of cells. Diseases could now be seen as disturbances of the chemical structure of the body and/or of its tissues or cells, and these changes could perhaps be directly accessed (fig. 23).

25 OPPOSITE Radiographic image by G. Leopold and T. Leisewitz, Dresden, 1908, showing the skeleton of a child born with two backbones and two heads. The accidental discovery of X-rays by Wilhelm Roentgen in 1895 prompted public fascination with 'shadow photographs' revealing bones (or needles or bullets) inside living flesh. WL, 17138i

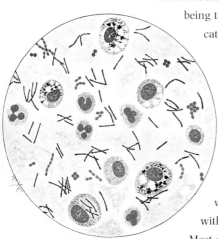

24 The causes of disease made visible? 'The characters of pathogenic micro-organisms': an illustration in Richard Muir, *Bacteriological Atlas*, Edinburgh, 1927. WL, QW17 1927M95b

Microscopy became popular from the 1830s, when Joseph Jackson Lister (the father of the famous surgeon) showed how to get rid of the coloured fringes which had been characteristic of objects seen through powerful lenses. By 1900, X-rays had appeared unexpectedly from the laboratory of a physicist; and electricians, photographers and a few doctors were exploring their utility for finding bullets in flesh, or fractures in bone. By that date, chemistry was accompanied by biochemistry – and a new range of apparatus – focusing on living processes and especially the roles of enzymes. And various instruments had been devised to 'read' the level of various substances in the blood. On the wards, thermometers were in general use, and in the new 'public health laboratories', specimens from patients, drains or dairies were being tested for bacteria – the microscopic plants newly implicated in the causation of infectious diseases (fig. 24).[15]

By 1950, immunological tests were routine, especially for blood transfusions; and chemical tests were beginning to be automated. By 2000, tissue-typing had been elaborated, and genetic testing and DNA analysis threatened to dissolve the line between normality and illness, making each of us into a set of characteristics and risks. And PET scanners were lighting up to show which bits of our brain were concerned with what; the phrenologist skulls of 1840 had been replaced with animated light shows.[16]

Most of these forms of analysis involved visualisation or measurement, often using special instruments – and much of 'medical technology' as usually defined is made up of such instruments. But analytical instruments were also used for action. The notion of disease as tissue lesions derived from surgical understandings of the body, and in turn supported attempts at surgical treatments, especially when the use of gaseous anaesthetics, first by dentists, gave insensibility to the patients and time to the surgeons. By about 1870, the sanitary application of creosote had been linked with 'germ theory' to produce Joseph Lister's antiseptic operative techniques, with which surgeons were emboldened to penetrate the body cavities. By 1900, surgical analysis and treatments were proliferating rapidly, aided by new kinds of scopes and by X-rays (fig. 25). Meanwhile, chemical analysis had produced a range of 'pure' medicines, which had often replaced 'nature's mixtures'.

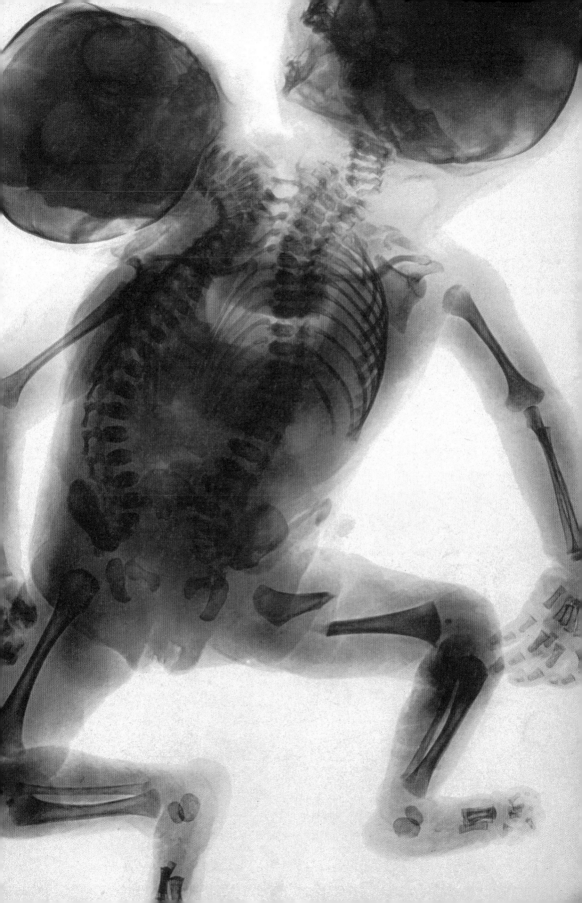

Much of the development was done in University laboratories rather than hospitals, for over the course of the nineteenth century, 'research' and the systematic improvement of industry, agriculture and medicine became recognised professions. In medical schools, especially in Germany, research often meant working on animal bodies – in life or just after their death – and many of the analytical instruments applied to humans were invented or developed for laboratory experiments and demonstrations. Such analyses provided means of seeing animal bodies as similar to humans, and demonstrably controllable in the laboratory.

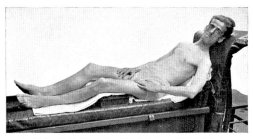

A CASE OF DIABETES MELLITUS TREATED BY

INSULIN.

I. —H.L.W. on Feb. 26th, 1925. Two days after admission to a London Hospital. Weight : 6 st. 3 lbs. 7 ozs.

II.—H.L.W. on July 2nd, 1925, after 4¼ months' Insulin Treatment.   Weight : 7 st. 8 lbs. 8 ozs.
Gain ; 1 st. 5 lbs. 1 oz.   He left Hospital after 6 weeks' treatment and returned to work 5 weeks ago.

26 'A case of diabetes mellitus treated by insulin'. An illustration from a 1925 pamphlet published by the Research Defense Society, promoting the benefits of medical research (against the antivivisectionists). WL, L23344

Experiments, products and meanings

From that manipulation of 'normal' animals came experimental systems to create disease by the disruption of the body or by the introduction of presumed disease agents, so that remedies could be suggested and tried. And from some of the agents and processes so tested there came new medical commodities – new drugs, vaccines, prostheses – which were then tried on humans (fig 26).[17]

Over the twentieth century, through the conversion of experimental products into new industrial commodities, and the continued proliferation of analytical methods, there developed the complex social organisms of present-day 'techno-scientific medicine' – linking patients and doctors with hospital and university laboratories, with pharmaceutical and other medical manufactures, and with the government agencies set up to regulate and support these varied activities.[18]

This massive articulation of disparate organisations and processes is perhaps the leading characteristic of medicine around 2000. These complexes of companies, hospitals, universities, and government – and of natural history, analysis, experiment and techno-science – may be the medical 'period phenomenon' of our age. Patients, even for a single condition, may have several doctors and nurses, and behind them are world-wide nets of information, and lots of tests and products, each depending on the work of thousands of technical and other staff. Nor is the commercialisation and division of labour only a matter of high technology; many of the traditional forms of care – such as washing clothes or preparing meals – are also industrialised.[19]

We persist in seeing the cultures of medicine as akin to other, older arts. We have yet to learn how to also see them as parts of a huge industrial complex stretching across the globe.

If a new Henry Wellcome were now to collect the varieties of medicine, then commercial advertisements would surely be central. As he already knew better than his contemporaries, the products of laboratory experiment could be sold by 'psychology' and good design. And

27 'A wrinkled face is a starved face', from a 1913 pamphlet on 'Beauty and Health. How to attain and preserve them', published by the Oatine Company whose cosmetic products were said to nourish the skin. WL, L28854

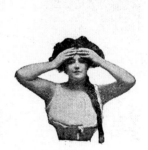

twist the head—move in straight lines. Apply more *Oatine* afterwards, the pores now being well opened, and finish by massage.

No. 6.—A wrinkled face is a starved face. Waste of tissue causes the lower skin tissue to contract and shrivel, leaving the outer covering like a loose mantle. To plump the tissues and eradicate wrinkles, apply *Oatine* with the finger tips until absorbed. Gently stroke the wrinkles crosswise with the tips of the fingers. Do this once a day for ten or fifteen minutes.

advertisements which now 'sell the benefit not the product' further shift our attention from the rationalised production of drugs to the cultural forms of wellbeing. As the preoccupations of puritanical health reformers merge with the magic of international business, almost anything can be sold as making you more healthy or beautiful (fig 27). Thus is techno-science folded back on itself, and advertisements come to seem the ritual presentations of our age.[20]

We live in a world where medical analysis, experiment, industrialisation and commercialisation increasingly shape our material culture and our understandings. It seems increasingly difficult to separate 'nature' from artefacts, or the 'environment' from the socio-economic systems in which we live. Or perhaps we should better say that those divisions of ours, so characteristic of 'modernity' for the last 350 years, are now blurring again. Our 'natural history' will not easily be separated from our human history; nor will the nature of human reproduction be independent of our individual and collective decisions about what it means to be human.[21]

Maybe that is the binocular answer to the questions prompted by this exhibition of Wellcome's objects – that whatever the medical elaborations of natural history, analysis, experiment and industry, and however they change our circumstances and possibilities, we should strive to envisage them as meaningful parts of human histories. If we can see the interwoven knowledges and practices of medicine as expressions of human aims and projects – in dynamic interaction with external constraints – then we may better understand both our present and our possible futures.

NOTES

1 Skinner, G.M. 1986. 'Sir Henry Wellcome's Museum for the Science of History' in *Medical History* 30, pp. 383–418.
James, R.R. 1994. *Henry Wellcome*. London: Hodder & Stoughton.

2 For an introduction by a past master, see Porter, R. 2002. *Blood and Guts. A Short History of Medicine*. London: Allen Lane. See also his longer work *'The Greatest Benefit to Mankind': A Medical History of Humanity*. London: HarperCollins, 1997. For recent multi-author guides, see Loudon, I. (ed.) 1997. *Western Medicine: An Illustrated History*. Oxford: Oxford University Press; or Porter, R. (ed.) 1996. *The Cambridge Illustrated History of Medicine*. Cambridge: Cambridge University Press.

3 See, for example, Porter, D. and Porter, R. 1989. *Patients' Progress: Doctors and Doctoring in Eighteenth-Century England*. Stanford University Press.

4 Pickstone, J.V. 2000/2001. *Ways of Knowing. A New History of Science, Technology and Medicine*. Manchester: Manchester University Press; Chicago: Chicago University Press.

5 For examples, see Helman, C. 1984. *Culture, Health and Illness. An Introduction for Health Professionals*. Bristol: Wright.

6 For examples, see ibid.

7 Ackerknecht, E. 1984. *Medicine at the Paris Hospital, 1794–1848*. Baltimore: John Hopkins University Press.
Foucault, M. 1983. *The Birth of the Clinic*. London: Tavistock Press.

8 Jewson, N. 1976. 'The disappearance of the sick man from medical cosmology' in *Sociology* 10, pp. 225–44.

9 Pickstone 2000/2001, Chapter 7.

10 Lawrence, G. (ed.) 1994. *Technologies of Modern Medicine*. London: Science Museum Publications.

11 Collingwood, R.G. 1938. *The Principles of Art*. Oxford: Oxford University Press.

12 Porter, D. 2000. 'The healthy body' in Cooter, R. and Pickstone, J. (eds), *Medicine in the Twentieth Century*. Amsterdam: Harwood Academic Publishers (paperback, London: Routledge, 2003).

13 For substantial introductions to ancient and early modern medicine see Conrad, L. et al. 1995. *The Western Medical Tradition: 800 BC to AD 1800*. Cambridge: Cambridge University Press.

14 For perspectives on non-Western medicine, see Kleinman, A. 1980. *Patients and Healers in the Context of Culture: An Exploration of the Borderland between Anthropology, Medicine and Psychiatry*. Berkeley: University of California Press.

15 For an overview see Bynum, W.F. 1994. *Science and the Practice of Medicine in the Nineteenth Century*. New York: Cambridge University Press. For the professional developments see Lawrence, C. 1994. *Medicine in the Making of Modern Britain, 1700–1920*. London and New York: Macmillan.

16 Reiser, S.J. 1981. *Medicine and the Reign of Technology*. Cambridge: Cambridge University Press.
Amsterdamska, O. and Hiddinga, A. 'The analysed body' in Cooter and Pickstone 2000.

17 Loewy, I., 'The experimental body' and Cooter, R., 'The ethical body' in Cooter and Pickstone 2000.

18 Blume, S., 'Medicine, technology and industry' and Goodman, J., 'Pharmaceutical industry' in Cooter and Pickstone 2000.

19 Pickstone 2000/2001, Chapter 7.

20 Porter, D., 'The healthy body' in Cooter and Pickstone 2000.

21 Latour, B. 1993. *We Have Never Been Modern*. Cambridge MA: Harvard University Press.

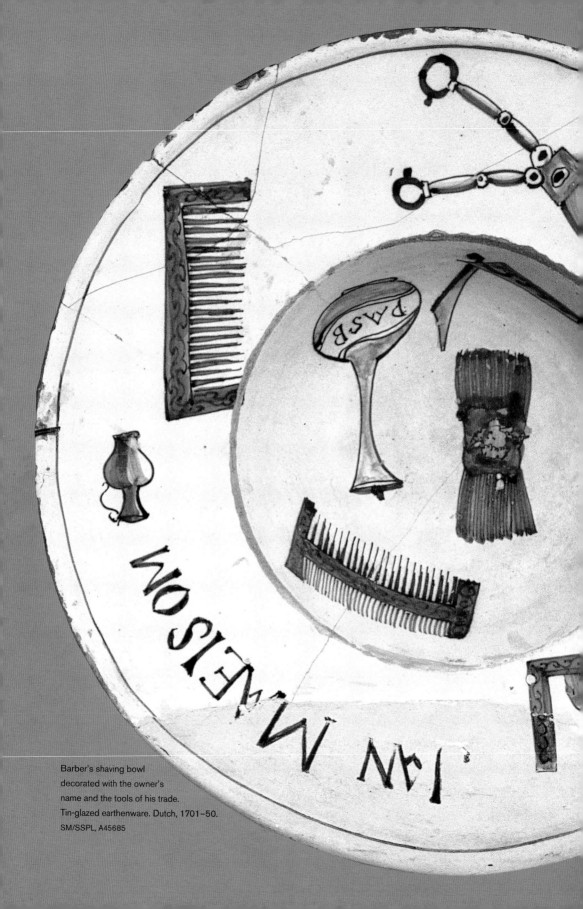

Barber's shaving bowl
decorated with the owner's
name and the tools of his trade.
Tin-glazed earthenware. Dutch, 1701–50.
SM/SSPL, A45685

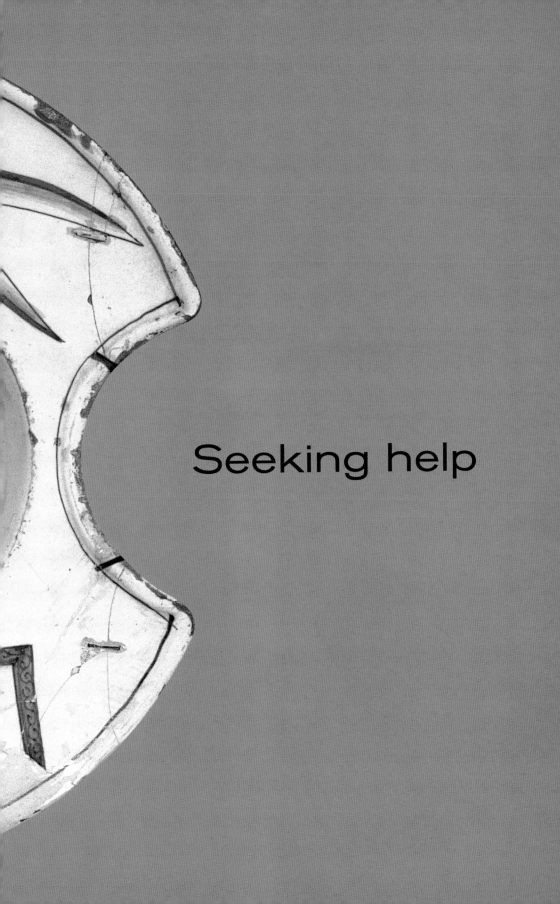

Seeking help

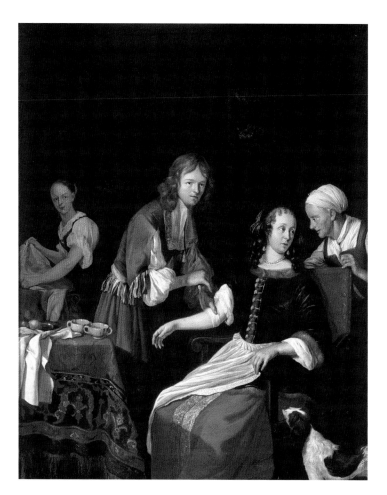

LEFT A surgeon binding up a woman's arm after blood-letting. Oil painting on copper by Jacob Toorenvliet. Dutch, 1666. WL, 44999i

RIGHT Leaf from a physician's folding calendar with 'Vein man' illustration above and lunar table below. 1463. WL, Western MS40

BELOW Tin-glazed earthenware bleeding bowl. 1700–70. SM, A43161

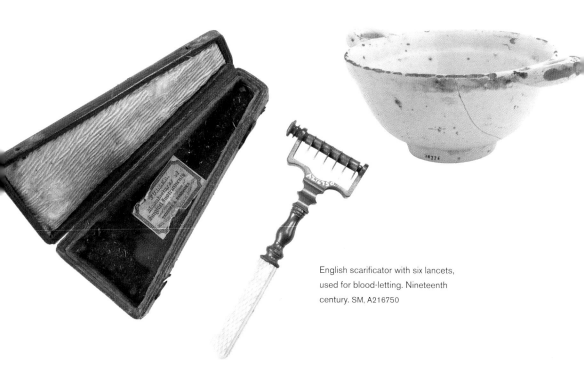

English scarificator with six lancets, used for blood-letting. Nineteenth century. SM, A216750

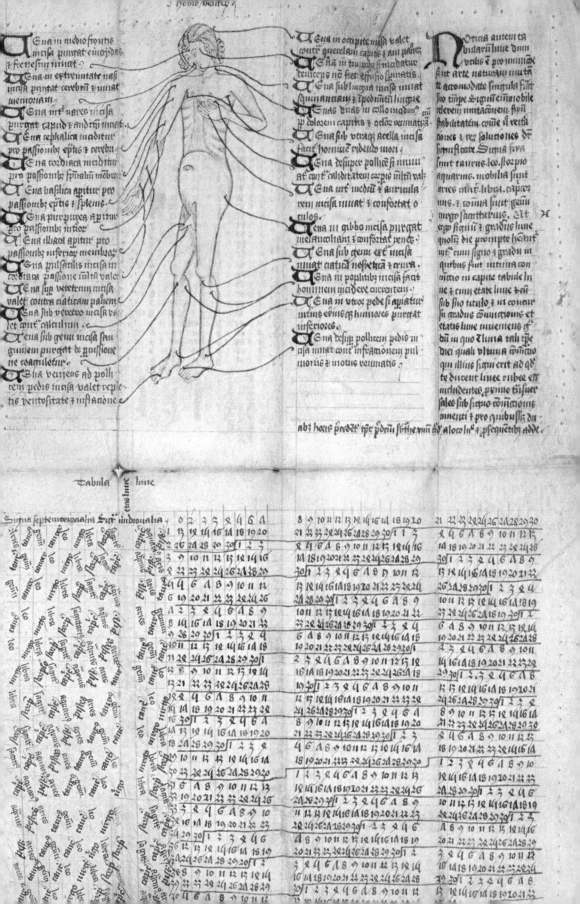

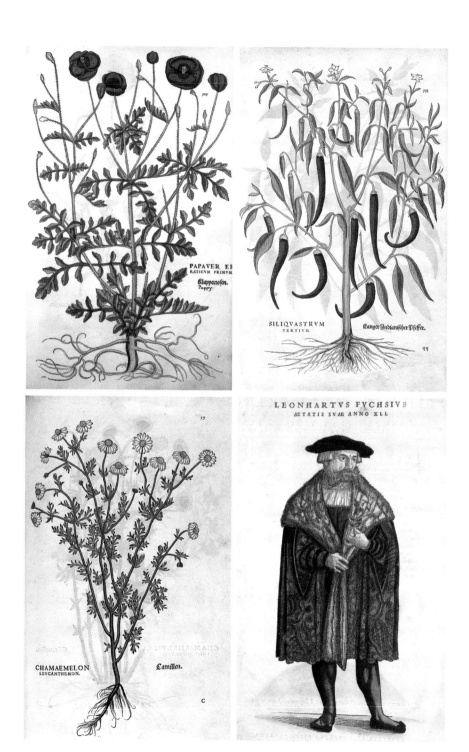

Illustrations from Leonhart Fuchs's encyclopaedia of medical plants, *De historia stirpium*, Basle, 1542. Clockwise from top left: a poppy plant, a red chilli plant, a portrait of Fuchs himself and a camomile plant. WL, EPB 2438/D

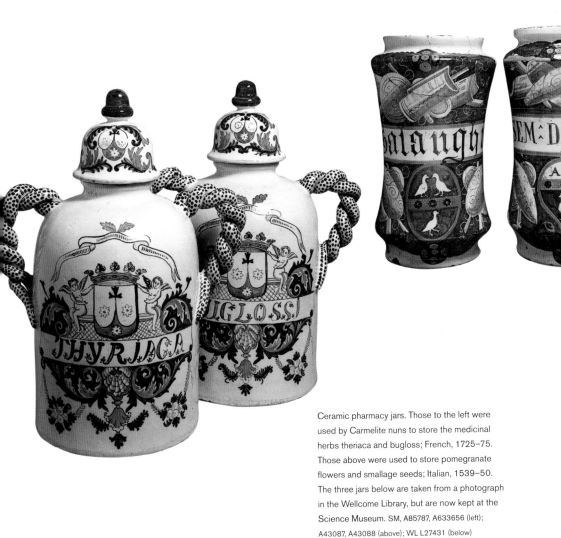

Ceramic pharmacy jars. Those to the left were
used by Carmelite nuns to store the medicinal
herbs theriaca and bugloss; French, 1725–75.
Those above were used to store pomegranate
flowers and smallage seeds; Italian, 1539–50.
The three jars below are taken from a photograph
in the Wellcome Library, but are now kept at the
Science Museum. SM, A85787, A633656 (left);
A43087, A43088 (above); WL L27431 (below)

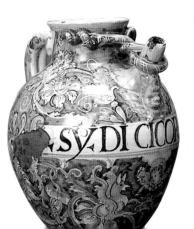

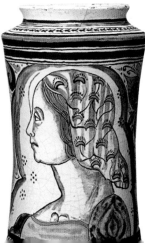

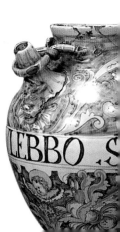

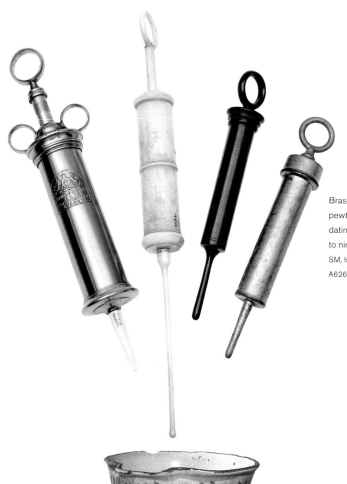

Brass, ivory, ebony and
pewter enema syringes,
dating from the seventeenth
to nineteenth centuries.
SM, from left to right: A626202,
A626932, A640607, A606384

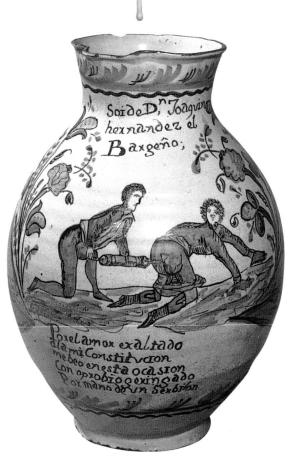

Spanish jug which illustrates an enema being
administered and includes the following
inscription: 'I am Don Joaquin Hernandez's
jar. Through intense devotion to my
constitution I find myself on this occasion
shamefully syringed at the hands of a serf'.
Tin-glazed earthenware with polychrome
decoration. Possibly seventeenth century.
SM/SSPL, A643327

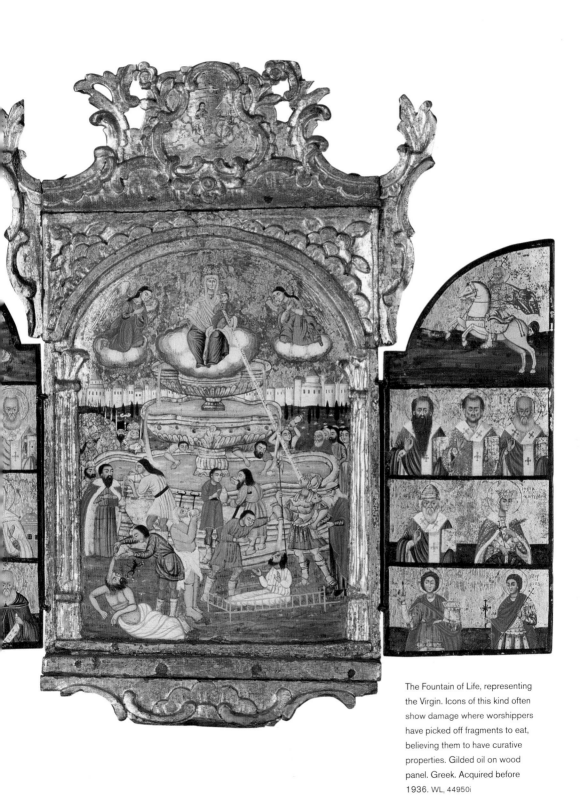

The Fountain of Life, representing the Virgin. Icons of this kind often show damage where worshippers have picked off fragments to eat, believing them to have curative properties. Gilded oil on wood panel. Greek. Acquired before 1936. WL, 44950i

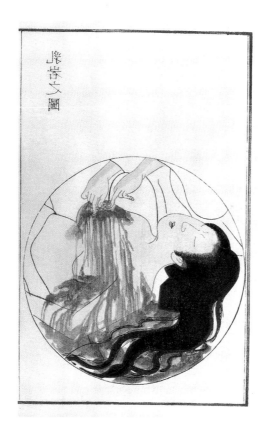

Page from Kamata Keishū's *Geta Kihai*, a surgical treatise published in Japan in 1851. The illustration shows the excision of a cancerous growth from a woman's breast. This operation was first carried out by Keishū's teacher, Hanaoka Seishū in 1804. Seishū operated on his wife and it was the first operation in the world conducted under a general anaesthetic. WL, Japanese Collection No. 18

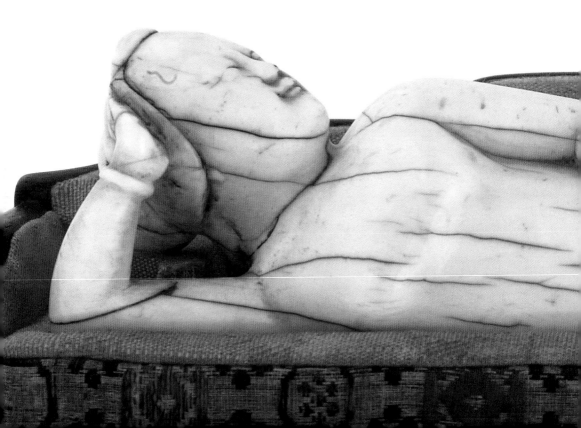

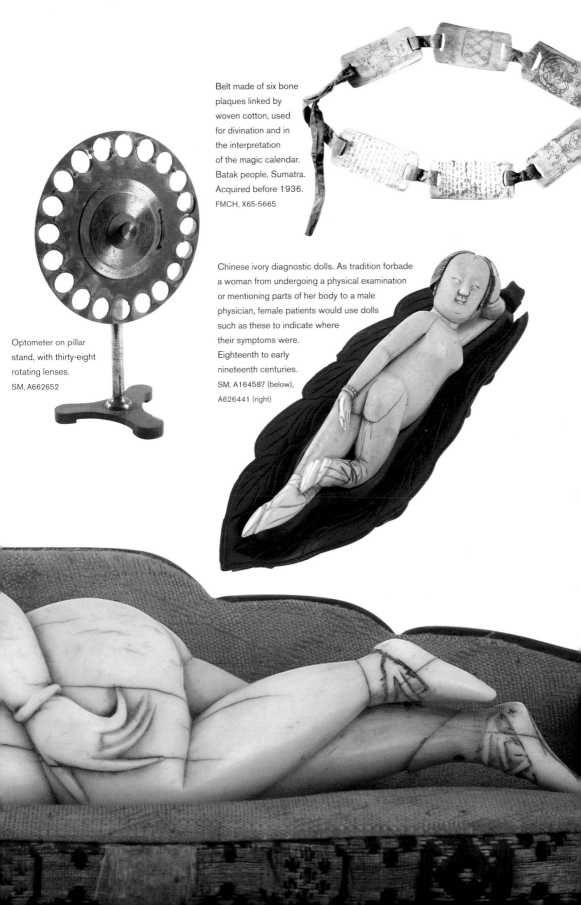

Belt made of six bone plaques linked by woven cotton, used for divination and in the interpretation of the magic calendar. Batak people, Sumatra. Acquired before 1936.
FMCH, X65-5665

Optometer on pillar stand, with thirty-eight rotating lenses.
SM, A662652

Chinese ivory diagnostic dolls. As tradition forbade a woman from undergoing a physical examination or mentioning parts of her body to a male physician, female patients would use dolls such as these to indicate where their symptoms were. Eighteenth to early nineteenth centuries.
SM, A164587 (below),
A626441 (right)

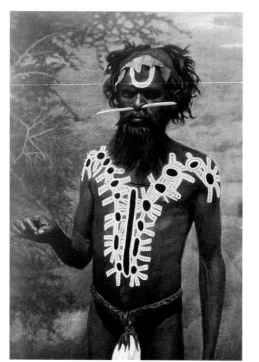
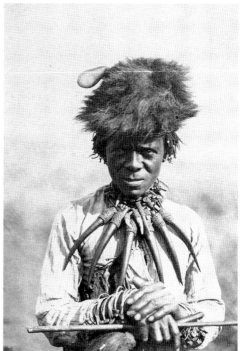
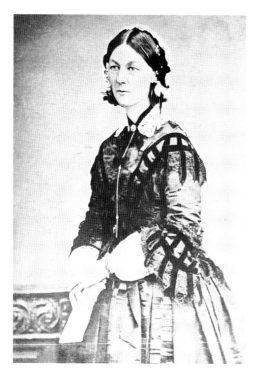
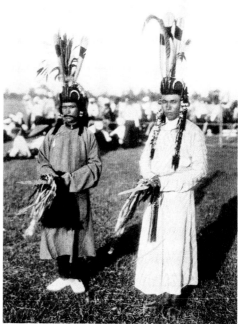

CLOCKWISE, FROM TOP LEFT Aboriginal medicine man of the Worgaia tribe, Australia, featured in S.G.B. Stubbs' and E.W. Bligh's *Sixty Centuries of Health and Physick*, 1931. Medicine man wearing necklet of horns and fur headdress (date and provenance unknown). Burmese Kachin medicine men. Photo by R.W. Marshall, date unknown. Florence Nightingale. Portrait taken by the London Stereoscopic Company, at the request of Queen Victoria, 1856. WL BA/STU, WL, 21318I, WL, M1008, WL, 13279i

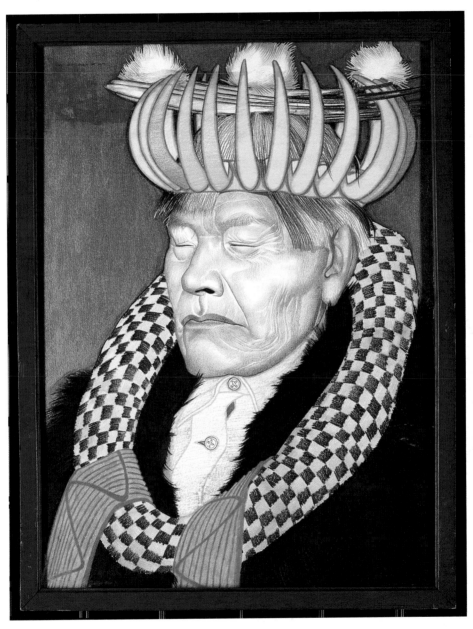

Captain Jack or Grizzly Bear Paw, medicine man of Kispiox, British Columbia, Canada.
Pastel by William Langdon Kihn. c. 1930–36. WL, 45895i

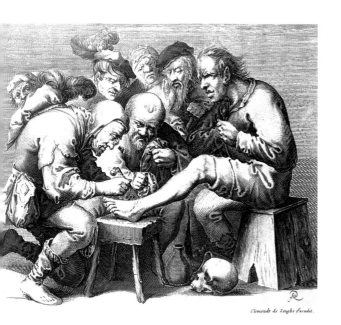

ABOVE A surgeon treating a patient's foot, watched by a crowd of onlookers. Line engraving by Pieter Jansz Quast (1606–47). Dutch, seventeenth century.
WL, 22561i

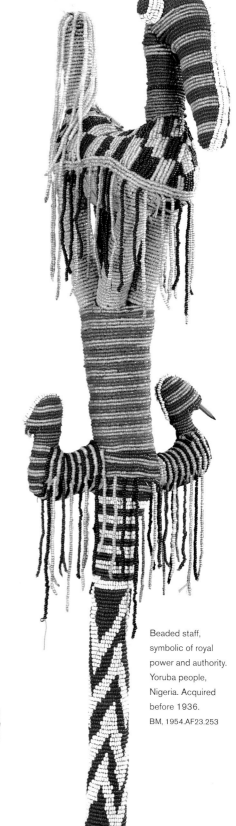

Funerary reliquary in which have been placed the bones (usually vertebrae) of the deceased. Figures such as these were designed both to protect ancestors from evil forces and to help the living communicate with and appeal to their ancestors for good health and success in hunting. Upper Ogowe, Gabon, 1870–1920. SM, A657377

Beaded staff, symbolic of royal power and authority. Yoruba people, Nigeria. Acquired before 1936. BM, 1954.AF23.253

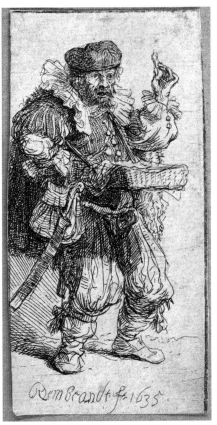

An itinerant street hawker selling
medicines (?). Etching by Rembrandt
van Rijn (1606–69). 1635. WL, 20476i

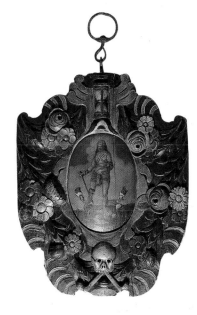

Barber surgeon's sign
painted with an image of
a wounded pirate whose
blood is being let by four
surgeon's hands. Above
and below are carved
symbols of time and
death respectively.
English, 1680–1830.
SM/SSPL, A631340

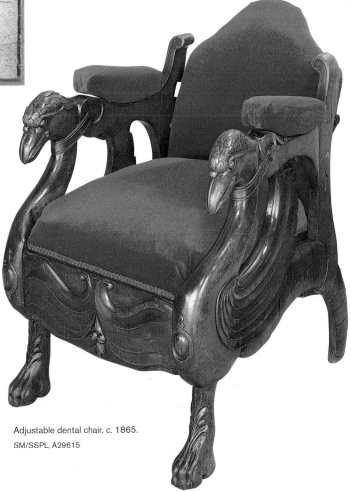

Adjustable dental chair. c. 1865.
SM/SSPL, A29615

A.1.

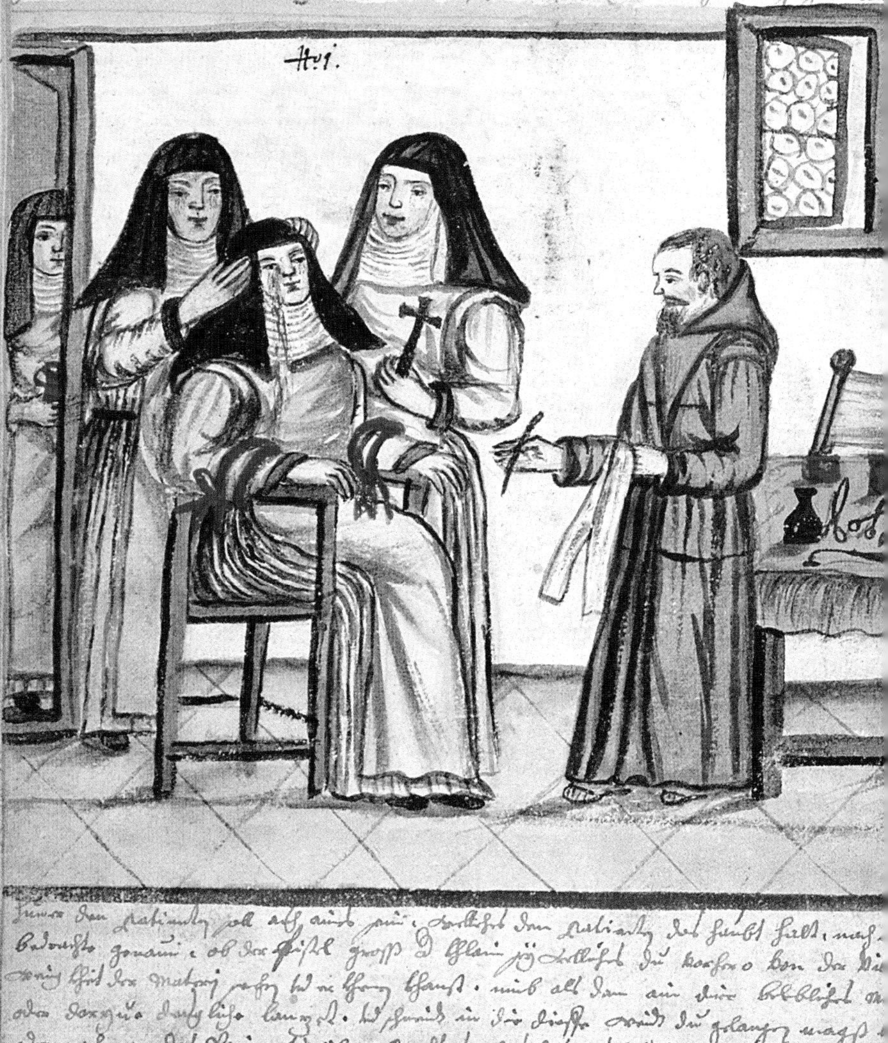

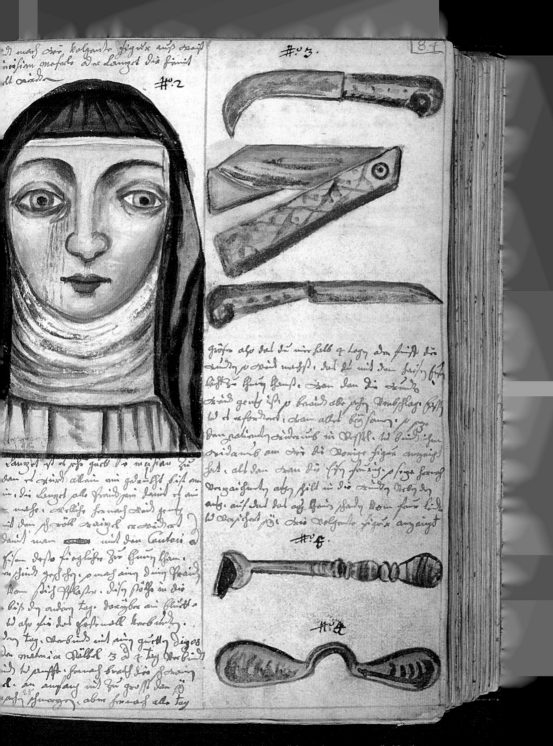

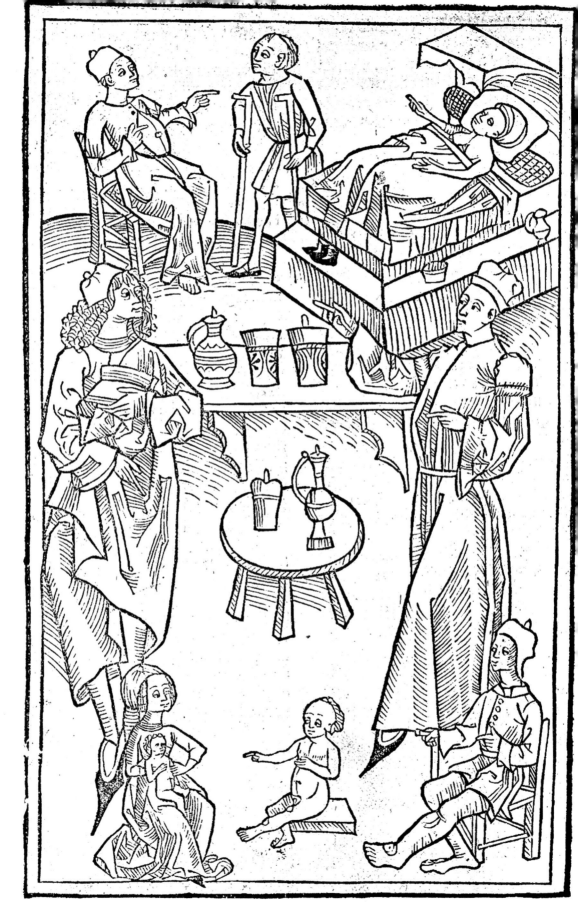

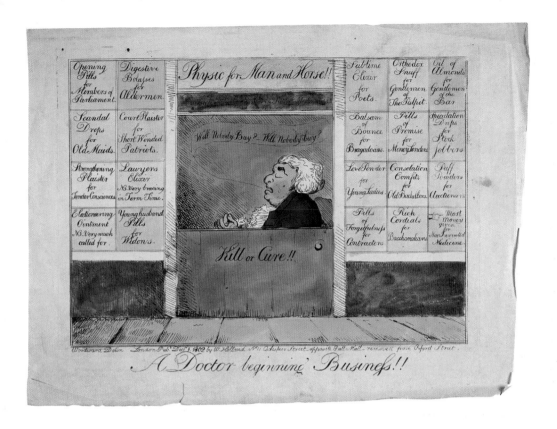

ABOVE This caricature by G.M. Woodward represents a quack doctor opening for business. Etching with watercolour. English, 1802. WL, 10932i

A donkey, representing Galinsoga, physician to the Queen of Spain, checks the pulse of a dying patient. The inscription reads, 'From which malady will he die?' Aquatint with etching by Francisco Goya (1746–1828). Spanish, c. 1797. WL, 18056i

LEFT *Ortus sanitatis*, or *Garden of Health*, Mainz, 1491. The woodcut shown here is taken from a chapter on uroscopy, a method of analyzing a patient's urine to diagnose disease. WL, EPB 3326

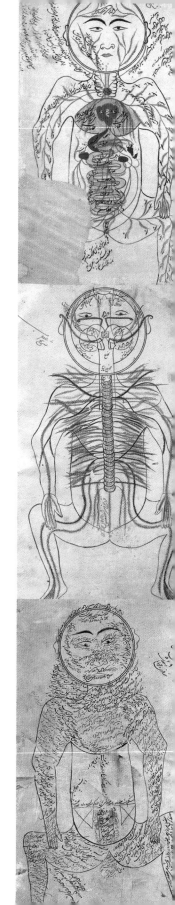

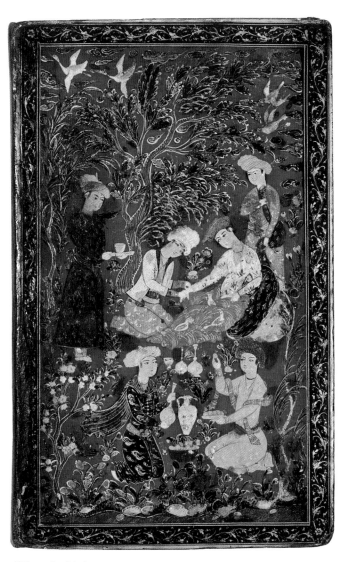

Al-Qānūn fī-ṭ-ṭibb. A 1632 manuscript copy of the *Canon of Medicine* of Avicenna
(980–1037), one of the key texts of medieval Arabic medicine. The cover shows a
physician taking a woman's pulse. His diagnosis is that she is suffering from love
sickness. The three leaves to the right illustrate (from top to bottom) arteries and
viscera, the nervous system and the muscular system. WL, Arabic MS Or. 155

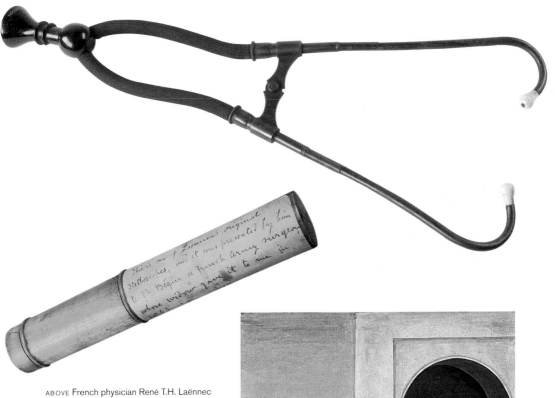

ABOVE French physician René T.H. Laënnec (1781–1826) invented the stethoscope in 1819. At first, when examining patients, he used a roll of paper to conduct the sound to his ear. He then had wooden versions made like the one shown here (above, c. 1820). Later these were modified with bell-shaped ends and flexible tubing for both ears (top, c. 1858, made by Scott Alison).

SM/SSPL, A106078 (above), SM, A625100 (top)

Physician taking a pulse, by a Delhi painter. c. 1830. This was not part of Henry Wellcome's collection, but was acquired by the Wellcome Library in 1992. WL, 5113i

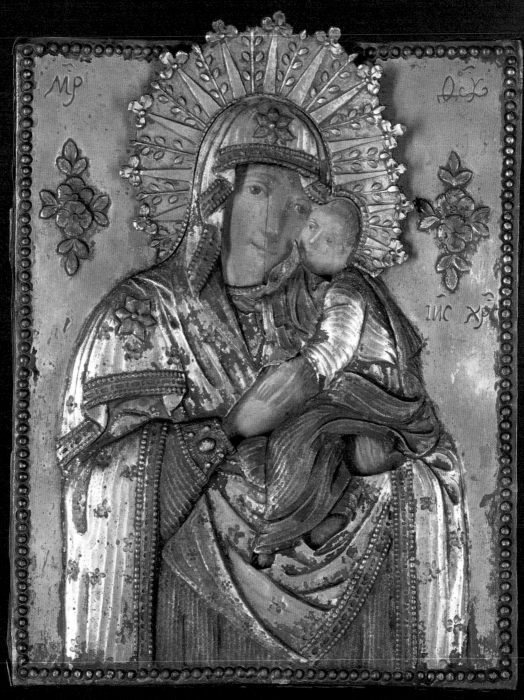

Icon of the Virgin and Child, carried by a Russian soldier in the Crimean War. The Russian text on the reverse of this piece indicates that its owner was 'Staff Captain Constantine Meshcheriakoff. Died in the Marine Hospital Sevastopol of Disease in the month of May 1855'. Oil painting and formed metal on wood. Nineteenth century. WL, 44966i

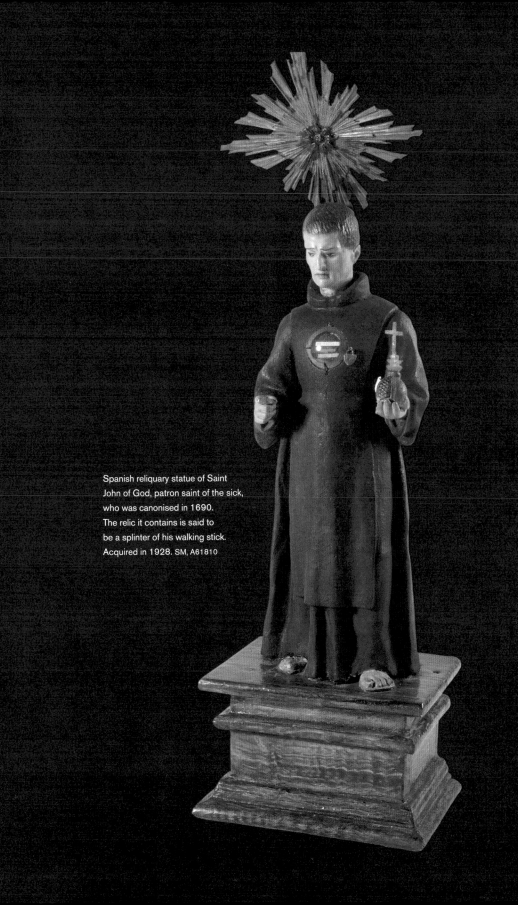

Spanish reliquary statue of Saint
John of God, patron saint of the sick,
who was canonised in 1690.
The relic it contains is said to
be a splinter of his walking stick.
Acquired in 1928. SM, A61810

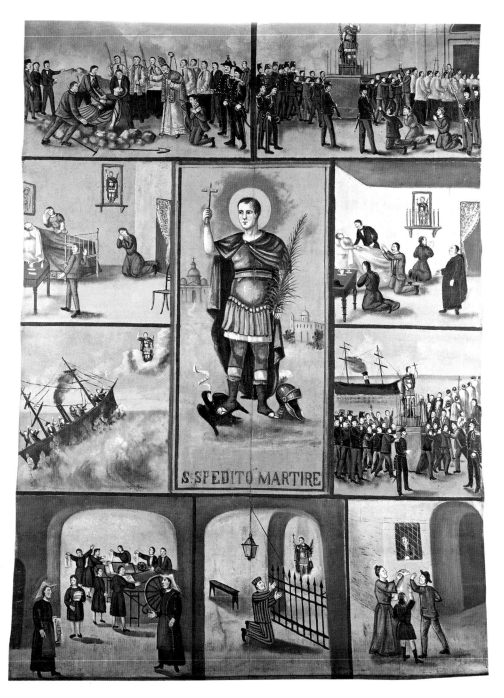

Saint Expeditus. Oil painting by a painter of Palermo, mid-nineteenth century. Two of the depicted scenes show patients in bed with bystanders in prayer to Saint Expeditus. WL, 47484i

RIGHT The Virgin and Child of Guadalupe. Oil painting by a Mexican painter, 1745. The Virgin of Guadalupe is one of the most revered figures in Mexican Catholicism. WL, 44828i

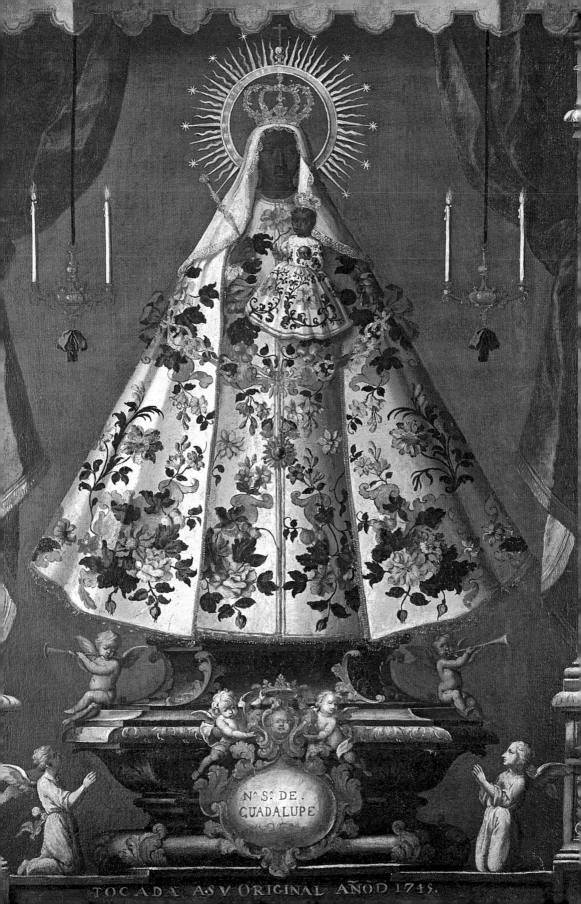

N.ª S.ª DE.
GUADALUPE

TOCADA A SV ORIGINAL AÑO D 1745.

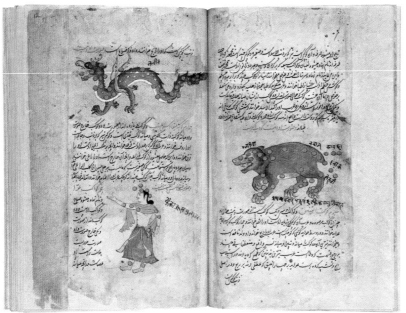

RIGHT Saint Elizabeth visiting a hospital. The subject of the picture is Saint Elizabeth of Marburg (1207–31) who, after her husband's death, gave away her worldly possessions and turned the income from her dowry over to the building and running of a hospital in Marburg, in which she personally cared for the sick, the poor and the homeless. Oil painting on copper by Adam Elsheimer (1578–1610). German, c. 1598. WL, 44650i

ABOVE Persian astronomical and astrological manuscript from India, seventeenth century. These pages illustrate the constellations of Ursa Major (left) and Draco and Cepheus (right). The golden dots inside the constellations represent the stars. WL, Persian MS 373

Shaman's mask with human features and a removable bird's beak. Haida people, Queen Charlotte Islands, British Columbia, Canada. Acquired before 1936. SM, A645087

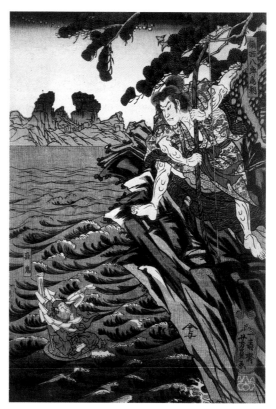

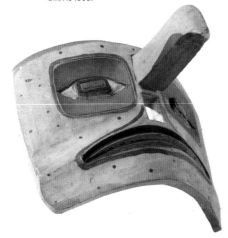

Tametomo repelling the demon of smallpox from the island of Oshima. Tametomo was a powerful historical figure of the twelfth century to whom many legendary feats were attributed. Woodcut by Utagawa Yoshikazu. 1847–52. WL, 565203i

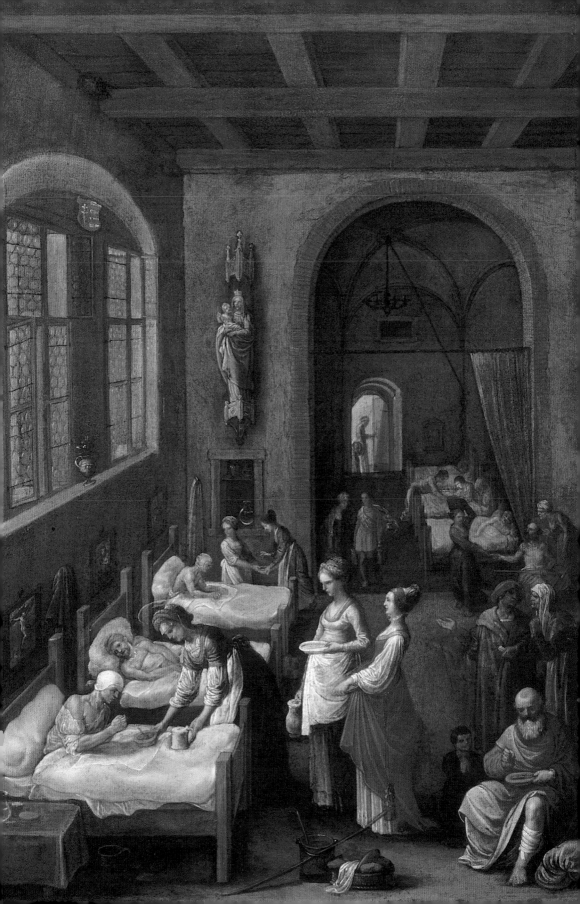

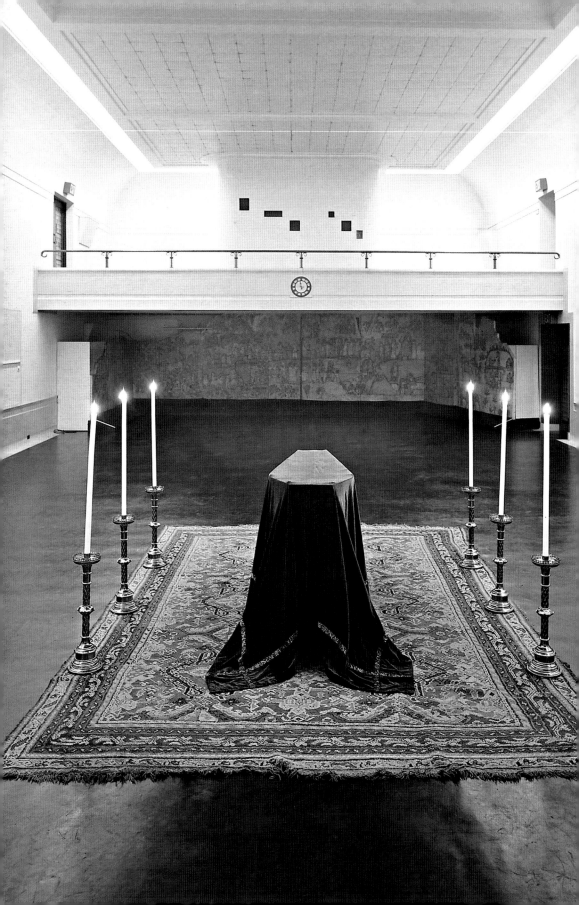

Henry Wellcome's body
lying in state at 183 Euston Road,
28 July 1936.

'One of the things about

Sir Henry was that he never

thought he would die.'

W.J. BRITCHFORD, EMPLOYEE FOR FORTY-TWO YEARS.

LETTER DATED 29 APRIL 1975.

Human Remains

Ruth Richardson

Accommodation

For years I've been a reader in Henry Wellcome's great library of
books and manuscripts, gazer at his pictures, Fellow of his Institute,
beneficiary of his munificence. But really only now, after having spent
genial time in one of the museum stores which house his collection,
have I learned to respect and admire this enigmatic man, whose
surname is a byword to anyone with a love of medical history.

The museum store itself is cool and dark. Its vaults exclude city
sounds. The slam of heavy doors sounds along chilly corridors, and
the jangle of keys awaits its echo. An emporium of artefacts is to be
found here, shelf upon shelf, cabinet beside cabinet, lying silently and
still in room after room. At first, I was surprised, but my astonishment
soon verged on bewilderment at the sheer abundance of *things*
(Wellcome called them 'curios') so thoughtfully gathered and placed.

In the store's locked rooms, large objects stand on the floor, or are
raised on enormous racks, but most simply rest directly on shelves.
Some occupy new-ish storage boxes: acid-free cardboard, or airtight plastic. Some have by them small containers in which shed
shards or shreds – fragments of whatever material has flaked or
crumbled away – are saved for future attempts at analysis or repair.

So although the place itself is cool and clean, and sunlight is
resolutely excluded, rubber perishes, wax cracks, leather flakes,
paper brittles and browns, as timebound processes of decay progress
imperceptibly.

Yet there's a curious sense of timelessness here, too. The business
of collection stopped dead at Wellcome's death in 1936. Although
some things have since been added by modern curators, and many
more dispersed, the whole project – the *things* these rooms contain,
those already on display, and all the thousands of books and manuscripts and images I know are elsewhere – the whole achievement,
seems rather like a geological formation: a fossilised stratum of

multitudinous forms . . . washed up from all human time and habitation: left safely high and dry.

This great collection serves as a pledge for Henry Wellcome's intended Historical Medical Museum, which though never completed, nevertheless abides as an intention. His is the presiding phantom of the place, and all visitors are therefore in a sense his guest.

Invitation

If you would care to accompany me, it would give me pleasure to share with you some of the things I've found in Mr Wellcome's collection. I shall look first at their documentation, then at generation and gestation, illustration, anatomical tokens of heavenly invocation, the demonstration of human anatomy in medical teaching, the mitigation of bodily losses by prosthetic substitution or supplementation, and the preservation of actual body parts. Three themes counterpoint this perambulation: endurance of the human condition, the embodiment of human ingenuity in the evolution of objects, and the recollection of the dead by forms of memorialisation.

Documentation

1 Part of the archive documenting the Wellcome Historical Medical Museum.

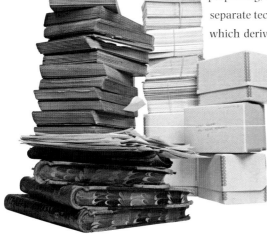

As I study these assembled things, I become increasingly interested in the process by which they were accumulated, and seek more avidly the available documentation. This in itself savours of an archaeological enquiry. The current museum computer records (so perplexing, that access is confined to trained personnel) allude to separate technical reports, and refer back to older paper records, which derive from data dating back further still – an old index card system which relates directly to the bulging (and crumbling) accession registers, in which the derivation of curios as gifts or purchases from individuals or at auction were recorded in Wellcome's day. A multitude of correspondence files, invoices, notebooks, receipts and accounts, chronicle these transactions (fig. 1). Documentary records are held at more than one location. When compared, they do not invariably concur. Nor, indeed, can they always be found: some, having never been cata-logued, lack shelfmarks, and even archivists doubt their existence.

Yet when the older records are sent for, and eventually found, and systematically examined, disappointment reigns. In most cases the records are painfully thin. All that was routinely recorded at acqui-sition was a transcription of sales catalogue entries, or brief descrip-tions sufficient to establish identity. Records rarely preserve information concerning an object's past history, use, or meaning.

Collecting was prosecuted, it seems, with rather an archaeological ardour. 'Finds' in archaeology at that time were cleaned on site, and shipped to museums to be classified later for explication and display.

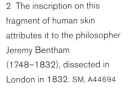

2 The inscription on this fragment of human skin attributes it to the philosopher Jeremy Bentham (1748–1832), dissected in London in 1832. SM, A44694

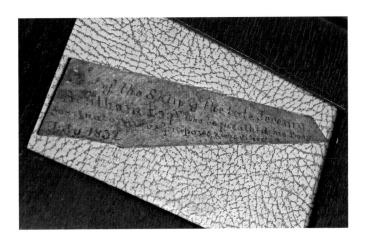

Many objects acquired for the Wellcome collections were treated as 'finds', already cleaned and shipped, as it were, but lacking source data. They have no stories, no recorded provenance. Although most had been created or collected within living memory, information crucial to an understanding of their history which might have been ascertainable at the time of acquisition, was not sought. The idea of recording the genealogy of an object, or at least recording how or where a donor or collector came by it, seems to have been mostly lacking. Historical knowledge having been lost, the explication and display which was intended to occur at a later stage is dependent on further research, which in most cases has yet to be done.

The deficiency of the original data is perpetuated from the acqui-sition registers to index cards, then to larger paper records, and eventually into the computer, which, apart from a search facility, appears to possess few advantages over the older paper records. In one case – a framed fragment of Jeremy Bentham's skin (fig. 2) – computerisation has transformed a thin record into a fallacious one. The computer indicates that Bentham's dissection took place *in France*, a misreading for 'in frame' on the paper record from which it was mis-transcribed (the error is now corrected).

The poverty of documentation for some of the objects I want to know more about dismays me. Yet museum staff seem unsurprised when I describe my sense of witnessing a kind of malnutrition in the midst of plenty. The Wellcome collection, it seems, is not dissimilar in this respect to other collections of its era.

Juxtaposition

Only the residuum of Wellcome's accumulated acquisitions is held in store, but its abundance and splendour somehow provokes an intense perception in this witness of the sustained enthusiasm and intelligence with which over many years the collection was assembled. Why these objects should convey this sense more pungently than, say, the books,

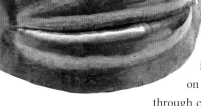

or the prints, is mysterious. It perhaps relates to the prodigious *diversity* of the things: the variety of their shapes, ages, colours, materials, derivation; and perhaps, too, their actuality: the space they occupy, the immediacy of their presence, their materiality, tangibility, their solid objectivity.

Originally, identification numbers were neatly hand-inscribed on obscure surfaces of the objects themselves; later, on little tags tied carefully around convenient protuberances, or through clefts. More recently, a slip of card bearing the appropriate long number for an article is hand-written in ink and tucked slightly underneath or beside it.

3 Beaten gold lips, found in Cyprus, supposed to be a Mycenaean amulet. SM, A3483

An object from ancient Mycenae lies on grey metal, alongside something a thousand years younger (fig. 3). Flint tools and human bones lie beside bowls, bead aprons, bottles and amulets, all neatly numbered, and respectfully separated by an appropriate measure of elbowroom. Sometimes juxtapositions seem incongruous, but more often reveal attempts to group like with like. Shelves, drawers, cabinets, walls, indeed entire rooms, are organised by theme.

My own historical work being in the history of anatomy – the use of the dead to the living, the fate of human remains, most particularly the history of dissection and of medical museums – there is much here to catch my eye.

'Human remains' usually signifies bodily evidences of the dead – bones, skeletons, cremated ashes – but in the context of the museum store, and of the breadth of Wellcome's collecting, it is often difficult not to perceive every object as in some sense representing remains of humanity. After all, every item derives from and is imbued with human activity, embodies human ingenuity; and although this might be said of all artefacts in all museums, this one primarily celebrates the corporeal nature of the human condition: the cycle of human bodily life, birth, maturity and death; the vulnerability of the human body to infection, disease, accident, malfunction, damage, disability; and, not without its own curious interest, the capacity of the human body itself to become artefact.

Most of the objects in the store are hand-made, and even items originally manufactured by mass production partake in odd ways of the identity of individual owners/users, or reflect an intrinsic eccentricity which derives from their own specific history, or from having been selected to represent their kin. That an object occupies a space in the store indicates, too, the investment of other forms of human industry – selection, collection, evaluation, acquisition, relocation, conservation, curation, devotion.

So although this great repository is shut off from the world, profoundly hushed and still, occasionally the bustle of other times becomes a din to the imagination, since every labelled object has a history, or rather a series of human stories, relating to its creation, its use, its manner of survival over time, its presence here. The store-rooms are redolent with histories, most of which will never be known. Our confrontation with them is only their most recent episode.

Generation

The most memorable of the storerooms I've explored is devoted to childbirth. The room is a dark storeroom, no more. Yet the first time I stood at its threshold, I sensed a wail of pain issuing from within. An assortment of birthing chairs, of varying ages and designs, stands on the floor and on racks. Hundreds of obstetric forceps crowd the shelves, with other cold instruments of a more destructive nature (fig. 4). Examination of the contents of the room's closed cabinets moderates the initial reaction of recoil: Victorian equipment for the administration of blessed chloroform; early contraceptive sponges in their delicate silk nets; sterile twentieth-century 'accouchement sets' of bandages, thread, and umbilical dressings; incubators and other objects which indicate kindlier aspects of the history of generation.

There are many museums of war, but where is the museum which honours the countless women whose skirmishes with death contributed so much to the survival of the species?

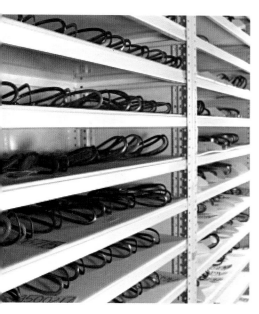

4 Stacks in the Obstetrics storeroom, showing part of the forceps collection.

Birthing chairs were used when germs were unknown, from ancient times to the nineteenth century – so they are quite unlike modern delivery tables. Some have padded seats, backs and arm-rests in fabric or leather, and space for cushions. They express both practicality and domesticity. The chairs are bespoke, sturdily constructed of wood, sometimes foldable for portability, and comely, carved, with shapely legs and finials (fig. 5). Handles and foot-rests are appropriately placed for the mother to pull/push upon in the course of her efforts to give birth. Back and foot-rests adjust to suit the mother's comfort. Doubtless, were a DNA expert to examine these chairs, they might yield a goodly supply of blood products and noxious organisms.

The centre of gravity of these old birthing chairs is low, for the convenience of the mother, to allow her to squat and be supported at the same time. More modern examples stand high off the ground, for the convenience of attending personnel. Though they may possibly be more hygienic, their metal surfaces look cold and uncomfortable, their posture immodest, demeaning, and their fixed stirrups unyielding.

Much of the history of medical intervention in birth shares this bittersweet quality. In cases of obstructed labour before the invention of forceps, there was little hope. Experienced midwives might turn a baby manually. But for *experience*, of course, we have no exhibits. Caesarean section was effectively a death sentence for a mother in such a case, the only option being the destruction of the child. Before forceps, flexible whalebone 'fillets' were used to assist birth, and it is believed that it was from a curved lever, the 'vectis', that the idea for the forceps was derived. If these contrivances failed, craniotomy hooks and knives (mentioned by Hippocrates *c.* 400 BC and in still earlier texts) were brought into use to destroy the child, in the hope of saving the mother. Many such tools lie here on the shelves: instruments of murder, yet of deliverance.

The obstetric forceps, which permitted the survival of both mother and child, seems to have been invented by the Chamberlen family,

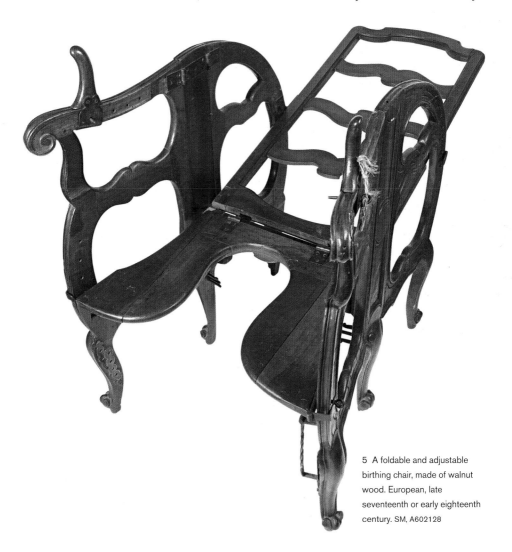

5 A foldable and adjustable birthing chair, made of walnut wood. European, late seventeenth or early eighteenth century. SM, A602128

Huguenots of Essex. Four generations practised midwifery between the late sixteenth and the early eighteenth centuries, each of whom may have influenced the design, which seems to have undergone significant evolution in their time. The family's rise from refugees to physicians to the royal family within a generation was doubtless assisted by their invention, which they diligently kept a family secret. Thus the self-interest of these clever men ultimately brings them shame.

Although Henry Wellcome's collection lacks the Chamberlen instruments themselves, others are abundant, among them several

6 An etching from William Smellie's *Sett of Anatomical Tables*, London, 1754, showing his forceps in use. WL, EPB F.587

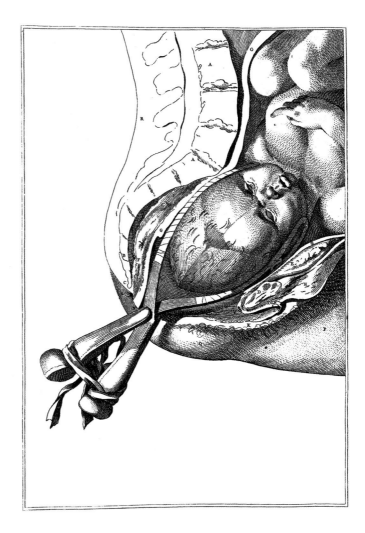

which probably date from the Chamberlen era: contemporary doctors in Britain and Europe (particularly in Essex) developed their own designs independently, probably after hearing of the Chamberlen secret, or getting sight of a pair. By the mid-eighteenth century, several men-midwives, or accoucheurs (as obstetricians were then known) like William Smellie, were designing their own forceps. Smellie tried boxwood ones, then short-handled leather and/or linen-covered iron ones, and scandalised the medical profession by teaching female anatomy to large mixed classes of men and women at his midwifery school in London. Poor women served as teaching material in return for free treatment. The desperate danger of spreading puerperal sepsis on obstetric instruments was not appreciated, and may explain the swift rise in maternal deaths mentioned at the time by one of Smellie's students.[1]

Illustration

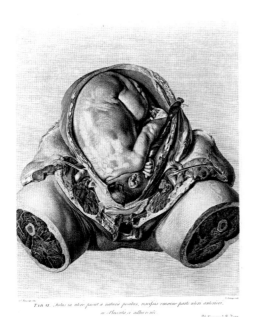

7 Jan Van Rymsdyk's magnificent Plate 6 from William Hunter's anatomical atlas of pregnancy, *Anatomia uteri humani gravidi tabulis illustrata* (*The anatomy of the human gravid uterus exhibited in figures*), Birmingham, 1774. WL, EPB F.438a

A copy of Smellie's remarkable book on complications of childbirth is in the Wellcome collection, in which the use of his forceps is shown diagrammatically by the artist Jan Van Rymsdyk (fig. 6).[2] Etching was chosen for the illustrations because characteristically Smellie wanted his book to be affordable. In the information explosion concerning human gestation and generation which occurred in the second half of the eighteenth century, Van Rymsdyk was a pivotal figure. Three important atlases of pregnancy appeared in this era: all of them with illustrations by him.

The finest of these books is William Hunter's *Gravid Uterus* (1774) (fig. 7).[3] The only reliable anatomical images of gestation before modern imaging techniques, were created from corpses. Hunter's great work had taken twenty-five years to assemble. It records explorations of the corpses of fourteen women he had managed to procure during that period, probably from bodysnatchers. Each was carefully injected for preservation, and meticulously dissected. Plastercasts (now in the Hunterian collection in Glasgow) were made which embody the form of these dead women with their babies *in situ*: the mischance of their fate configured in the physiology they reveal. Observance of the customary sorrowful interval between death and burial is manifest in the softness of the tissues on the day they were cast, still evident in the plaster.

The perfection of the dissections – Hunter acknowledged his brother John's assistance in his Preface – is preserved in that of the illustrations, which display clinical detachment on the part of the artist (and of the many superb engravers who worked to bring the enormous illustrations to the press) no less than the dissector. Thighs sectioned across, the layers of flesh and fat like butchered meat; entire bodies sliced across above the diaphragm (including vertebrae) so these mothers now lack heads, hearts and arms. Identity excised. Almost photographic in their detail, 'only from immediate observation', the earnest focus is the womb within, now opened to view.

Van Rymsdyk's meticulous recording of the humane (from the particularity of a baby's finger-crease, the tenderness of tiny testicles, even to the window reflected in the waters within the translucent membranes) parallels the Hunters' exploration of the structures of gestation from full-grown death in the womb, right back to the bubble of a five weeks' conceptus. The resolution to comprehend such calamitous deaths wrought from them hope of future amelioration.

I said a moment ago that for experience we have no exhibits. Perhaps Thomas Rowlandson's cartoon, *A Midwife going to a Labour* (1811) offers us a glimpse (fig. 8).[4] Rowlandson's midwife rushes out at night to attend a birth, in vile weather, on high metal pattens to raise her clear of the mud and dirt of the streets. The bottle she clutches looks convincingly alcoholic, which suggests that years before anaesthesia, simple expedients served to ease the pains of childbirth. Facially, this midwife looks as if she likes a drink, too, but we shouldn't take this too seriously, as Rowlandson rarely created a figure (male or female) *without* grotesque features, witness the night-watchman and young chimney-sweep here. The archetypal drunken midwife Sarah Gamp created later by Dickens has been shown to have been a propaganda figure, atypical of her real-life counterparts.[5]

This midwife carries her equipment tied up in a cloth. Her bundle looks too small to have contained forceps, so what equipment might

8 *A Midwife going to a Labour*. Hand-coloured etching by Thomas Rowlandson (1756–1827), published by Tegg, London, 1811. WL, 16984i

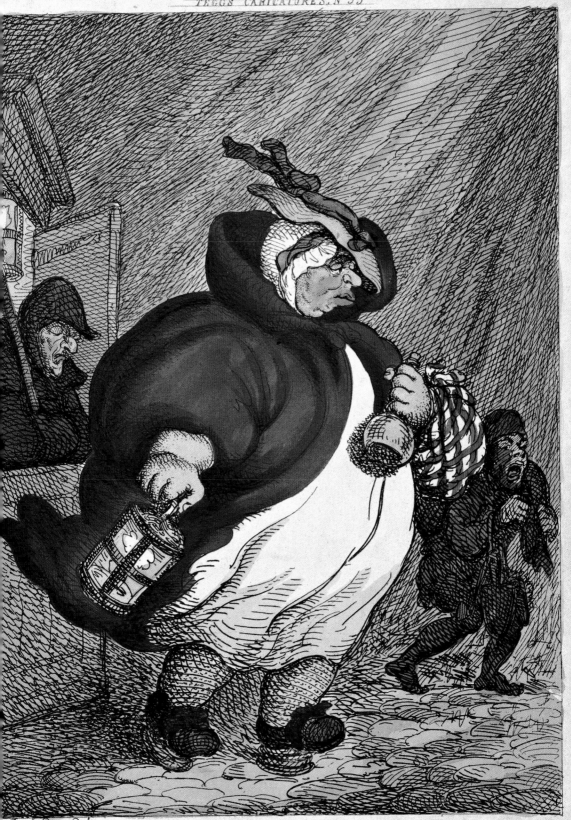

Rowlandson Del

A MIDWIFE GOING TO A LABOUR.

Pub.d Feb.y 12 1811 by Tho.s Tegg N° 111 Cheapside. Price One Shilling

she have been carrying? ('Midwifery bags' in the Wellcome collection are of no assistance here, being more modern leather 'Gladstone' bags for forceps.) Her bundle probably contained thread, linen strips and scissors, and possibly whalebone fillets (a female expedient, in all likelihood, born of necessity and fabricated from the traditional stiffeners for stays) which in an emergency could slip through the dilated cervix and loop around the baby. Intelligence and experience this woman carried elsewhere. Her clothing, and parts of her bundled cloth, are bright white (apparently in deliberate contrast to the sweep) which suggests cleanliness was important to her. The cry for hot water from the delivery room is proverbial – what *was* it all for?

The history told of 'untrained' midwives has been malign: rooted perhaps in professional jealousy. A midwife was as trained in her field as the contemporary general practitioner, who served a conventional apothecary's apprenticeship, was in his. It has been demonstrated that the affluent classes, who were more likely to use doctors, were more likely to die in childbirth than were the poor.[6] Rates of death in childbirth remained calamitously high in Britain until early antibiotics became available in the mid-1930s.[7]

Invocation

The tenderness of pregnancy is recorded in a beautiful clay figurine from Roman Britain.[8] The figure is of a naked pregnant woman whose lovely rounded belly and bosom are echoed by her surviving hand and arm. The tenderness of gesture and the vulnerability of her body have been modelled with a sensitivity and affection which seem to nullify time.

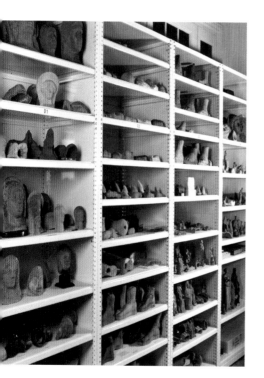

9 Part of the Wellcome collection of votive objects.

She was probably created as a votive figure, to be deposited as a prayer token at an appropriate shrine, or in a sacred pool (see Chapter 4), a custom widely observed in the ancient Greek and Roman worlds, 400 BC–AD 400.[9] Surviving ancient votive objects are usually terracotta, but occasionally wood or metal; and it seems that analogues in bread or cake could substitute. The Wellcome collection has a prodigious number of terracotta votives, mainly of external body parts from temples dedicated to Aesculapius and other health-giving gods. There are shelves of feet, legs, heads, faces, hands, eyes, ears, breasts and penises with and without testicles (figs 9 and 10). They are all well made, apparently from moulds, and mostly in good condition. The variety of their clay-colouration, shapes, and sizes, suggests the diversity of their sources of manufacture, and perhaps a wide timespan. Paint traces suggest that originally some were marked with realistic wounds or personal inscriptions.

10 A tray of votive penises.

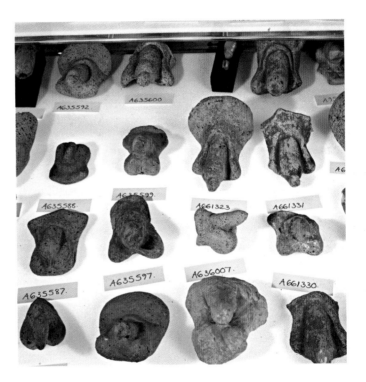

The invocation these things imply remains active: altars in Europe and in South America are still sometimes hung with miniature votive limbs and other body parts. In a play by W.B. Yeats a character asks: 'Would you be cured or would you be blessed?' and lists some of the objects people left beside an Irish holy well.[10] Wishes are still made at the toss of a coin in the water of pools and fountains; while Great Ormond Street Hospital for Children fundraises under its 'Wishing Well Appeal'.

It is strange to see so many quite realistic body parts standing about like sculpted amputations. Even more puzzling are the shelves of things resembling exotic limbless lobsters archaeologists believe to represent wombs (fig. 11). Some have a small balloon-like appendage, or a double orifice, believed to indicate the bladder. Representations of intestines are anatomically semi-convincing, in contrast to these wombs. The supposition is that dissection being uncommon, their design derives from a lost medical textbook, copied to unintelligibility.[11]

The survival of large numbers of these objects suggests they were popular, probably because they served for any of the many gynaeco-logical problems to which female flesh is heiress (from pain and flooding during menstruation, to infertility or over-fecundity, preg-nancy, miscarriage, birth, post partum problems, cancer, prolapse, fibroids, and various infections) for which there were few treatments and perhaps no cures.

Pregnant and breast-feeding female figurines are often found clustered at the shrines of Artemis, protectress of women in labour, who also received gifts of clothes, and (interestingly) of keys.[12] But we cannot know what prayer each votive object betokens, just as we cannot know who placed them – be it women for themselves, parents, husbands or friends – petitioning for fertility, safe pregnancy or easy birth, possibly in thanksgiving for a safe delivery, or a beautiful baby: perhaps all these, and others at which we can only guess.

Votive body parts manifest lay apprehensions of anatomy, the limits of contemporary medicine, the encounter of the human and the mysteries of divinity in the quest for the amelioration of corporeal ills: invocation, supplication, veneration, celebration. Although we are largely ignorant of their contexts and the particularity of their application, these body parts possess an uncommon potency. Like Keats's famous urn, they tease us out of thought.

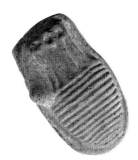
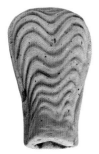
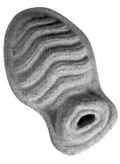

11 Clay-baked wombs from the votive objects collection, probably Roman 200 BC–AD 200. SM, from top to bottom: A636165, A636107, A636076

Perturbation

Lay notions of anatomy are also to be found in the collection's *memento mori*. One waxwork is a *vanitas* tableau of a life-size head, half fleshed (resembling Queen Elizabeth I) the other half skull, with attendant insects and reptiles, the whole in poor condition (fig. 12). Its biblical text survives: 'Vanity of vanities, all is vanity'.[13] Another, a pair of exquisite miniature figurines, male and female, only inches high, seem to be made of painted, waxed and varnished fine cloth and paper, perhaps French, dressed in the high fashion of the Napoleonic/Regency period (fig. 13). These too, are split vertically – dress, flesh and skeleton – and want repair.

12 *Vanitas* tableau. European, possibly eighteenth century. SM, A99821

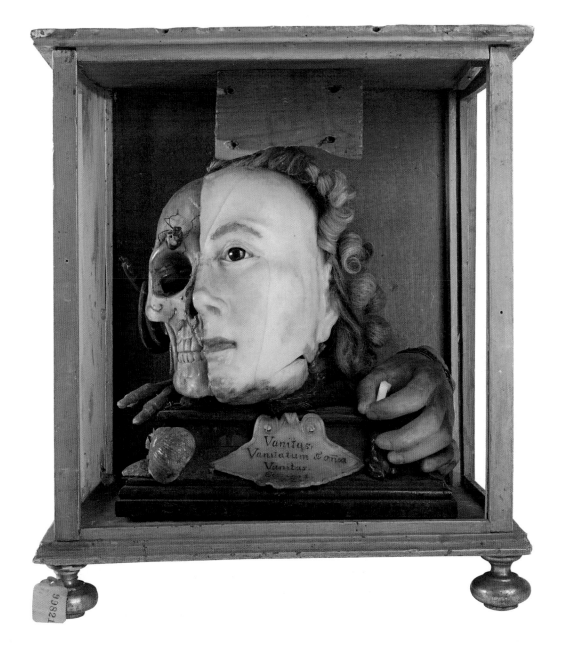

Wellcome collected a number of small coffin-shaped boxes containing skeletons or decomposing corpses, objects which were probably not intended for anatomical teaching but for spiritual contemplation. These *memento mori* figures may have been created for a similar purpose, though their effect today accords with that Gothic *frisson* so relished and so ridiculed by contemporary readers of Anne Radcliffe's gothic novel *The Mysteries of Udolpho* (1794), in which the discovery

13 A pair of delicate *memento mori* figurines. European, *c.* 1800. SM, A78827 (left), A78828 (right)

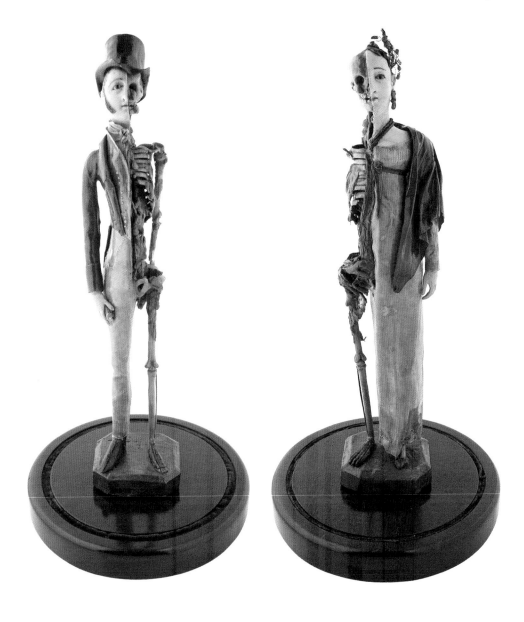

of a life-size tableau of human decomposition impels the heroine to swoon.[14]

Come to think of it, the dark corridors of the museum store partake somewhat of the Gothic, nowhere more so than where the bodily remains of real human beings are found interspersed among the objects.

Opening a cupboard in one of the ethnography rooms, a complete Peruvian mummy, crouched knees to chin, sat facing me on an upper shelf. That such a thing should have been collected can be understood historically; but that it should continue to be kept seems a molestation of the culture from which it derives, and an indignity to our own.

Demonstration

The collection is home to all sorts of anatomical curiosities, like the life-size plaster *écorché* of a strong man's back, showing the musculature in such particularity that it seems almost real.[15] Only if you are aware of the history of anatomical teaching might you recognise the likelihood that this *is* the cast of a real man, flayed after death, possibly after his execution, like the crucifixion which still hangs in the schools of the Royal Academy of Art in London.[16]

On another shelf sits the cast of an umbilical cord, the vessel which connects a baby in the womb to its placenta, formed into a perfect knot.[17] The baby must have looped-the-loop in the waters of the womb, and someone must later have been struck with the perfection of the knot. Cord knots can damage a child, starving it of oxygen and sustenance. Here the vessels seem patent, so one hopes the knot was not a post-mortem finding.

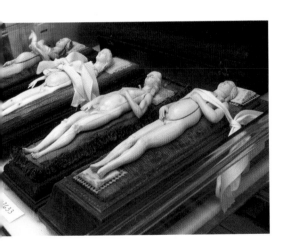

14 Carved ivory manikins of expectant women in the Anatomy storeroom. European, sixteenth–eighteenth centuries.

Wellcome collected numerous dissecting tools and teaching materials: muscle men, anatomical models, teaching skeletons, casts, wax body parts sporting the florid lesions of smallpox and other diseases, and a considerable number of tiny carved ivory manikins of expectant women designed to reveal inner layers of anatomy, and eventually the foetus curled up in its diminutive home (fig. 14). They are said to have been used in the education of students, midwives and young married women.[18] The passage of centuries is evident less in any evolving understanding of anatomy they exhibit, than in the stylistics of the carvings, which manifest their historical age in the body-type transiently fashionable in their era.

Mitigation

The stylistics of corporeality are evident, too, in prosthetics. Dispersed through most of the themed divisions of the collection are things designed to mitigate the physical deficiencies of innumerable unknown people: we have their false ears and noses, their spectacles, their false teeth and limbs, their crutches, braces, sticks, stump-sticks and nipple-shields (fig. 15). There are cupboards of equipment for the construction of dentures, for the testing and amelioration of the

15 Nipple-shields in silver, ivory and glass. The silver one is hallmarked to the reign of George III (1786–1821). SM, from left to right: A641255, A606830, A606829

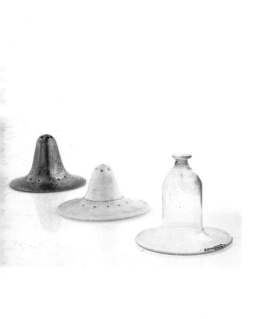

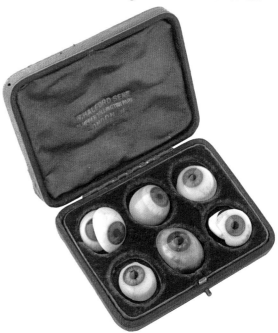

16 ABOVE RIGHT A small case of false eyes, white glass, with blood vessels in red glass, and vari-coloured irises. W. Halford, London, c. 1890. SM, A680646

shortcomings of human eyes (and indeed their substitution, in glass eyes of every likely hue) and a diversity of objects designed to straighten or support their bodies, from wheeled chairs and calipers to orthopaedic corsets (fig. 16).

These prostheses form in some ways a companion collection to the votives. In their substance, both groups embody their own time-bound aesthetics, and the artistry of the handiwork they preserve.

While the votives evidence a spiritual quest for assistance with physical ills, prosthetics encapsulate human efforts at physical mitigation or restitution. Both symbolise the ameliorative impetus Wellcome sought to document.

Most of them are hand-made, for individuals. Bespoke spectacles, lorgnettes, monocles, reading glasses, sunglasses, snowglasses, corrective eyeglasses of all kinds: hundreds of them, all different. Blue-lensed, green-lensed, with and without flaps, with broad or narrow bridges, folding or hooked wire earpieces; eye-glasses with mixed abilities, some of which fold down to the dimensions of long-decayed pockets: all these many adjustments created by individual artificers to suit individual clients, all of them (like Wellcome) now expired (fig. 18).

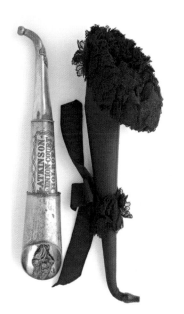

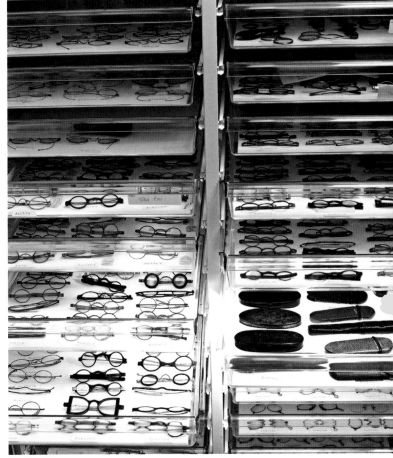

17 ABOVE Two Victorian ear trumpets, one collapsible in tin, the other swathed in black silk and lace mourning. SM, A602553 (left), A129677 (right)

18 RIGHT Stacks of spectacles in the Ophthalmic storeroom.

Bespoke ear-trumpets, formed for one or for both ears, curved in tortoiseshell, folding telescopically in tin, engraved with the owner's address, or trimmed with black lace to suit an old grief (fig. 17). What sounds passed along them we know not. Bespoke teeth, for Etruscan jaws in gold, younger ones in ivory, wood and bone, with wires to attach to other teeth long gone, and worn by mastication. Bespoke shoes, built up by dextrous leather-workers, to accommodate withered legs long since departed. Bespoke corsets – designed to straighten and support withered spines, twisted spines, weak backs – their metallic lace and leather straps sit up with trim symmetry, hinged for stepping into, perforated for the escape of ill-humours. Having a twisted spine (scoliosis) myself, I found myself regretting my inability to seek out the fabricator of an exceptionally fine one (fig. 19) to forge another, in the hope of returning to a historic shapeliness.

Perhaps the most poignant of these things are the limbs. Legs (sometimes hinged at the knee, or to allow toe flexion) terminate in feet designed to fit real shoes. Now their secret parts are visible: not only the sites of bumps and indentations, but those parts from which we can impute the original site of amputation. Parts designed to function invisibly under garments are now nakedly revealed with their metal struts, leather straps, hinges, joints, buckles, cuffs, rivets, casings, lacings, loops, studs, pads, swivels, slots and prongs; and revealed to our eyes, too, are the poignant evidences of sufferers'

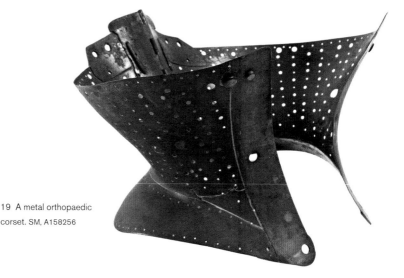

19 A metal orthopaedic corset. SM, A158256

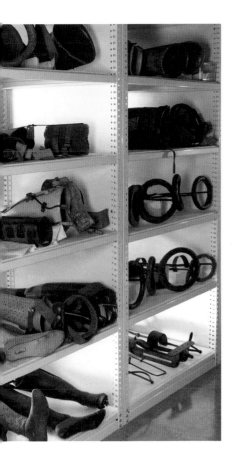

20 Leg and foot prostheses in the Orthopaedics storeroom.

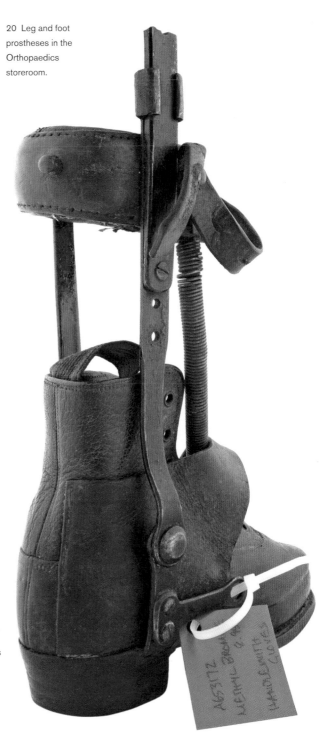

21 A Victorian child's shoe and leg caliper, in leather and steel.
SM, A653172

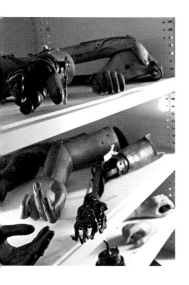

discomfort – in the soft scarves and wisps wound round to bandage the chafing-places (figs 20 and 21).

Arms, articulated at elbow, wrist or knuckle, with painfully pragmatic hooks like Hook's hook at their extremity; or hands, realistic by the notions of their day, carved with fingernails in wood, moulded in plastic, or in steel designed to be discreetly hidden by leather gloves (figs 22 and 23). Hands made by hand rest on their shelves, beckoning attention with empty gestures.[19]

Preservation

Stylistics change in anatomical teaching, too. Whereas today we might use computer technology, in the past real body parts were dissected for display, and preserved by wax-injection, desiccation and

22 Arm and hand prostheses
in the Orthopaedics
storeroom.

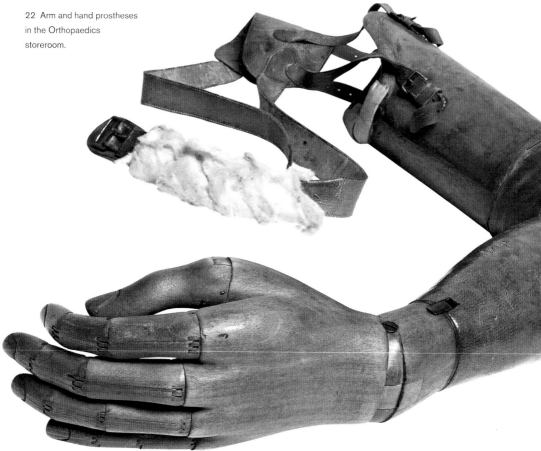

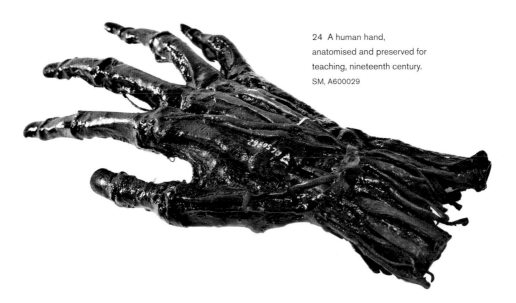

24 A human hand,
anatomised and preserved for
teaching, nineteenth century.
SM, A600029

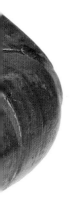

23 LEFT A beautiful artificial
left arm and hand, in leather
and wood, jointed at elbow
and wrist, with articulated
fingers and sprung thumb.
European, nineteenth century.
SM, A653499

varnishing, or in spirits (fig. 24). For much of the century from 1750 to 1850 medical students in Europe were expected to dissect well, and to learn preservation techniques. The collection in the museum store has almost no wet specimens in bottles and jars. There are however many skulls, several dried brains, a tongue, half a man's skin, skeletons, vertebrae and other bones, several dried penises, lung tissues, and some dried arms and hands, ligaments and blood vessels complete, now blackened with age.

An injected human stomach, fanned out like a seaweed[20] reveals also the stylistics of museology. Together with a piece of trepanned skull,[21] it was collected because it was originally preserved by Edward Jenner, pioneer of medical vaccination.

One of Wellcome's categories for the classification of objects was 'relics': not the religious variety, but things previously belonging to notable medical men, evidently esteeming them as in some way saintly enough to consecrate belongings. In only one case, however, did I find one which was self-composed: among a group of mourning rings the bezel of one commemorates the great Quaker doctor, John Coakley Lettsom (1744–1815), pivoting to reveal a panel of his hair, plaited in basketweave. Other figures represented by hair in the collection include George Washington, George III, Napoleon Bonaparte, the Duke of Wellington, Grace Darling, and an extinct native aboriginal of Tasmania, whose name is unrecorded (fig. 25).

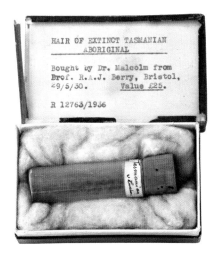

HAIR OF EXTINCT TASMANIAN
ABORIGINAL

Bought by Dr. Malcolm from
Prof. R.A.J. Berry, Bristol,
29/5/30.   Value £25.

R 12765/1936

25 Glass phial containing
a sample of hair from an
unnamed native inhabitant of
Tasmania, said to represent a
'now extinct race'. Purchased
from Professor R.A.J. Berry
in 1930. SM, A79800.

26–8 OPPOSITE Human skull
with painted features and
cowrie shell eyes. The hair is
real. Said to have been used in
rituals associated with ancestor
worship. Papua New Guinea,
probably nineteenth century.
SM, A656000
Human skull inscribed with
prayers for the deceased.
Collected by Robert Baden-
Powell's Asante (Ghana)
expedition, 1895. SM, A666427
Human skull inscribed for
'phrenological demonstration'.
One half accords with Gall's
theories, the other, Spurzheim's.
Probably French, nineteenth
century. SM, A25407

Relics of murderous bodysnatchers are to be found here, too: the brain of Burke, of Burke and Hare, executed in Edinburgh in 1829, and skin belonging to Williams, of the 'London Burkers' Bishop and Williams, executed in London two years later.[22]

The presence in Wellcome's collection of souvenirs of famous and infamous body parts testifies to a European preoccupation, which perhaps spread to North America. The Wellcome Library houses a small notebook said to be bound in the tanned skin of the man who sparked the American War of Independence.[23] To us such objects partake of that fetor emanating from the commissioners of lampshades for the Third Reich.

These things occupy the intersection of corporeality, mortality and morality: trophies of triumphalist power exercised without restraint by the living over the dead.

The sense of curious assortment and assiduous care in the preservation of the identity of these parts is unmistakable, but so too is the knowledge that much of their significance is endowed by inscription. They resonate by association. Without attribution, they would be cryptic indeed: uniquely human perhaps, but undistinguished from all other possible locks of hair or body parts. We take their authenticity on trust, just as Wellcome did.

Some curios have inscriptions which inhere: bones deformed by leprosy or rickets, or fused by osteo-arthritis; shrunken heads; a remarkable collection of (mainly French) tattoos cut from the dead and kept in airtight plastic lunch boxes; the ink-inscribed irregular skin fragment said to derive from the body of Jeremy Bentham;[24] and a number of skulls inscribed with museum numbers as well as their original inscriptions: skulls commemorative, phrenological, and ceremonial, the latter said to have been prepared for 'ancestor-worship' (figs 26–8). We utilise such terms to classify things held dear to others, of other times and places, yet resist their applicability to our own.

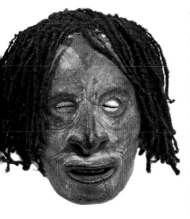

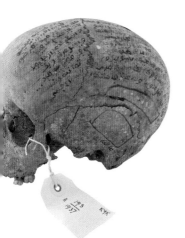

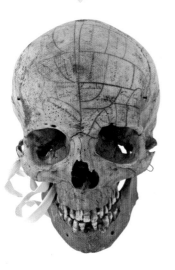

Conclusion

Henry Wellcome's artefacts communicate something akin to what the novelist Elizabeth Bowen once described as the 'electrical-imaginative current' she found in short stories.[25] The importance of these objects lies partly in their nature, and partly in their collected amplitude. A major impetus behind Wellcome's urge to collect so broadly seems to have been an understanding that although health is fundamental to the survival of the human species, the ways in which it has been sought and maintained are as diverse as are human communities and civilisations. From his curiosity concerning the variety of human reactions to adversity, developed the wider understanding that the history of medicine fundamentally informs the history of humankind.

The exhibits are embedded with other people's thought, other people's endeavour, other people's efforts at the amelioration of other people's infirmity and suffering. They beg many questions: Whose ingenuity and skill/craft is manifested here? Whose ideas? What motive created this? How did this thing survive, to arrive here? *What stories does it hold?*

For most objects in the Wellcome collection such questions can receive only imperfect answers, or none at all. Yet nonetheless the collection resonates with what Italo Calvino has called 'the convergence of infinite relationships'.[26] We sense the hands behind hands, growing paler and paler[27] these things imply.

Wellcome's curios exist, substituting in strange and unaccountable ways for perishable things which they to some extent embody: care, human effort, ingenuity, capacity, creativity, skill, industry, thought, pain, grief, sadness, physicality, infirmity, deprivation, vanity, even cruelty; and yet, too, resilience, love, faith, kindness, concern, joy and hope.

Phantoms, vestiges, remnants of perishables, amassed.

NOTES

1 Glaister, J. 1894. *Dr William Smellie and his Contemporaries*. Glasgow: Maclehose. Douglas, W. 1748. *A Letter to Dr. Smellie*. London: Roberts.

2 Smellie, W. 1754. *A Sett of Anatomical Tables*. London: Smellie. Thornton, J.L. 1982. *Jan van Rymsdyk*. Cambridge: Oleander.

3 Hunter, W. 1774. *The Anatomy of the Human Gravid Uterus*. Birmingham and London: Baskerville.

4 Rowlandson, T. 1811. *A Midwife going to a Labour*. London: Tegg. Etching and hand applied watercolour.

5 Summers, A. 1988–9. 'The mysterious demise of Sarah Gamp: the domiciliary nurse and her detractors' in *Victorian Studies* 32, pp. 365–86.

6 Loudon, I. 1997. 'Midwives and the Quality of Maternal Care' in *Studies in the Social History of Medicine*, pp. 180–200.

7 Loudon, I. 1992. *Death in Childbirth*. Oxford: Oxford University Press.

8 Accession no. A634992.

9 Jackson, R. 1988. *Doctors and Diseases in the Roman Empire*. London: British Museum Press, pp. 86–111, 157–69.
Edlund, I. 1987. '*Mens Sana in Corpore Sano*' in Linders, T. and Nordquist, G. (eds), *Gifts to the Gods. (Proceedings of the Uppsala Symposium, 1987)*. *Acta Universitatis Uppsaliensis* 15: pp. 67–75.
Thompson, C.J.S. 1922. *Graeco-Roman votive offerings for health in the Wellcome Historical Medical Museum*. London: Hazell Watson & Viney.
Turfa, J.M. 1986. 'Anatomical Votive Terracottas from Etruscan and Italic Sanctuaries' in Swaddling, J. (ed.), *Italian Iron Age Artefacts in the British Museum*. London: British Museum Publications, pp. 205–13.

10 Yeats, W.B. 1966. *The Cat and the Moon*. New York: Macmillan (Variorum edition), line 198.

11 Jackson 1988.

12 Helen King and Judith Swaddling (personal communication).

13 Ecclesiastes I:2.

14 Radcliffe, A. 1794. *The Mysteries of Udolpho*. London: Robinson.

15 Accession no. A127719.

16 Llewellyn, N. 1991. *The Art of Death*. London: Reaktion Books, p. 40.

17 Accession no. A661132.

18 Thompson, C.J.S. 1924–5. 'Anatomical Manikins' in *Journal of Anatomy* 59, pp. 441–5.
Crummer, L.R. 1927. 'Visceral Manikins in Carved Ivory' in *American Journal of Obstetrics and Gynaecology* 13, pp. 26–9.
Cannon, R. 1938. 'Ivory Apes and Angels' in *Coronet*, March 1938, pp. 99–106.

19 'Empty gestures' derives from an observation by the medical historian Hilary Morris (personal communication).

20 Accession no. A600030.

21 Accession no. A683007.

22 Richardson, R. 2000. *Death, Dissection and the Destitute*. Chicago: University of Chicago Press, pp. 142–4.

23 Wellcome EPB Special Bindings (Human Skin), purchased at auction 1929. It seems there is now (2002) some doubt (despite the label and shelfmark) that the skin used in binding is human.

24 Accession no. A44694.

25 Elizabeth Bowen, quoted in Lee, H. (ed.) 1999, *The Mulberry Tree: writings of Elizabeth Bowen*. London: Vintage, p. 128.

26 Calvino, I.; trans. Creagh, P. 1996. *Six Memos for the next Millennium*. London: Vintage, p. 107.

27 Hardy, T. 1974. 'Old Furniture'. *Collected poems of Thomas Hardy*. London: Macmillan, p. 456.

ACKNOWLEDGEMENTS

I would like to thank above all Danielle Olsen, Ken Arnold, Christine Bradley, and the other contributors to this volume, who have made this project a great pleasure on which to work.

Staff at the Science Museum and at the British Museum including Tim Boon, Stewart Emmens, Ralph Jackson, Judith Swaddling, David Thomas, and especially Geoff Bunn are due thanks for help when it was needed; as also are Andrew Crook at the Royal Veterinary College, and Library staff at the Wellcome Trust and at the British Library, St Pancras. Conversations with fellow historians Nikki Harrison, Helen King, Hilary Morris and Jane Wildgoose helped me formulate ideas, and Susan Armstrong and my family gave me important support. This essay is dedicated to Brian Hurwitz and our son Joshua Richardson.

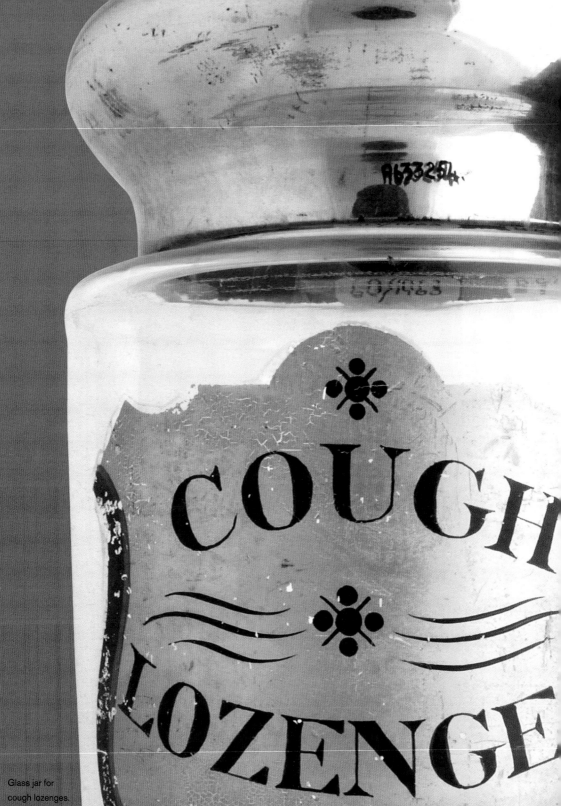

Glass jar for
cough lozenges.
English, late
nineteenth century.
SM, A633254

Treating yourself

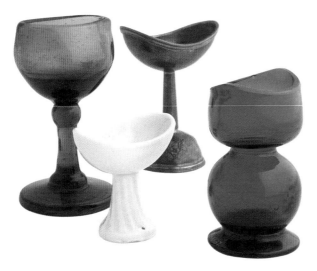

Selection of porcelain, glass and silver eye baths. Nineteenth century. SM, from left to right: A606637, A606638, A627014, A606660

Napoleon Bonaparte's toothbrush with silver-gilt handle, engraved on the rear with Napoleon's coat of arms. 1790–1820. SM/SSPL, A600139

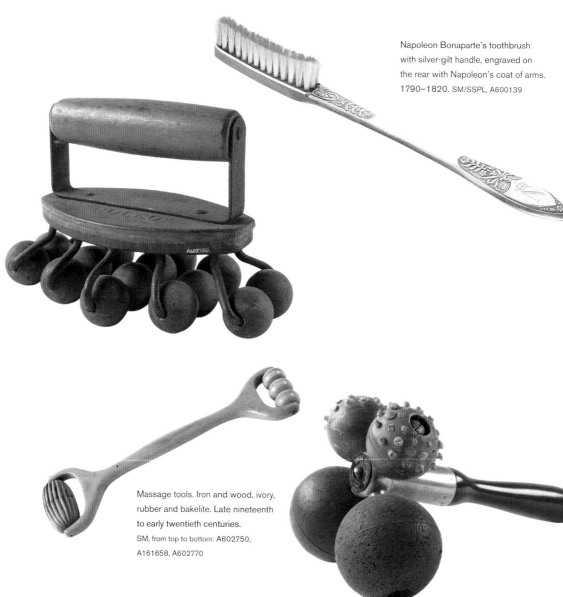

Massage tools. Iron and wood, ivory, rubber and bakelite. Late nineteenth to early twentieth centuries. SM, from top to bottom: A602750, A161658, A602770

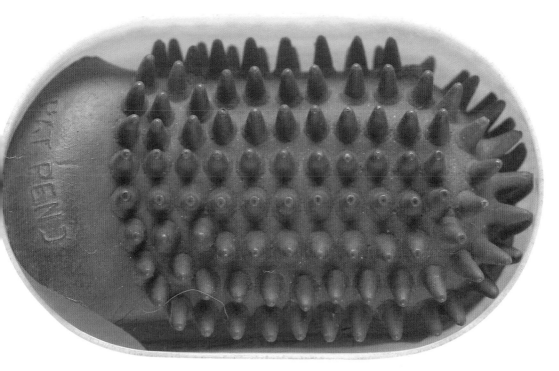

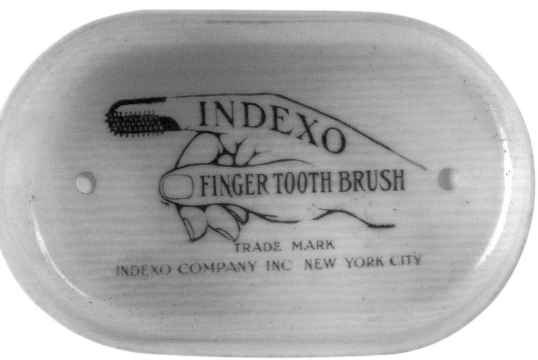

'Indexo' finger toothbrush and its plastic box (below). 1901–25. SM, A619222

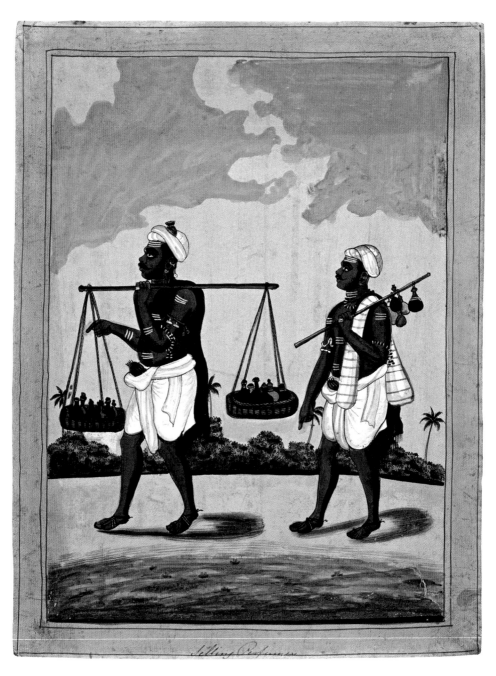

Indian perfume sellers. Gouache drawing
in Tanjore (Thanjayur) style, South India.
1840–60. WL, 29047i

RIGHT A guide to pressure points for use in shiatsu massage from a pressure
massage manual, c. 1850. This was not part of Henry Wellcome's collection,
but was acquired by the Wellcome Library more recently. WL, Thai MS

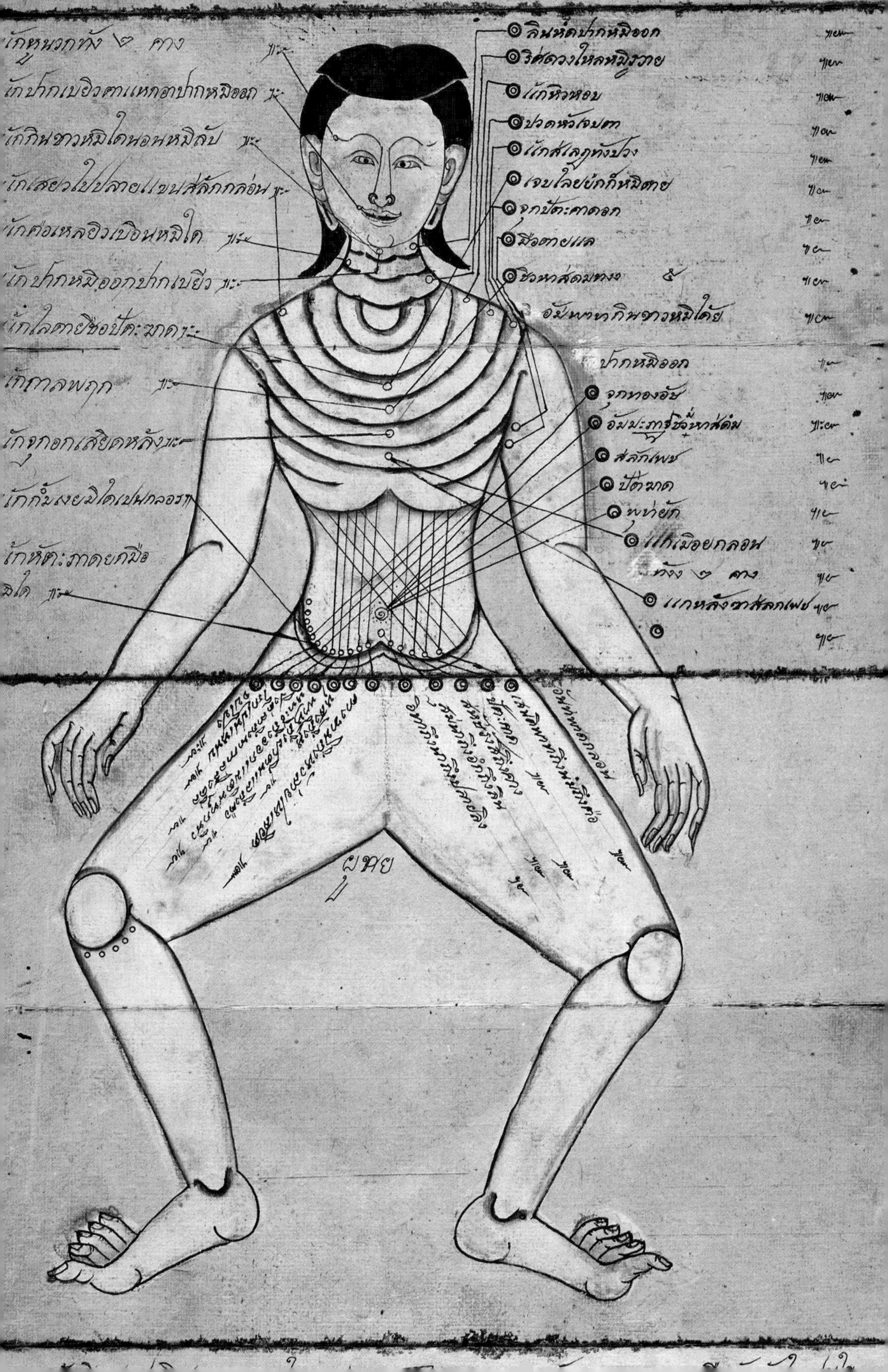

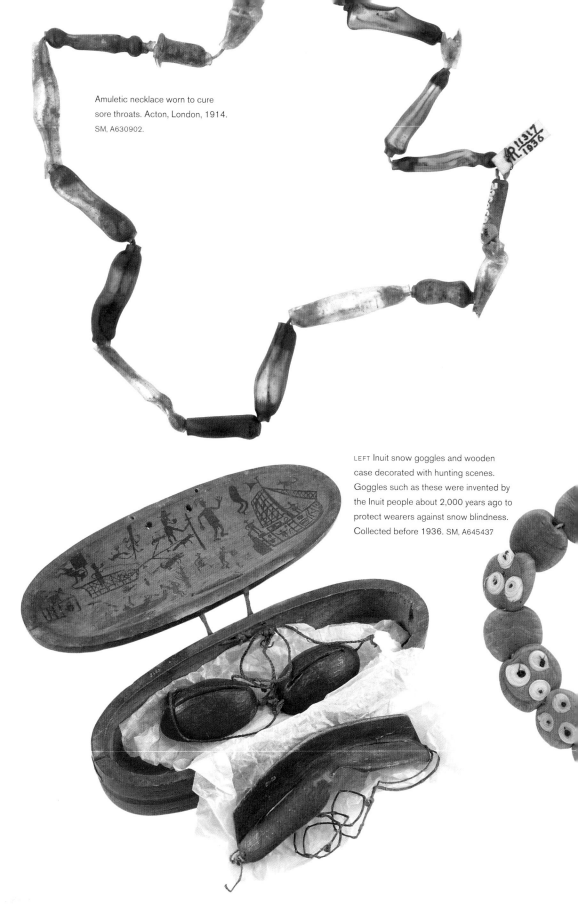

Amuletic necklace worn to cure sore throats. Acton, London, 1914. SM, A630902.

LEFT Inuit snow goggles and wooden case decorated with hunting scenes. Goggles such as these were invented by the Inuit people about 2,000 years ago to protect wearers against snow blindness. Collected before 1936. SM, A645437

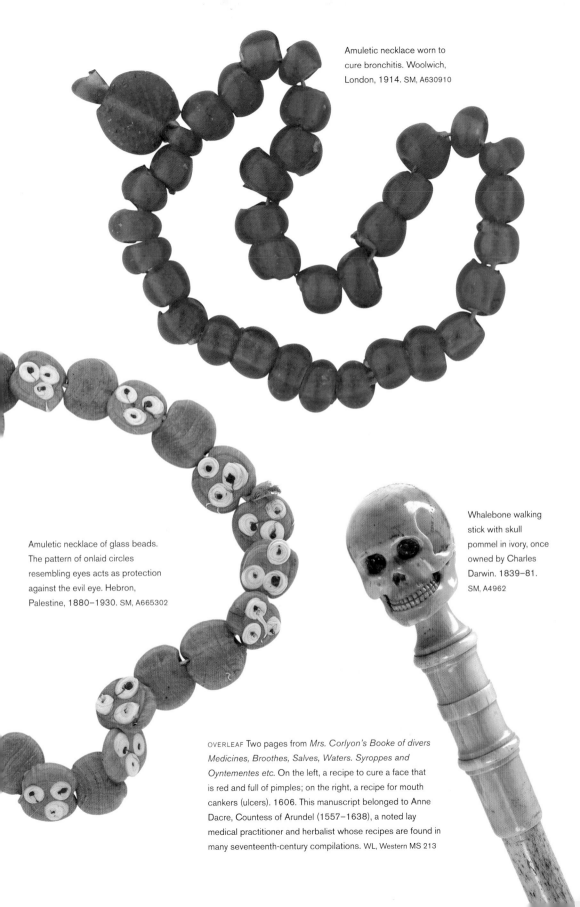

Amuletic necklace worn to cure bronchitis. Woolwich, London, 1914. SM, A630910

Amuletic necklace of glass beads. The pattern of onlaid circles resembling eyes acts as protection against the evil eye. Hebron, Palestine, 1880–1930. SM, A665302

Whalebone walking stick with skull pommel in ivory, once owned by Charles Darwin. 1839–81. SM, A4962

OVERLEAF Two pages from *Mrs. Corlyon's Booke of divers Medicines, Broothes, Salves, Waters. Syroppes and Oyntementes etc.* On the left, a recipe to cure a face that is red and full of pimples; on the right, a recipe for mouth cankers (ulcers). 1606. This manuscript belonged to Anne Dacre, Countess of Arundel (1557–1638), a noted lay medical practitioner and herbalist whose recipes are found in many seventeenth-century compilations. WL, Western MS 213

A Medecine to cure a face that is Redd, and full of Pimples.

Take two penny worthe of Quicksiluer, putt it in a littl glasse add thereto so much fasting, Spitle as will seru to kill it, then shake them well togeather, and the quicksiluer when it is killed will looke like auste: Then take such a Stone as Paynters do grynde theire coulors vppon, beyng cleare washed, and take of the Oyle of Bayes the quantity of a good Aple, Grinde your Quicksyluer and it togoather vppon the Stone, and temper it still with woodbynde wate and so grynde it vntill the Oyntement do looke very graye then putt it in a Boxe, and annoynte your face therewit euery euening and morning for the space of 14. dayes keto ping your selfe cloose in your chamber all that tyme, and vsing the drinck following. one weeke before you applye the Oyntement, all the tyme you do apply it, and one weeke after viz. Take a quantity of new Brane and to euery tenn gallons take halfe a pounde of Madder, stirr these well togeather and putt them in a vessell and when it is stale drinck thereof both morning and euoning and diuers tymes in the daye. These beyng vsed as is aforesaid will by Gods helpe heale it. But for a Seuennighte your face will looke worse then before, vntill such tyme as the humor be killed, that is betwixte the fleshe and the skinn.

twelue howers, and continue it as you shall see occasion: to
much heate of the fyer is hurtefull, to those that haue the Palsye
but competent warmeth is good.

A Medecine for a Canker in the mouthe.

Take a pinte of white wine, and as much of fayre water
then take of the litle slyppes of Rosemary of Hearbegrasse,
otherwise called Rewe, and of Sage of eche of these halfe an
handfull, and of woodbynde leaues and Plantyn leaues of eche
of these an handfull, and when your Lyquor doth boyle, then putt
in all those hearbes cleane washed and so lett them boyle softly
vntill the hearbes beginn to Looke yeollowe Then putt thereto so
much Allome as will make it to Looke yeollowe and to tast
very sweete then skumm it cleane, and so take it of and
putt it altogeather into a pott and vse it as followeth
Take a Sawserfull of this water with some of the Loaues of
Sage woodbynde and Plantyne, and when it is warme take
a cleane clothe, and lapp it about your forefyngar, then wett it
in the Lyquor, and rubb therewith your mouthe and gummes and
vnder your tounge and then spitt it out, and Lay of the loaues
about the gummes and vnder the tounge lettyngo them Lye
there a litle while then spitt them out. you must dresse it
thus in the morning fasting, about fower of the clocke in the
after noone and againe when you goe to Bedd. If the disease
be in the throote Lapp your clothe about thende of a flatt Sticke
and lett it hange an Inche ouer the Ende of the Sticke, then

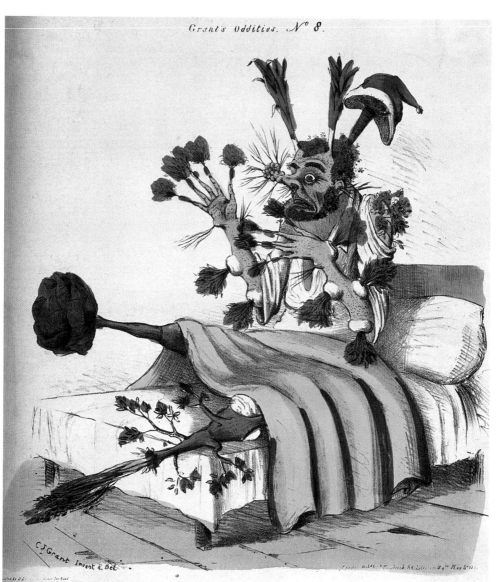

C.J.Grant Invent & Del.

SINGULAR EFFECTS OF THE UNIVERSAL <u>VEGETABLE</u> PILLS ON A GREEN GROCER! *A FACT!*

Who <u>Green'un</u> like was order'd to live for the space of one Month upon <u>Vegetable</u> Diet & to Take during that time 132 Boxes of <u>Vegetable</u> Pills for the Cure of a Gan<u>green</u>. & Being caught in a Shower of Rain in the <u>Green</u> Fields in the evening of the 1st of April last, was put to Bed mid'st <u>Shooting</u> pains, & in the Morning presented the above Phenomenon of a Moving Kitchen Garden !!!

Query — Is he not one of the **Productive** Classes .

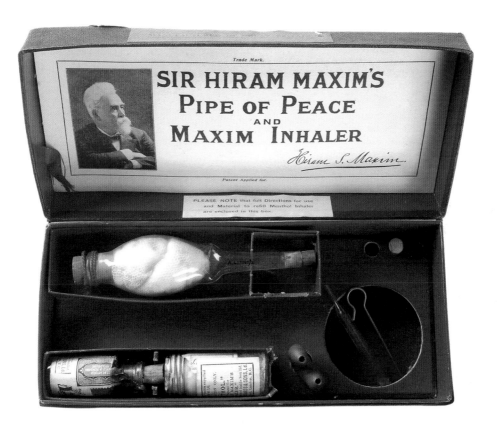

Hiram Maxim (1840–1916), friend of Henry Wellcome and inventor of the machine gun, patented this 'Pipe of Peace' which he devised to treat his bouts of bronchitis. SM, A629585

LEFT A man in bed with vegetables sprouting from all parts of his body as a result of taking J. Morison's Vegetable Pills. Morison's pills were made from vegetable extracts by the Englishman James Morison (1770–1840) who said they were free from the side-effects of the conventional drugs of the time. Coloured lithograph by C.J. Grant. 1831. WL, 11852i

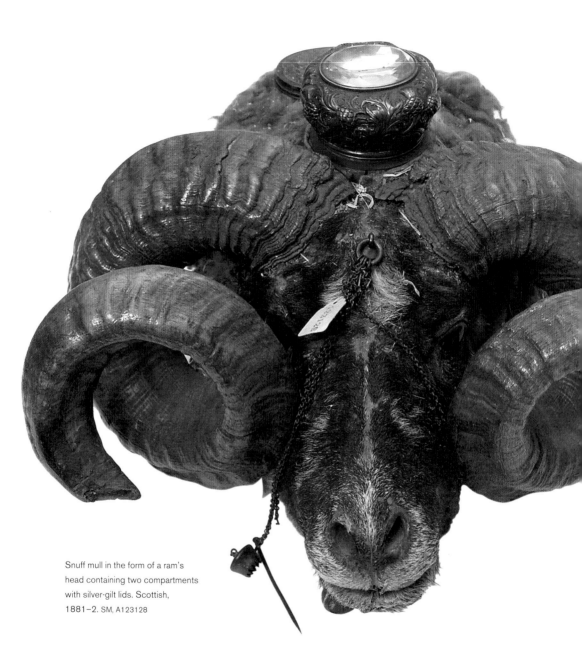

Snuff mull in the form of a ram's
head containing two compartments
with silver-gilt lids. Scottish,
1881–2. SM, A123128

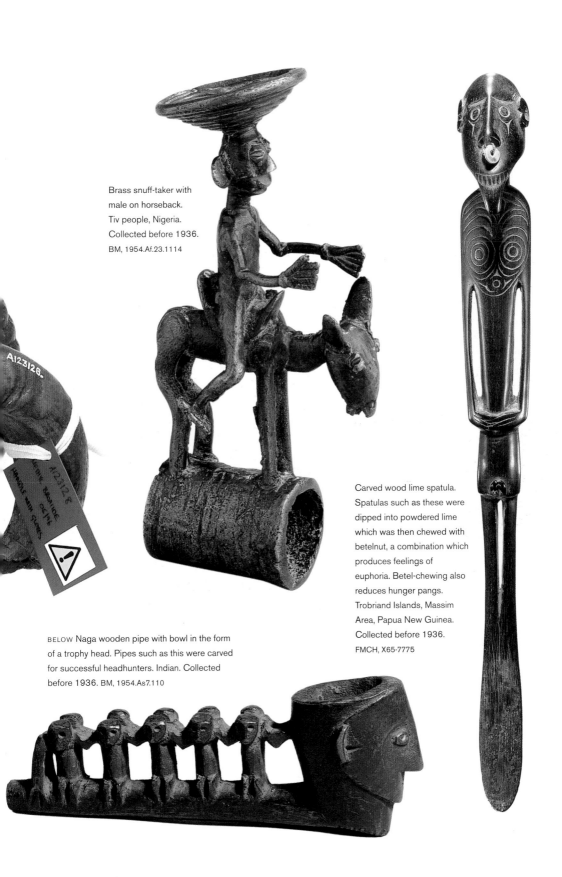

Brass snuff-taker with male on horseback. Tiv people, Nigeria. Collected before 1936. BM, 1954.Af.23.1114

Carved wood lime spatula. Spatulas such as these were dipped into powdered lime which was then chewed with betelnut, a combination which produces feelings of euphoria. Betel-chewing also reduces hunger pangs. Trobriand Islands, Massim Area, Papua New Guinea. Collected before 1936. FMCH, X65-7775

BELOW Naga wooden pipe with bowl in the form of a trophy head. Pipes such as this were carved for successful headhunters. Indian. Collected before 1936. BM, 1954.As7.110

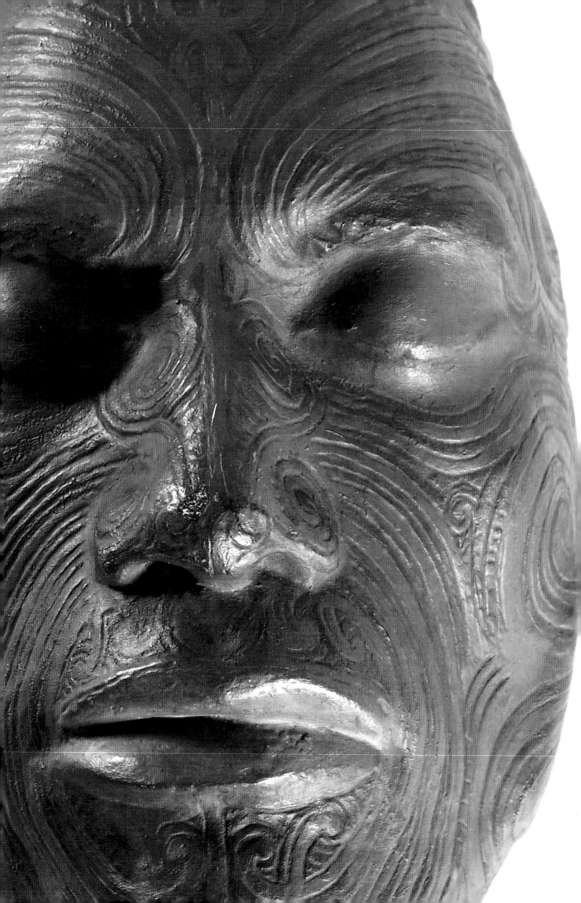

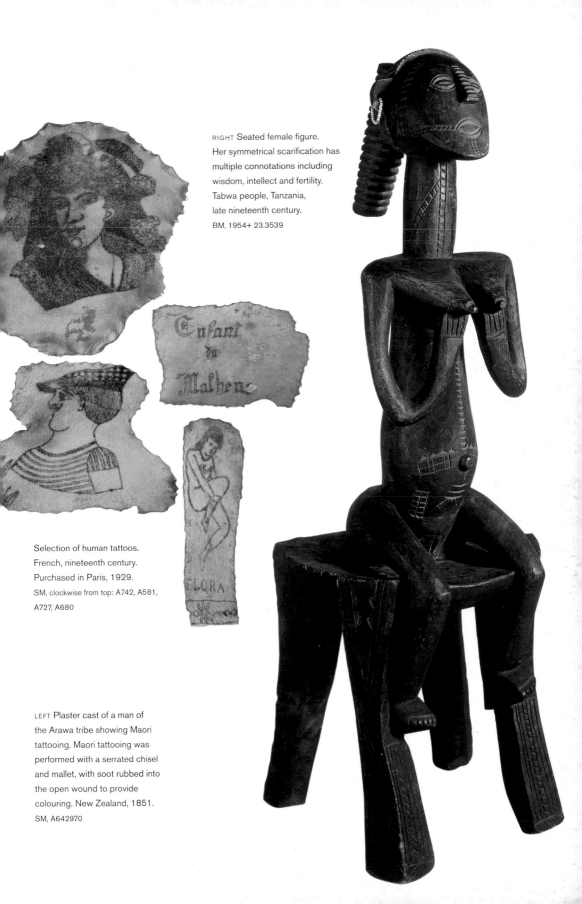

RIGHT Seated female figure.
Her symmetrical scarification has
multiple connotations including
wisdom, intellect and fertility.
Tabwa people, Tanzania,
late nineteenth century.
BM, 1954+ 23.3539

Selection of human tattoos.
French, nineteenth century.
Purchased in Paris, 1929.
SM, clockwise from top: A742, A581,
A727, A680

LEFT Plaster cast of a man of
the Arawa tribe showing Maori
tattooing. Maori tattooing was
performed with a serrated chisel
and mallet, with soot rubbed into
the open wound to provide
colouring. New Zealand, 1851.
SM, A642970

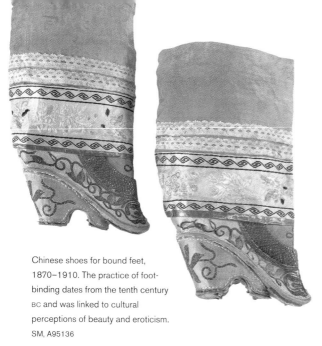

Chinese shoes for bound feet,
1870–1910. The practice of foot-
binding dates from the tenth century
BC and was linked to cultural
perceptions of beauty and eroticism.
SM, A95136

Brass corset used to minimise
the waist. Probably English,
1800–1880. SM, A158256

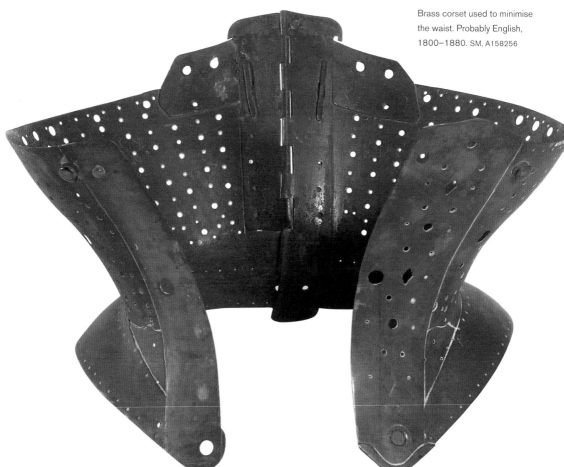

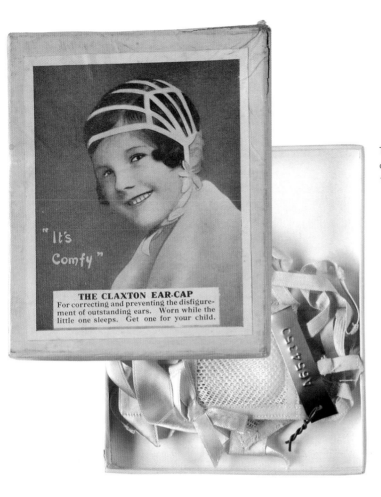

The 'Claxton' earcap, designed to correct 'outstanding' ears. English, 1925–36. SM, A654350

THE CLAXTON EAR-CAP
For correcting and preventing the disfigurement of outstanding ears. Worn while the little one sleeps. Get one for your child.

"It's Comfy"

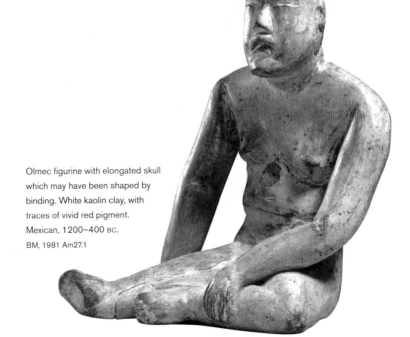

Olmec figurine with elongated skull which may have been shaped by binding. White kaolin clay, with traces of vivid red pigment. Mexican, 1200–400 BC. BM, 1981 Am27.1

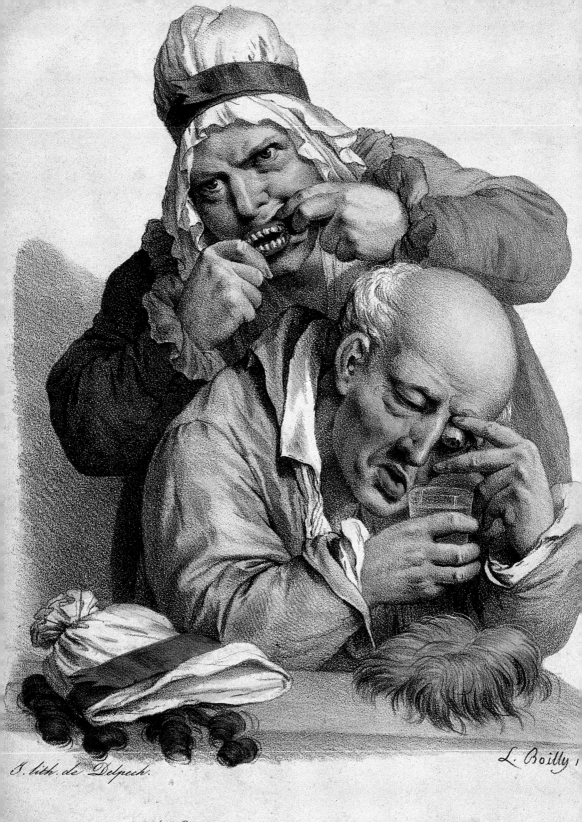

lith. de Delpech.

L. Boilly 1

Les époux assortis.

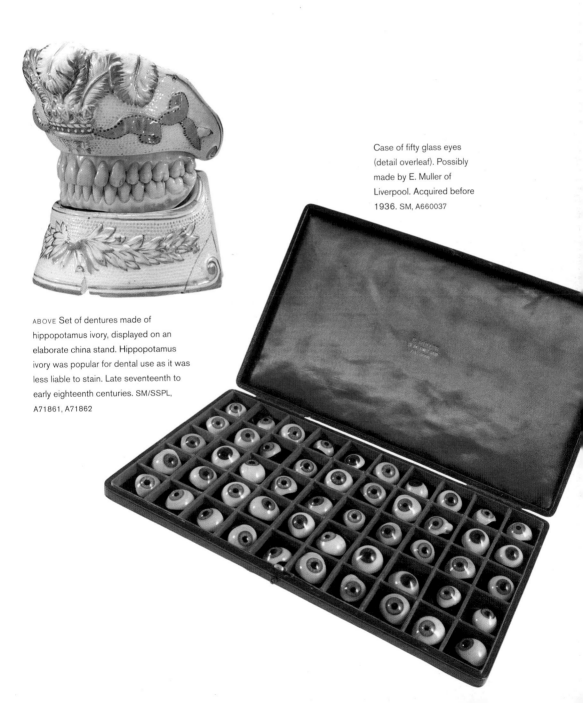

LEFT A couple assemble their false body parts: false teeth, a glass eye and wigs. Coloured lithograph by F.-S. Delpech after L. Boilly. French, 1825. WL, 16329i

ABOVE Set of dentures made of hippopotamus ivory, displayed on an elaborate china stand. Hippopotamus ivory was popular for dental use as it was less liable to stain. Late seventeenth to early eighteenth centuries. SM/SSPL, A71861, A71862

Case of fifty glass eyes (detail overleaf). Possibly made by E. Muller of Liverpool. Acquired before 1936. SM, A660037

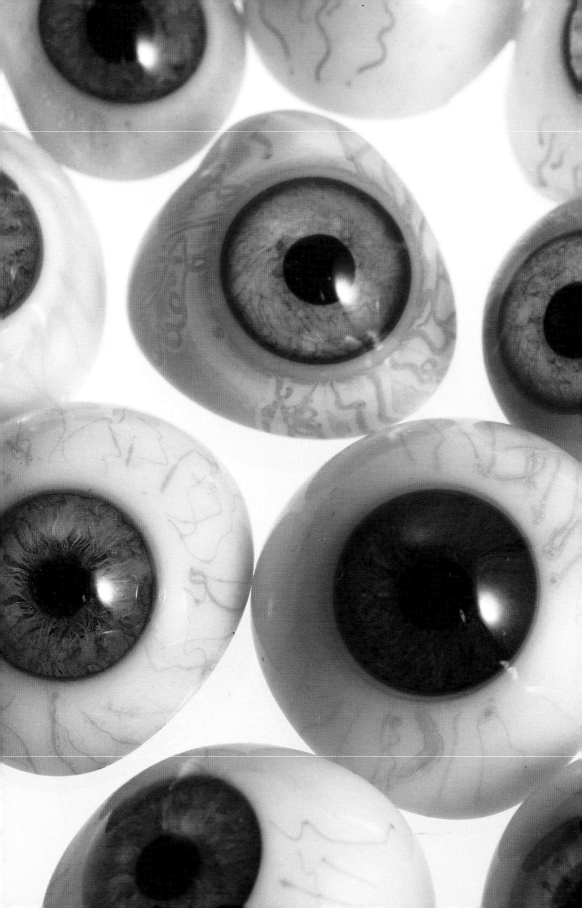

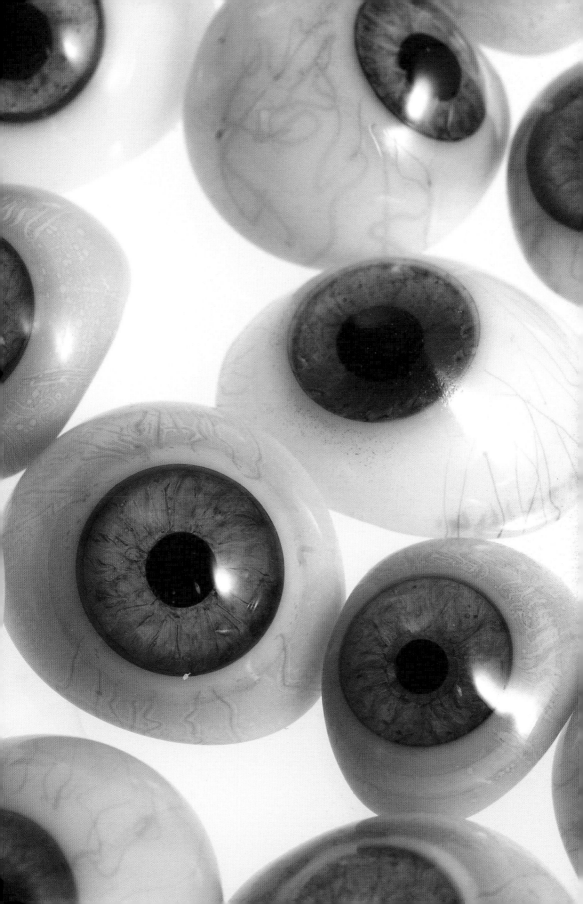

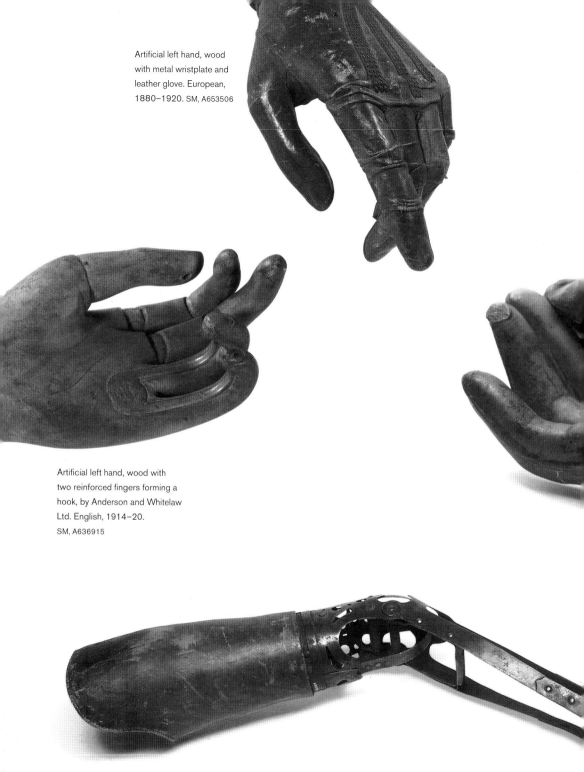

Artificial left hand, wood
with metal wristplate and
leather glove. European,
1880–1920. SM, A653506

Artificial left hand, wood with
two reinforced fingers forming a
hook, by Anderson and Whitelaw
Ltd. English, 1914–20.
SM, A636915

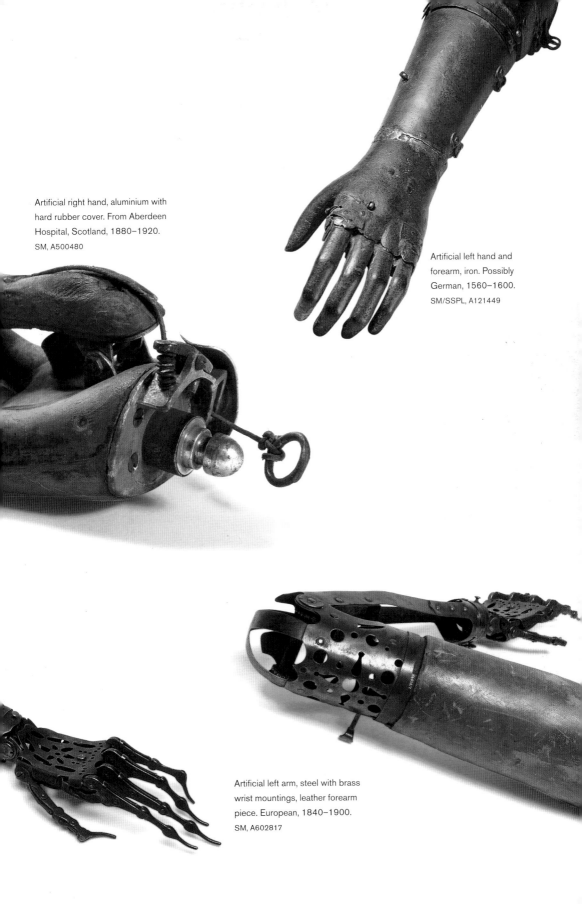

Artificial right hand, aluminium with
hard rubber cover. From Aberdeen
Hospital, Scotland, 1880–1920.
SM, A500480

Artificial left hand and
forearm, iron. Possibly
German, 1560–1600.
SM/SSPL, A121449

Artificial left arm, steel with brass
wrist mountings, leather forearm
piece. European, 1840–1900.
SM, A602817

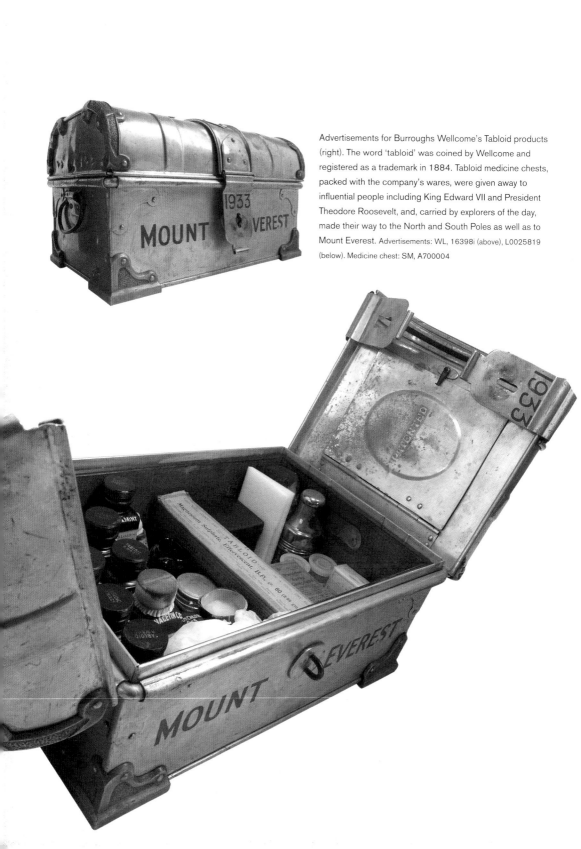

Advertisements for Burroughs Wellcome's Tabloid products (right). The word 'tabloid' was coined by Wellcome and registered as a trademark in 1884. Tabloid medicine chests, packed with the company's wares, were given away to influential people including King Edward VII and President Theodore Roosevelt, and, carried by explorers of the day, made their way to the North and South Poles as well as to Mount Everest. Advertisements: WL, 16398i (above), L0025819 (below). Medicine chest: SM, A700004

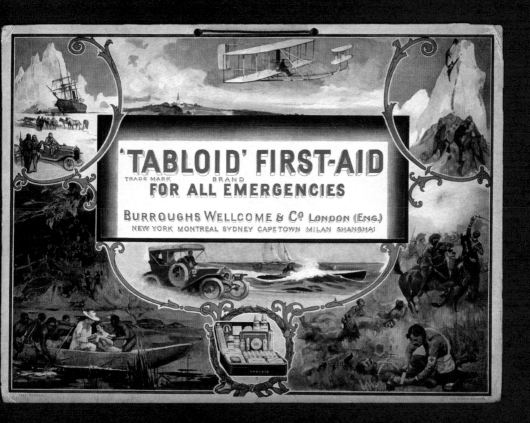

'TABLOID' FIRST-AID
TRADE MARK BRAND
FOR ALL EMERGENCIES
BURROUGHS WELLCOME & Co LONDON (ENG.)
NEW YORK MONTREAL SYDNEY CAPETOWN MILAN SHANGHAI

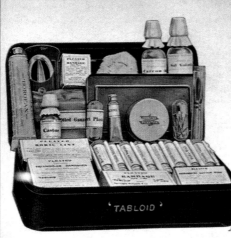

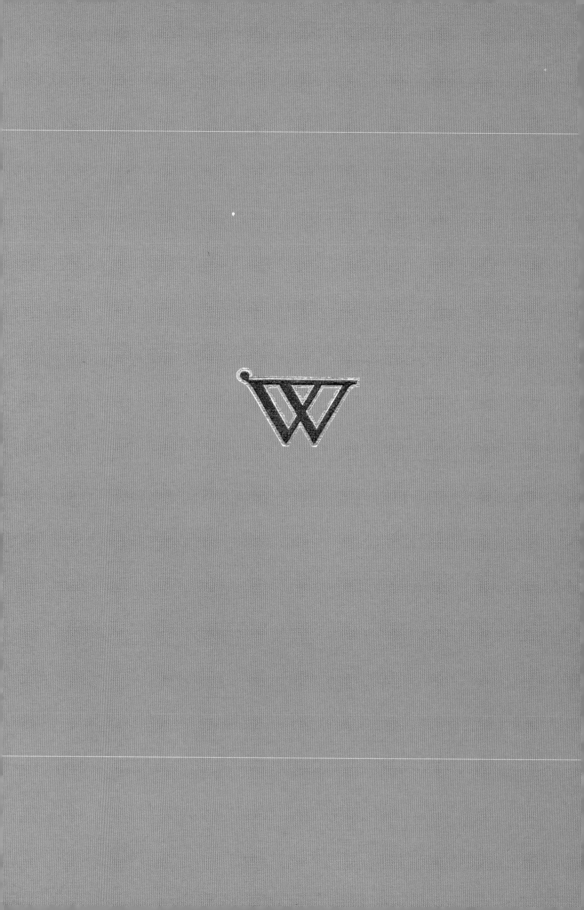

'Never tell anyone

what you

propose to do

until you've done it.'

HENRY WELLCOME, QUOTED IN A.W.J. HAGGIS,

THE LIFE AND WORK OF SIR HENRY WELLCOME,

TYPESCRIPT, 1942.

The *Medicine Man* Exhibition

As this book will outlive the exhibition it accompanies, we have included a list of the objects in the exhibition and a brief description of how they were displayed.

Focus objects
The first room of the exhibition presents just six objects (or, in two cases, object groups), and focuses on the idea that every object could tell a variety of different stories. The audio interpretation of each of these objects, produced by Hannah Andrassy, presents three different voices giving three different commentaries.

Narrative and mass groupings
The second room presents clusters of objects in two radically different styles. Six showcases explore broad narrative themes through the arrangement of heterogeneous elements. For example, one of the showcases – 'Understanding the body' – shows how the body has been observed in different cultures and at different times through such juxtapositions as an eighteenth-century Armenian astrological manuscript and a seventeenth-century Chinese acupuncture figure. These selections take deliberately diffuse topics around which to group objects from across history and around the globe. The selection of images presented as visual essays in between the chapters of this book indicates the approach taken here.

In another style of presentation, within eight groupings, homogeneity is employed instead of heterogeneity, with showcases housing massed arrays of pharmaceutical glassware, surgical metalwork in the form of obstetrical forceps and amputation saws, terracotta votive offerings, ex-voto pictures, artificial limbs, photographs, oil paintings and masks. More respectful of the development of museum collections over the last century and a half, these arrays enable us to reflect a central aspect of Wellcome's collecting habits within the exhibition – namely that he collected collections as much as objects.

Brothers Quay film
The last room of the exhibition is completely empty of objects. A commissioned film by the Brothers Quay provides an eerie, comical, beautiful, troubling and occasionally erotic journey through the storerooms of one particular part of Wellcome's collections – those kept by the Science Museum in their West London storerooms. The film also deftly plays with the possibility that the objects are at their best only after the last visitor has left the gallery, when anatomical models spring into a bizarre form of after-life and birthing chairs go through their obstetrical motions.

Medicine Man, then, is shown through four different modes of looking at things: individual pieces to which a number of stories are attached; juxtapositions of mixed exhibits that variously illuminate broad themes; massed groupings that appear similar, but that also suggest progression and variation through incremental change; and, finally, objects in their storerooms, animated on film.

Focus objects

Shrunken head (*tsantsa*) with long hair, decorated with birds' heads and feathers. Shuar people, Upper Amazon, Ecuadorian/Peruvian borders. SM, A36674

L'Homme à la Pipe: Portrait du Docteur Gachet. Etching by Vincent van Gogh. Dutch, 1890. WL, 3418i

Appliances from Mr George Thomson's 'Mechanical Substitute for the Arms', with notebook of writing practice. Scottish, 1919. SM, A683067

A lock of hair said to be from King George III (1760–1820). SM, A1315

Histoires Prodigieuses, a compendium of prodigies and freaks of nature drawn from ancient authorities, by Pierre Boaistuau. Paris, 1559. WL, Western MS 136

Nineteen amulets from the Hildburgh Collection, The Pitt Rivers Museum, University of Oxford:

Jewish Kabbalistic amulet. Paper and tin. Algerian. Acquired 1906. 1985.50.1360

Silver gilt hand amulet. Algerian. Acquired 1906. 1985.50.1028

Cornelian stone amulet. Tunisian. Acquired 1906. 1985.50.1197

Bone, blackwood and coral amulet. Algerian. Acquired 1906. 1985.50.992

Lizard brooch amulet. Brass, glass and enamel. Algerian. Acquired 1906. 1985.50.1146

Jewish silver amulet chain. Algerian. Acquired 1906. 1985.50.1133

Belt buckle amulet. Gilt metal, glass and enamel. Algerian. Acquired 1906. 1985.50.961

Belt buckle amulet. Gilt metal, imitation turquoise. Algerian. Acquired 1906. 1985.50.959

Cornelian stone amulet. Tunisian. Acquired 1906. 1985.50.1294

Shark's tooth amulet. Italian. Acquired 1912. 1985.50.312

Reliquary amulet containing relics of numerous saints. Silver, glass, paper and textile. Italian. Acquired 1902. 1985.50.164

Human tooth amulet. Italian. Acquired 1906. 1985.50.707

Silver cross amulet. Italian. Acquired 1908. 1985.50.897

Heart-shaped amulet containing incense, salt and olive leaves. Textile, metal, beads and sequins. Italian. Acquired 1914. 1985.50.15

Seahorse amulet on chain. Silver. Italian. Acquired 1919. 1985.50.639

Silver fish amulet. Italian. Acquired 1906. 1985.50.685

Plastic baby doll amulet. Italian. Acquired 1914. 1985.50.39

Heart-shaped pendant amulet containing a pressed four-leafed clover. Green glass bound with brass. Italian. Acquired c. 1901–2. 1985.50.93

Group of thirteen amulets including a fish, a heart, and a mandolin. Silver. Italian. Acquired 1906. 1985.50.871

The beginning of life

Obstetric phantom. Leather and wood. Italian, eighteenth century. SM, A600052

A collection of sexual aids including penis sheaths, penis rings, bells and a dildo. Made by Arita Drug and Rubber Goods Co., Kobe, Japan, 1930–35. SM, A641105

Ivory figurine in the form of a man and woman engaged in sexual foreplay. Chinese. Acquired before 1936. SM, A641137

Stone statue in form of male and female copulating. Possibly South American. Acquired before 1936. SM, A79472

Male anti-masturbation device. Metal and leather. British, late nineteenth century. SM, A641285

Iron chastity belt with red velvet lining. Possibly sixteenth century. SM, A641274

Silver-bound hinged cowrie shell containing a painting of a man unlocking the chastity belt of a reclining woman. Acquired before 1936. SM, A641131

Porcelain fruit containing representations of a couple engaged in sexual foreplay. Far Eastern. Acquired before 1936. SM, A641133, A641134, A641135

Still life of roses with concealed erotic scenes. Oil painting by Sommonte. Italian, nineteenth century. WL, 47297i

Epa mask. Wood and paint. Yoruba people, Nigeria. Acquired before 1936. FMCH, X65-7432

Phallic amulet. Bronze. Graeco-Roman, 100 BC–AD 400. SM, A154056

Phallic amulet. Alabaster and bronze. Roman, from Pompei, 100 BC–AD 100. SM, A67895

Phallic amulet. Bronze. Graeco-Roman, 100 BC–AD 400. SM, A97578

Ceremonial sword linked to Hevioso, the pantheon of thunder deities. Wood and metal. Republic of Benin. Acquired before 1936. BM, 1954 +23.2692

Wooden 'Akua ba' figure. Asante people, Ghana. Acquired before 1936. BM, 1954 +23.3579

Wooden 'Akua ba' figure. Asante people, Ghana. Acquired before 1936. BM, 1954 +23.3580

Puppet figure made of vegetable fibre moulded with earth. South-west Malekula, Vanuatu. Acquired before 1931. FMCH, X65-8800

Mary Tofts duping several distinguished surgeons, physicians and male midwives into believing that she is giving birth to a litter of rabbits. Etching by William Hogarth. British, 1726. WL, 17342i

Thirteen diagrams of a child in the womb in various positions, two obstetrical chairs and several obstetrical instruments. Etching by Francesco Sesone. Italian, 1749. WL, 17074i

Obstetrical forceps. Steel and wood. Belgian, c. 1726. SM, A615661

Kitāb-i vilādet-i Iskandar, 1411. Iranian manuscript showing the position of the heavens at the moment of Iskandar's birth on 25 April 1384. WL, MS Per.474

Infant identification set. J.A. Deknatal & Son Inc., USA, 1925. SM, A626425

A birth scene. Oil painting, possibly by a French painter, 1800. Acquired in Åbo, Sweden (now Turku, Finland). WL, 44694i

Wooden statue depicting child-birth. Bazombo people, Angola. Acquired before 1936. SM, A642971

A pregnant woman depicted in a fifteenth-century English anatomy text. Pseudo-Galen. WL, Western MS 290

Ivory anatomical model of a pregnant female, with removable parts. Possibly German, c. seventeenth century. SM, A127699

Ivory anatomical model of a pregnant female, with removable parts. Possibly German, seventeenth to early eighteenth centuries. SM, A642631

Sioux Indian protective amulet said to contain a child's umbilical cord. Leather, beads and quill. Northern Plains, USA, 1880–1920. SM, A230279

Sioux Indian protective amulet said to contain a child's umbilical cord. Leather and beads. Northern Plains, USA, 1880–1920. SM, A51675

Sioux Indian protective amulet said to contain a child's umbilical cord. Leather, beads and quill. Northern Plains, USA, 1880–1920. SM, A121191

Sioux Indian protective amulet said to contain a child's umbilical cord. Leather and quill. Northern Plains, USA, 1880–1920. SM, A47761

Soft leather beaded cradle with wooden board. Plateau region, Rocky Mountains, USA, 1880–1910. BM, 1954 W.Am5.962

Ivory netsuke. Japanese, eighteenth or nineteenth century. SM, A641100

A fashionable mother wearing a dress with slits across the breasts in order to feed her baby before she dashes off to the carriage. Coloured etching by James Gillray. British, 1796. WL, 17465i

Glass nipple-shield. British, 1786–1821. SM, A606829

Ivory nipple-shield. British, nineteenth century. SM, A606830

Silver nipple-shield. British, 1786–1821. SM, A641255

Roman teething charm. Bronze, first century AD. SM, A33500

Japanese porcelain feeding bottle. c. 1800. SM, A42325

Roman feeding bottle. Glass, mid-third to mid-fifth century AD. SM, A170402

Neolithic infant feeding cup. Earthenware. Excavated at Jebel Moya, Sudan, 1000–400 BC. SM, A602006

Helmet mask. Wood and raffia fibre. Mende people, Sierra Leone, nineteenth century. NMS, A.1953.343

Carved wooden face-mask. Songye people, Kinshasa, Democratic Republic of Congo, late nineteenth to early twentieth centuries. NMS, A.1953.336

The end of life

Peruvian mummified male. c. 1200–1400. SM, A31655

Wooden mask-head. Bamileke kingdoms, Cameroon, nineteenth century. FMCH, X65-5820

Guillotine blade, used during the French Revolution at the execution of Carrier in 1794. SM, A79526

Carved ivory skeleton in ebony coffin. Possibly eighteenth century. SM, A641345

Gold pendant in the form of a coffin which opens up to reveal a skeleton. European, possibly eighteenth century. SM, A641823

Carved wooden statue of a dead man, in a miniature wooden coffin. Italian, sixteenth century. SM, A629458

Bronze miniature skeleton. Roman. SM, A629420

Miniature oil painting contrasting life and death in a young woman's face, possibly Florentine. The costume is seventeenth-century Italian but the date of the painting could be later. WL, 45064i

Painted wooden double-faced mask. Rawhide covering on crown. Tsimshian people, British Columbia, Canada, c. 1900. FMCH, X65-8554

White-faced carved statue. Wood, paint, and pigment. Mbole people, Democratic Republic of Congo. Acquired before 1936. FMCH, X65-7486

Life of Buddha. Burmese manuscript, c. 1850–85. WL, Burmese MS 22

Baked clay memorial head. Akan people, Ghana, 1890–1920. SM, A657221

Elephant mask of cloth with beadwork and cowrie shell. Bamileke kingdoms, Cameroon. Acquired before 1936. BM, 1954+23.3446

Memento mori gold brooch. Set with garnets and pearls with plaited hair at the centre. Acquired before 1936. SM, A71928

Memento mori brooch containing a graveyard scene made from hair. Metal and glass. Acquired before 1936. SM, A642442

Memento mori brooch containing gold thread, pearls and hair. Acquired before 1936. SM, A642443

Memento mori slide containing entwined hair and an illustration of a skeleton. Gold and glass. 1689. SM, A642143

Mask with movable eyes, with a whale's tail made of black cloth hanging from mouth. Wood, cloth and pigment. Kaigani-Haida people, Prince of Wales Island, Alaska, c. 1875. FMCH, X65-4280

'Korwar' ancestor figure. Carved wood, partially wrapped in cloth, with glass eyes. Geelvink Bay, Irian Jaya. Acquired before 1936. FMCH, X65-4562

Watercolour of a dead child. Vienna, 1846. WL, 45065i

Mask with beard of human hair, headdress hair and barkcloth, cloak of blue-black wood pigeon feathers. New Caledonia, late nineteenth century. FMCH, X65-7799

Lead mortuary cross. Replica of a seventeenth-century original. London. SM, A115565

Lead mortuary cross from the grave of a plague victim. London, c. 1348. SM, A654846

Lead mortuary cross from the grave of a plague victim. London, c. 1348. SM, A654851

Lead mortuary cross from the grave of a plague victim. London, c. 1348. SM, A654853

Limestone jackal-headed canopic jar. Egyptian. Excavated between 1850 and 1894. SM, A635038

Limestone human-headed canopic jar. Egyptian. Excavated between 1850 and 1894. SM, A635039

Glass funerary urn with fragments of bones. Roman, AD 1–200. SM, A28417

Resuscitator for reviving 'persons apparently dead'. Royal Humane Society, England, 1774. SM, A640992

Kiśordās's vernacular translation and commentary of the Sanskrit *Bhagvadgītā*. Indian, c. 1820–40. WL, Panjabi MS 255

Thai manuscript illustrating the Buddhist story of the monk Phra Malai and his journeys to Heaven and Hell. c. 1860–70. WL, Thai MS 1

Marker for the grave of children. Wrought iron with oil painting. Austrian or German, late eighteenth to early nineteenth centuries. WL, 47295i

Carved and painted wood spirit board. Hohao people, Papua New Guinea. Acquired before 1936. FMCH, X65-7786

Carved and inlaid wooden reliquary chest containing relics of several saints. Possibly Spanish, eighteenth century. SM, A634987

Guardian figure ('mbulu-'ngulu). Wood, sheet brass and copper. Kota people, Gabon. FMCH, X65-3801

A woman with the muscles of her upper body and her viscera exposed. Colour mezzotint attributed to Jacques-Fabien Gautier d'Agoty (c. 1717–85). French. WL, 225i

Anatomical specimen, dissected and prepared by Edward Jenner (1749–1823). SM, A600030

Fragment of skin of Jeremy Bentham (1748–1832), with a handwritten inscription. 1832. SM, A44694

A woman covers her eyes as she steals the teeth of a hanged man. Aquatint with etching by Francisco Goya. Spanish, c. 1797. WL, 18059i

Wax death mask of Benjamin Disraeli taken six hours after his death in 1881. SM, A652234

Gall bladder stuffed with rice, taken from an executed Chinese criminal. Acquired before 1936. SM, A642965

Small black notebook bought because it was allegedly bound in human skin. The actual material is camel, horse, or goatskin. c. 1770–1850. WL, EPB – Spec Binding

Nepalese ceremonial headdress incorporating a human skull. Coral beads and cloth, eighteenth or nineteenth century. SM, A22073

Understanding the body

Chinese wooden acupuncture figure. Seventeenth century. SM, A604024

Wooden female anatomical figure with removable parts. German, c. 1700. SM, A118272

Three anatomical figures drawn on cloth. Tibetan. Acquired in 1920. WL, Tibetan catalogue no. 53

De humani corporis fabrica libri septem by Andreas Vesalius. Basle, 1543. WL, EPB 6560

Wood and ivory figure group representing an anatomical demonstration, based on Rembrandt's 1632 painting, *The Anatomy Lesson of Dr Nicholaas Tulp*. Dutch, eighteenth century. SM, A119917

Tashrīḥ-i Manṣūrī (*Mansur's Anatomy*). Persian eighteenth-century manuscript copy. WL, Persian MS 449

Anatomical fugitive sheet, *Tabula exhibens insigniora / maris viscera*. Wittenberg, Germany, 1573. WL, EPB 297

Anatomical fugitive sheet, *Tabula foeminae member / demonstrans*. Wittenberg, Germany, 1573. WL, EPB 298

Model of human ear. Ivory and leather. Eighteenth century. SM, A600028

Plaster model of a sectioned human eye. French, 1870. SM, A661186

Exercitatio anatomica de motu cordis et sanguinis in animalibus (*An Anatomical Study of the Motion of the Heart and of Blood in Animals*) by William Harvey. German, 1628. WL, EPB 3069/B

Ancestor mask (Tatanua type). Wood, fibre, textiles, paint, chalk or lime. New Ireland, Papua New Guinea. Acquired before 1936. FMCH, X65-4362

Carved Ikenga figure. Wood and paint. Ibo people, Nigeria. Acquired before 1924. FMCH, X65-3807

Skull inscribed in French with phrenological markings. European, nineteenth century. SM, A25407

Wooden case containing sixty small plaster phrenological heads by William Bally. Dublin, 1831. SM, A642804

Three perspectives on the head of an ox and three on the head of an ox-like man. Etching. French, c. 1820, after Charles Le Brun. WL, 34139i

Chart of a head containing over thirty images symbolising the phrenological faculties. Coloured wood engraving by Henri Bushea after Orson Squire Fowler. English, c. 1845. WL, 27923i

A comparison between Daniel Lambert and Charles James Fox, two obese men. Etching with watercolour by Charles Williams. English, 1806. WL, 854i

Claude Ambroise Seurat, a man weighing 77lb and known as the 'Human Skeleton'. Stipple engraving by George Cruikshank. English,1825. WL, 1811i

Daisy and Violet Hilton, conjoined twins, being wooed by two young men. Black and white photograph, USA, c. 1927. WL, 33703i

Wooden Ibeji figure representing one of a set of twins. Glass bead and metal jewellery. Yoruba people, Nigeria, 1871–1910. SM, A655924

Wooden Ibeji figure representing one of a set of twins. Glass bead and metal jewellery. Yoruba people, Nigeria, 1871–1910. SM, A655927

Compound monocular microscope with green, tooled leather body tube and ornate base. German or Italian, c. 1700. SM, A56283

Micrographia: or some physiological descriptions of minute bodies made by magnifying glasses. Robert Hooke, London, 1665. WL, EPB 29309/C

Glass X-ray tube. 1896. SM, A201

Skeleton of a mature child. Collotype by Rommler and Jonas after a radiograph by G. Leopold and T. Leisewitz, Dresden, 1908. WL, 17137i

A skeleton of a child born with two backbones and two heads. Collotype by Rommler and Jonas after a radiograph by G. Leopold and T. Leisewitz, Dresden, 1908. WL, 17138i

The injected arterial vessel system of a nine-month-old foetus. Collotype by Rommler and Jonas after a radiograph by G. Leopold and T. Leisewitz, Dresden, 1908. WL, 17141i

Brass astrolabe. Italian, 1572. SM, A629481

Armenian astronomical manuscript. 1795. WL, Armenian MS 7

Ars computistica by Heymandus de Veteri Busco. Holland, 1488. WL, Western MS 349

Chinese manuscript illustrating recipes on acupuncture. Early eighteenth century. WL, Chinese MS 71

Nail figure (Nkisi). Wood and nails. Kongo people, Democratic Republic of Congo, nineteenth century. SM, A197491

Arzneibuch. A physician's handbook of practical medicine, with notes on medical astrology, blood-letting, uroscopy etc. German, 1524–50. WL, Western MS 93

Illustration of a meditator showing *chakras* and *kundalinī*. Gouache and gold leaf on paper. c. late eighteenth to early nineteenth centuries. WL, Indic MS beta 511

Pair of fakir's sandals, with iron spikes through the soles and wooden toe pegs. Indian, 1871–1920. SM, A23375

A man walking on his hands. Black and white photogravure, Eadweard Muybridge, USA, 1887. WL, 27829i

A man performing a forward flip. Black and white photogravure, Eadweard Muybridge, USA, 1887. WL, 27827i

De Motu Animalium by Giovanni Alfonso Borelli. Naples, 1734. WL, EPB 14628/B

The body under attack

Kareau figure of carved and painted wood. Nicobar Islands, Bay of Bengal, 1880–1925. SM, A655619

Gilded wooden figure of Saint Michael, patron of soldiers and the sick. Spanish, 1700–1850. SM, A156108

Ancestor bird figure (*Tenyalang*). Carved wood, paint, wool and cloth. Iban Dayak people,

Borneo. Acquired before 1936. FMCH, X65-5653

Bullet extractor. Metal. Sixteenth century. SM, A647839

Bullet extractor. Steel and brass. English, nineteenth century. SM, A619874

Karo Batak amulet inscribed on buffalo bone. Indonesian, probably nineteenth century. WL, Batak MS 331834

German artillery manual. 1559. WL, Western MS 87

Shield of woven fibre decorated with a pattern of pearl shell inlaid on black resin. Central Solomons, Solomon Islands. Acquired before 1860. BM, 1954.Oc.6.197

War shield. Wood, paint and pigment. Papua New Guinea. Acquired before 1936. FMCH, X65-4325

Ceramic amulet depicting a saint worn by a Russian soldier in the First World War. SM, A79980

Ceramic amulet depicting saints worn by a Russian soldier in the First World War. SM, A79981

Paper amulet in the form of a cat worn by an English soldier in the First World War. SM, A79978

Metal amulet in the form of a soldier worn by an English soldier in the First World War. SM, A79977

Amulet in the form of a tiny compass set into a cowrie shell. Possibly worn by a Japanese soldier in the First World War. SM, A79972

First aid kit used during the First World War. German. SM, A652170

First World War gas mask. German, 1918. SM, A51114

Oil painting by Ugo Matania depicting the transport of wounded First World War soldiers. 1916. WL, 45949i.

An account of two successful operations for restoring a lost nose from the integuments of the forehead in the cases of two officers of His Majesty's Army; to which are prefixed historical and physiological remarks on the nasal operation; including descriptions of the Indian and Italian methods. Joseph Constantine Carpue, London, 1816. WL, EPB 16856/C

Artificial ivory nose. Seventeenth to eighteenth centuries. SM, A641030

Woodcuts from *Instrumenta chyrurgiae et icones anatomicae.* Ambroise Paré, Paris, 1564. WL, EPB 4818/B

German manuscript *Apocalypsis S Johannis cum glossis et vitas Johannis: ars moriendi* with an illustration of 'Wound man'. *c.* 1420. WL, Western MS 49

Carved wooden Bulul figure. Igorot people, Philippines. Acquired before 1936. BM, 1954.As7.274

Antelope horn, surmounted by human jaw bone. Nigerian, 1880–1910. SM, A127047

Silver gilt pomander. Acquired after 1936. SM, A629413

Gold spherical pomander with square cut diamonds. Sixteenth century. SM, A629434

Wooden leper's clappers. English, reproduction of seventeenth-century version. SM, A635021

Small goa stone and silver stand. Possibly seventeenth century. SM, A642467

Oval goa stone and gold stand. Eighteenth–nineteenth centuries. SM, A642470

Carved wooden ancestor figures (*adu zatna*) lashed together to a bamboo slat. Nias Island, Indonesia. Collected before 1907. FMCH, X65-5679

Monster Soup. Etching by William Heath. English, 1828. WL, 12079i

Compendium rarissimum totius Artis Magicae sistematisatae per celeberrimos Artis hujus Magistros. Possibly German, *c.* 1775. WL, Western MS 1766

Iron scold's bridle. Belgian, 1550–1800. SM, A13704

Copy of a canvas and leather strait-jacket. English, *c.* 1930. SM, A130344

Trepanned skull. New Ireland, Papua New Guinea, *c.* 1890. SM, A650847

The sleep of reason produces monsters. Etching by Francisco Goya, Spanish, 1796–98. WL, 36752i

A Portugese watercolour drawing of a woman with scales on her upper body and grossly enlarged lower limbs. 1695. WL, 87i

Bronze statue depicting male with elephantisis of the scrotum. Yoruba people, Nigeria, nineteenth century. SM, A221402

Bronze statue depicting female with a goitre-like growth. Yoruba people, Nigeria, nineteenth century. SM, A67081

Carved wooden effigy said to show gigantism or possibly elephantisis of the foot. Possibly Basonge people, Democratic Republic of Congo or Zaire, 1880–1910. SM, A652610

Carved wooden effigy said to show macroglossia (enlargement of the tongue). Possibly Basonge people, Democratic Republic of Congo or Zaire, 1880–1910. SM, A114489

A swollen and inflamed foot; gout is represented by an attacking demon. Coloured soft-ground etching by James Gillray. British, 1799. WL, 10507i

An Inquiry into the Cases and Effects of the Variolae Vaccinae by Edward Jenner. London, 1798. WL, EPB 30385/C

Ophthalmodouleia by George Bartisch. Dresden, 1583. WL, EPB 697/D

A man vomiting after overeating and drinking. Engraving by J.J. Kleinschmidt after Jan van de Velde the younger. Augsburg, Germany, eighteenth century. WL, 27165i

Reports of medical cases, vol. 1, by Richard Bright. London, 1827. WL, EPB 15395/D/2

Seeking help

Adjustable dentist's chair. Velvet covering and mahogany frame. *c.* 1865. SM, A29615

Saint Elizabeth visiting a hospital. Oil painting on copper by Adam Elsheimer. German, *c.* 1598. WL, 44650i

Icon of the Virgin and Child. Oil painting and formed metal on wood. Russian, nineteenth century. WL, 44966i

Pottery statue of Saint John of God. Spanish. Acquired in 1928. SM, A61810

Ancestor figure (*Adu*). Wood. Nias Island, Indonesia. Acquired before 1936. BM, 1954.As7.144

Ancestor figure (*Adu*). Wood. Nias Island, Indonesia. Acquired before 1936. BM, 1954.As7.145

Persian astronomical and astrological manuscript. Indian, seventeenth century. WL, Persian MS 373

Standing figure of Chicomecoatl. Aztec, Mexico, AD 1300–1521. BM, 1954.Am5.1479

Sandstone block statue of an official with naos containing a figure of Ptah. Egyptian, Dynasty XIX. Petrie Museum of Egyptian Archaeology (PMEA), UC 8739

Limestone seated statue of Imhotep as a priest with a papyrus roll. Egyptian, Late Period. PMEA, UC 8709

Bronze figure of Isis and Horus. Egyptian, Ptolemaic Period. PMEA, UC 8060

A donkey, representing Galinsoga, physician to the Queen of Spain, checks the pulse of a dying patient. Aquatint with etching by Francisco Goya. Spanish, *c.* 1797. WL, 18056i

Quack doctor open for business. Etching with watercolour by George Moutard Woodward. English, 1802. WL, 10932i

An itinerant street hawker. Etching by Rembrandt van Rijn. Dutch, 1635. WL, 20476i

Beaded crown. Yoruba people, south-west Nigeria or Benin. Acquired before 1936. BM, 1954.Af.23.261

Beaded staff. Yoruba people, south-west Nigeria or Benin. Acquired before 1936. BM, 1954.Af.23.253

Gold angel used as a touchpiece in the ceremony of healing by touch. English, 1553–58. SM, A641045

Loadstone reputedly used by Queen Anne as a touchpiece in the ceremony of healing by touch. English, 1702–14. SM, A641031

Doctor's signboard, inscribed and hung with human teeth. Wood. Chinese. Acquired before 1936. SM, A642963

Captain Jack or Grizzly Bear Paw. British Columbia, Canada. Pastel by William Langdon Kihn. American, *c.* 1930–36. WL, 45895i

Funerary reliquary containing the bones of the deceased. Wood, hide, copper, brass wire and plastic buttons. Upper Ogowe, Gabon, 1870–1920. SM, A657377

Pair of leather moccasins said to have been worn by Florence Nightingale during the Crimean War. 1850–56. SM, A96087

Arzneibuch. Compendium of popular medicine and surgery, receipts, etc. German, *c.* 1675. WL, Western MS 990

Glazed earthenware feeding cup. English, 1820–91. SM, A232180

Stethoscope made by René T.H. Laënnec. Wood and brass. French, *c.* 1820. SM, A106078

Stethoscope made by Scott Alison. Ebony, ivory and metal. English, *c.* 1858. SM, A625100

Al-Qānūn fī-ṭ-ṭibb. A 1632 manuscript copy of the *Canon of Medicine* of Avicenna (980–1037). WL, Arabic MS Or. 155

Optometer on metal pillar stand, with thirty-eight rotating lenses. Acquired before 1936. SM, A662652

Chinese ivory diagnostic doll. Eighteenth to early nineteenth centuries. SM, A164587

Chinese ivory and wood diagnostic doll. Eighteenth to early nineteenth centuries. SM, A626441

Belt made of six bone plaques linked by woven cotton. Batak people, Sumatra. Acquired before 1936. FMCH, X65-5665

Ivory enema syringe. European, seventeenth century. SM, A626932

Brass and ivory enema syringe. English, 1851–1900. SM, A626202

Plastic enema syringe. Acquired before 1936. SM, A640607

Pewter enema syringe. Eighteenth or nineteenth century. SM, A606384

Dental instrument set. European, 1501–1700. SM, A610718

A surgeon treating a patient's foot. Line engraving by Pieter Jansz Quast. Dutch, seventeenth century. WL, 22561i

Articulated iron manikin used to teach bone setting. Italian, seventeenth century. SM, A73318

The Fountain of Life. Gilded oil on wood panel. Greek. Acquired before 1936. WL, 44950i

A surgeon bandaging a patient's arm after bloodletting. Oil painting on copper by Jacob Toorenvliet. Dutch, 1666. WL, 44999i

Tin-glazed earthenware bleeding bowl. English, 1700–1770. SM, A43161

Physician's folding calendar, 1463. WL, Western MS 40

Scarificator with six lancets. Ivory, brass and steel. English, nineteenth century. SM, A216750

Geta Kihai, a surgical treatise by Kamata Keishū. Japanese, 1851. WL, Japanese MS 18

Barber's shaving bowl decorated with the owner's name and the tools of his trade. Tin-glazed earthenware. Dutch, 1701–50. SM, A45685

Coconut shell charm (*Lakakare*) carved to represent a swordfish. Coconut shell, fishbone and woven string. Papua New Guinea, 1890–1920. SM, A160938

De historia stirpium by Leonhart Fuchs. Basle, 1542. WL, EPB 2438/D

Treating yourself

Wheeled walking frame. Iron and leather. London, 1901–30. SM, A602319

Olmec clay figurine. Mexican, 1200–400 BC. BM, 1981.Am27.1

Brass corset. Probably English, 1800–1880. SM, A158256

Chinese shoes for bound feet. Wood, cotton and silk. 1870–1910. SM, A95136

The 'Claxton' earcap, designed to correct 'outstanding' ears. Net, ribbon and elastic. English, 1925–36. SM, A654350

Copper anklet. Ibo people, Nigeria, 1880–1930. SM, A161483

Set of fifty artificial glass eyes. Possibly made by E. Muller of Liverpool. Acquired before 1936. SM, A660037

Hippopotamus ivory dentures and porcelain stand. Late seventeenth to early eighteenth centuries. SM, A71861, A71862

A couple assemble their false body parts: false teeth, a glass eye and wigs. Coloured lithograph by F.-S. Delpech after L. Boilly. French, 1825. WL, 16329i

Carved female head with elaborate coiffure. Wood, skin, zinc and bone. Egbo people, West Africa. Acquired before 1936. SM, A32577

Carved wooden hair comb. Asante people, Ghana. Acquired before 1936. BM, 1954.+23.439

Seated wooden female figure. Tabwa people, Tanzania, late nineteenth century. BM, 1954+23.3539

Plaster cast showing Maori tattooing. New Zealand, 1851. SM, A642970

Human skin tattooed with a male bust and flower stem. French, 1850–1900. SM, A680

Human skin tattooed with a lady's face. French, 1850–1900. SM, A621

Incised and patterned pubic ornament. Pearl shell and earth pigment. Niol-Niol and Pidungu people, Western Australia, nineteenth century. NMS, A.1953.345

Incised and patterned pubic ornament. Pearl shell and earth pigment. Niol-Niol and Pidungu people, Western Australia, nineteenth century. NMS, A.1925.8894

Hip ornament. Wood, vegetable fibre and hair. Naga people, north-east India. Acquired before 1936. BM, 1954.As7.44

Ear ornaments. Wood, vegetable fibre, hair and beads. Naga people, north-east India. Acquired before 1936. BM, 1954.As7.62a&b

Chest ornament. Wood, cowrie shell, vegetable fibre and hair. Naga people, north-east India. Acquired before 1936. BM, 1954.As7.43

Leg ring amulet made of beetle wings. Amerindian people, Guyana. Acquired before 1936. SM, A642567

Double effigy ceramic vessel. Nazca people, Peru. 100 BC– AD 600. BM, 1954.Am5.805

Glass perfume bottle decorated with flowers. Acquired 1918. SM, A641961

Glass perfume bottle decorated with a gold pattern. Acquired 1919. SM, A641964

Glass perfume bottle decorated with flowers. Acquired before 1936. SM, A641765

Glass perfume bottle decorated with gilt paint. Acquired 1922. SM, A641656

Egyptian toiletry implements on a ring. Bronze. Acquired before 1936. SM, A634882

Steel cut-throat razor with horn handle said to have belonged to Lord Nelson. English, 1780–1805. SM, A650921

Incised wooden snow goggle case containing two pairs of snow goggles. Pine and rawhide. Inuit people. Acquired before 1936. SM, A645437

Spectacles with coloured glass and side-flaps. English, 1830–80. SM, A62428

Silver-rimmed spectacles with folding arms. English, c. 1790. SM, A682602

Folding, 'scissors-style' spectacles with tortoiseshell cover. Possibly English, 1800–80. SM, A682149

Blue glass eye bath. Probably English. Acquired before 1936. SM, A606637

Porcelain eye bath. Acquired before 1936. SM, A606638

Green glass eye bath. European, 1851–1920. SM, A627014

Silver eye bath. Acquired before 1936. SM, A606660

Napoleon Bonaparte's toothbrush with silver-gilt handle and horsehair bristles. French, 1790–1820. SM, A600139

'Indexo' finger toothbrush. Rubber. USA, 1901–25. SM, A619222

Koka-sāra. Nanda and Mukunda. Indian, eighteenth century. WL, MS Hindi 197

Advertisement for a Burroughs Wellcome Tabloid medicine chest. Print on hardboard. London, early twentieth century. WL, 16398i

Aluminium medicine chest used on the 1933 Mount Everest expedition. Burroughs, Wellcome and Co., London. SM, A700004

Sledge case medicine chest used on the 1924 Mount Everest expedition. Burroughs, Wellcome and Co., London. SM, A700026

Wooden massage tool in the form of a flat iron. Roleo, German, 1880–1920. SM, A602750

Ivory massage tool. Acquired before 1936. SM, A161658

Rubber ball massage tool. British, 1900–30. SM, A602770

Whalebone walking stick with skull pommel in ivory, once owned by Charles Darwin. Probably English, 1839–81. SM, A4962

Amuletic necklace of glass beads. Hebron, Palestine, 1880–1930. SM, A665302

Amuletic necklace for curing sore throats. Glass and brass. Acton, London, 1914. SM, A630902

Amuletic necklace for curing bronchitis. Glass beads. Woolwich, London, 1914. SM, A630910

Galvanic anti-neuralgic headband with instructions. Zinc and copper discs, felt band. English, 1870–80. SM, A656298

Feng Shui geometric compass. Chinese. Wood, glass and metal. Acquired before 1936. SM, A642257

Mather's earthenware fly paper plate to hold Mather's chemical fly papers. English, late nineteenth century. SM, A60562

Snuff mull in the form of a ram's head containing two compartments with silver-gilt lids. Scottish, 1881–2. SM, A123128

Cast brass snuff-taker, with male on horseback. Tiv people, Nigeria. Acquired before 1936. BM, 1954.Af. 23.1114

Wooden pipe with bowl in the form of a trophy head. Naga people, India. Acquired before 1936. BM, 1954.As7.110

Carved pipe with scene of a great dragonfly crest, bear and two figures. Argillite, Haida people, British Columbia, Canada. Late nineteenth to early twentieth centuries. BM, 1954.Am5.995

Ivory opium pipe. Chinese. Acquired before 1925. SM, A54680

Sir Hiram Maxim's 'Pipe of Peace' and Maxim Inhaler. English. Acquired before 1936. SM, A629585

Mrs. Corlyon's Booke of divers Medecines, Broothes, Salves, Waters. Syroppes and Oyntementes etc. English, 1606. WL, Western MS 213

A man in bed with vegetables sprouting from all parts of his body as a result of taking J. Morison's Vegetable Pills. Coloured lithograph by C.J. Grant. English, 1831. WL, 11852i

Anthropomorphic food bowl. Haida people, British Columbia. Acquired before 1936. FMCH, X65-7474

Wooden lime spatula. Massim area of Trobriand Islands, Papua New Guinea. Acquired before 1936. FMCH, X65-7775

Tin-glazed earthenware posset pot. English, 1630–1730. SM, A634395

Tin-glazed earthenware female urinal. Spode, English, 1820–91. SM, A625645

Tin-glazed earthenware chamber pot. Probably Dutch, 1651–1780. SM, A1189

Ex-voto paintings

A man being hit on the head by a falling flowerpot in Rome, Via del Nazzareno. Oil painting on canvas. Italian, c. 1890. WL, 44873i

A woman in bed, a second woman kneeling beside her in prayer to the Virgin and Child. Oil painting on canvas. Italian, nineteenth century. WL, 44881i

A woman expressing thanks to the Madonna del Parto for cure of insanity in the form of expelled devils. Oil painting on wood. Italian, nineteenth century. WL, 44882i

A woman praying for a child, with intercessors in a fire. Oil painting on wood. Italian, 1887. WL, 44883i

Antonino Caroselli run over by a coach. Oil on tin. Italian, 1860. WL, 44885i

A child in bed, its parents praying to the Madonna del Parto. Oil on wood. Italian, nineteenth century. WL, 44886i

A woman appealing to Christ, to Sansovino's Virgin and Child, and to Saint Nicholas on behalf of her child. Mixed media on paper. Italian, early nineteenth century. WL, 44888i

Four people praying to Sansovino's Virgin and Child for a woman in premature childbirth. Mixed media on paper pinned to wood. Italian, 1871. WL, 44891i

Lucia Manconi being cured of an injury or disease of the foot. Mixed media on paper. Italian, nineteenth century. WL, 44892i

Two men and a woman praying for the health of a child. Oil on canvas. Italian, 1890. WL, 44899i

A man in bed praying to the Virgin and Child and two Franciscan saints. Oil on wood. Probably Italian, nineteenth century. WL, 44903i

Dona Mercedes Velasco's recovery from a nosebleed after prayer to the Lord of the Abandoned, not after intervention of the physician. Oil on wood. Spanish, 1854. WL, 44910i

Francisco Wiedon and his wife praying for a cure for his pneumonia and pain in his side. Oil on wood. Spanish, 1864. WL, 44920i

José Maria Martinez in prison praying to the Virgin and Child of Guadalupe. Oil on canvas. Spanish, 1798. WL, 44935i

A woman in bed in a sickroom, attended by a physician, receiving the blessing of the Madonna del Parto. Oil on canvas. Italian, 1872. WL, 44870i

A woman praying to the Virgin and Christ crucified for a person in bed attended by physicians. Oil on millboard. French, 1846. WL, 47315i

A woman who has fallen down a well being rescued by a man praying to Sansovino's Virgin and Child. Watercolour. Italian, nineteenth century. WL, 44876i

A woman kneeling with crutches, praying to the Virgin and Child. Oil on canvas, laid on millboard. French, nineteenth century. WL, 47311i

Two women attending a man in bed and appealing to Sansovino's Virgin and Child. Oil on wood. Italian, 1888. WL, 44884i

A man praying to the Virgin as he is run over by a horse-drawn cart carrying textiles. Oil on canvas. Italian, nineteenth century. WL, 44887i

A man stabbing a woman with a stiletto. Oil on canvas. Italian, nineteenth century. WL, 44875i

A woman praying before a painting or tapestry of the Virgin and Child in glory. Oil on wood. French, 1829. WL, 47314i

A man praying to Sansovino's statue of the Madonna del Parto. Oil on wood. Italian, nineteenth century. WL, 44880i

Agata Paladino in a street accident. Oil on metal. Italian, 1843. WL, 44894i

Photographs

A Hong Kong artist at work. John Thomson, 1871. WL, 19843i

Manchu women being sold hair ornaments. John Thomson, 1869. WL, 19655i

A Cantonese boat-girl. John Thomson, 1869. WL, 19581i

Mandarin and son, China. John Thomson, 1869. WL, 19543i

Manchu lady having her hair styled. John Thomson, 1869. WL, 19667i

Manchu bride. John Thomson, 1869. WL, 19685i

A Pekinese chiropodist. John Thomson, 1869. WL, 19709i

Old Chinese woman with elaborate hairstyle. John Thomson, 1869. WL, 19579i

Portrait of A Mokwena, South Africa. Alfred Duggan-Cronin, early twentieth century. WL, 536884i

Gaberone, Chief of the Batholura, South Africa. Alfred Duggan-Cronin, early twentieth century. WL, 536874i

Portrait of Ama Fengu, a Fingo man. Alfred Duggan-Cronin, early twentieth century. WL, 540815i

A Pedi mother breastfeeding her child, South Africa. Alfred Duggan-Cronin, early twentieth century. WL, 536952i

A Tembu mother carrying her child, South Africa. Alfred Duggan-Cronin, early twentieth century. WL, 540868i

A Pedi girl, South Africa. Alfred Duggan-Cronin, early twentieth century. WL, 536953i

Portrait of a Bushman, South Africa. Alfred Duggan-Cronin, early twentieth century. WL, 541315i

AmaBomvana tribe members being painted, South Africa. Alfred Duggan-Cronin, early twentieth century. WL, 541220i

Pondo witch doctor taking snuff, South Africa. Alfred Duggan-Cronin, early twentieth century. WL, 541144i

A group of boys starting a fire, South Africa. Alfred Duggan-Cronin, early twentieth century. WL, 536956i

Peter Iron Shell, Omaha. Frank Rinehart and Adolf Muhr, c. 1898. WL, 557870i

A Kiowa tribe member, Omaha. Frank Rinehart and Adolf Muhr, c. 1898. WL, 557803i

Henry Wilson and wife, Mojave–Apache Indians, Omaha. Frank Rinehart and Adolf Muhr, c. 1898. WL, 557809i

Native American and squaw, Omaha. Frank Rinehart and Adolf Muhr, c. 1898. WL, 557813i

Portrait of Yellow Smoke, Omaha. Frank Rinehart and Adolf Muhr, c. 1898. WL, 557542i

Omaha dance bonnet and scalplock. Frank Rinehart and Adolf Muhr, c. 1898. WL, 557547i

Navajo Yebichai dancers. Matt brown toned silver platinum print. Edward S. Curtis, 1904. WL, Icv 39041

A Yebichai dancer representing the Navajo God Zahadolzha. Matt brown toned silver gelatin print. Edward S. Curtis, 1904. WL, 559067i

A Navajo medicine man. Edward S. Curtis, 1904. WL, 559250i

A Piegan Indian, Iron Breast, in ceremonial dress. Edward S. Curtis, 1900. WL, 559111i

Masks

Skin-covered wood headdress mask. Ekoi people, Nigeria. Acquired before 1936. BM, 1954. Af 23.892

Skin-covered wood headdress mask. Ekoi people, Nigeria. Acquired before 1936. BM, 1954.Af.23.1087e

Skin-covered wood headdress mask. Ekoi people, Nigeria. Acquired before 1936. BM, 1954. Af.23.1087f

Carved and painted wood mask with fibre fringe. Ibibio people, Nigeria. Acquired before 1936. BM, 1954.Af.23.826

Carved and painted wood mask with a fibre fringe. Ibibio people, Nigeria. Acquired before 1936. BM, 1954.Af.23.828

Carved and painted wood mask. Ibibio people, Nigeria. Acquired before 1936. BM, 1954.Af.23.840

Ekpo society mask which represents an elephant. Ogoni people, Nigeria. Acquired before 1936. BM, 1954.Af.23.877

Skin-covered wood headdress mask depicting a stylised human head. Ekoi people, Nigeria. Acquired before 1936. BM, 1954.Af.23.879

Skin-covered headdress mask depicting a stylised human head.

Ekoi people, Nigeria. Acquired before 1936. BM, 1954.Af.23.880

Skin-covered headdress mask depicting a human head. Nigeria. Acquired before 1936. BM, 1954.Af.23.882

Carved wood mask depicting a stylised face. Guro people, Ivory Coast, nineteenth century. NMS, A.1949.203

Helmet mask. Papua New Guinea, nineteenth century. NMS, A.1951.372

Leather helmet mask with beaded and shell decoration. Kuba people, Democratic Republic of Congo, early twentieth century. NMS, A.1953.335

Carved and painted wood mask depicting a character from a Kolam play. Sri Lanka, 1771–1920. SM, A100831

Carved and painted wood mask depicting a character from a Kolam play. Sri Lanka, 1771–1900. SM, A134254

Carved and painted wood mask depicting a skull. Bhutan, 1850–1920. SM, A193924

Carved and painted wood mask depicting a green human face. Sri Lanka. Acquired before 1936. SM, A19437

Carved and painted wood mask depicting a demon's face. Sri Lanka, 1771–1920. SM, A232391

Carved and painted wood mask depicting a character from a Kolam play. Sri Lanka, 1771–1900. SM, A30158

Carved and painted wood mask depicting a character from a Kolam play. Sri Lanka, 1771–1900. SM, A53679

Carved and painted wood boar's head mask depicting a character from a Kolam play. Sri Lanka, 1771–1900. SM, A53683

Carved and painted wood mask depicting a character from a Kolam

play. Sri Lanka, 1771–1900. SM, A53685

Carved and painted wood mask depicting a blue male face. Sri Lanka, before 1870. SM, A62943

Carved and painted wood mask depicting a yellow male face. Sri Lanka. Acquired before 1936. SM, A62947

Large carved and painted wood mask depicting a character from a Kolam play. Sri Lanka, 1771–1885. SM, A657020

Carved and painted wood mask depicting demonic faces surmounted by a crown of cobras. Sri Lanka. Acquired before 1936. SM, A8649

Mask thought to represent the spirit of sleep. British Columbia, Canada. Acquired before 1936. FMCH, X65-4266

Carved wood mask depicting a human face decorated with painted geometric patterns. Possibly Tsimshian people, British Columbia, Canada. Acquired before 1936. FMCH, X65-4273

Eharo mask. Elema people, Papuan Gulf. Acquired before 1936. FMCH, X65-4344

Mask used in complex mortuary ceremonies (*malangaan*). New Ireland, Papua New Guinea. Acquired before 1936. FMCH, X65-4360

Carved and painted wood mask. Oani District, Gabon. Acquired before 1936. FMCH, X65-5270

Carved and painted wood face mask with basketry horns and grass collar. Yaka people, Democratic Republic of Congo. Acquired before 1936. FMCH, X65-5447

Skin-covered headdress mask depicting a human head. Ekoi people, Cross River, Nigeria. Acquired before 1936. FMCH, X65-8235

Carved wood headdress mask depicting an abstract face with cylindrical eyes. Possibly Urhobo people, Nigeria. Acquired before 1936. FMCH, X65-9041

Skin-covered headdress mask depicting a human head with three long curled horns. Possibly Ekoi people, Nigeria. Acquired before 1936. FMCH, X65-9043

Headpiece of an 'egungun' mask depicting an ancestral hunter. Yoruba people, Nigeria. Acquired before 1936. FMCH, X65-9051

Carved and painted wood Gelede mask depicting a human face with scarification on the cheeks. Yoruba people, Nigeria. Acquired before 1936. FMCH, X65-4742

Artificial limbs

Artificial right foot and ankle with lace-up leather boot. 1891–1930. SM, A500474

Artificial lower left leg with leather strapping for attachment. 1901–40. SM, A500465

Artificial lower right leg with flesh-coloured thigh socket. 1901–40. SM, A500472

Artificial lower left leg with laced leather sheath over thigh. English, 1861–1920. SM, A603149

Artificial lower leg known as a 'peg leg'. 1850–1900. SM, A205286

Artificial left hand and forearm. Possibly German, 1560–1600. SM, A121449

Artificial left arm. English, 1937. SM, A500475

Artificial forearm with upper arm socket. European, 1840–1900. SM, A602817

Artificial right hand with leather arm sheath. 1880–1920. SM, A653501

Artificial left arm. European, 1850–1910. SM, A653499

Artificial left arm and hand with

shoulder strap. English, 1927.
SM, A653498

Artificial right hand, known as the
McKay, after the inventor. Scottish,
1880–1920. SM, A500480

Artificial left hand. English,
1914–20. SM, A636915

Artificial left hand with glove.
European, 1880–1920.
SM, A653506

Oil paintings

A seated female dissected figure
holding a dissected baby. In the
style of Jacques-Fabien Gautier
d'Agoty, c. 1770. WL, 44575i

Lateral view of a dissected
pregnant female with arms
upraised. In the style of Jacques-
Fabien Gautier d'Agoty, c. 1770.
WL, 44574i

Standing male figure, posterior
view, showing superficial muscles
and tendons. In the style of
Jacques-Fabien Gautier d'Agoty,
c. 1770. WL, 44567i

Standing male figure showing
superficial muscles and tendons.
In the style of Jacques-Fabien
Gautier d'Agoty, c. 1770.
WL, 44566i

Anterior view of skeleton with
tendons. In the style of Jacques-
Fabien Gautier d'Agoty, c. 1770.
WL, 44564i

Skeleton, left ribs removed, with
some nerves and viscera. In the
style of Jacques-Fabien Gautier
d'Agoty, c. 1770. WL, 44565i

A standing dissected figure,
posterior view, with separate
sections of the brain. In the style
of Jacques-Fabien Gautier d'Agoty,
c. 1770. WL, 44573i

Glass

Glass apothecary bottle,
possibly used to store potassium
citrate. English, 1840–1900.
SM, A634337

Glass apothecary bottle,
possibly used to store tincture of
cardamom. English, 1840–1900.
SM, A634463

Glass apothecary bottle,
possibly used to store tincture
of catechu. English, 1840–1900.
SM, A634462

Glass apothecary bottle,
possibly used to store tincture
of bryony. English, 1840–1900.
SM, A634033

Glass apothecary bottle,
possibly used to store tincture
of saffron. English, 1840–1900.
SM, A634038

Glass apothecary bottle,
possibly used to store tincture of
cinchona. English, 1840–1900.
SM, A634037

Glass apothecary bottle,
possibly used to store tincture of
capsicum. English, 1840–1900.
SM, A634032

Glass apothecary bottle,
possibly used to store tincture of
cantharides. English, 1840–1900.
A634464

Glass storage jar for nail
brushes. English, 1850–1900.
SM, A633227

Glass storage jar for 'Delectable
Lozenges'. English, 1850–1900.
SM, A633246

Glass storage jar for powder
puffs. English, 1850–1900.
SM, A633252

Glass storage jar for corn
plasters. English, 1850–1900.
SM, A633249

Glass storage jar for cough
lozenges. English, 1850–1900.
SM, A633254

Glass storage jar for voice
jujubes. English, 1850–1900.
SM, A633248

Glass storage jar for aromatic
pastilles. English, 1850–1900.
SM, A633247

Glass apothecary bottle,
possibly used to store sodium
tartrate. SM, A660618/5

Glass apothecary bottle used
to store ammonium compound.
SM, A660618/7

Glass apothecary bottle, possibly
used to store potassium sulphate.
SM, A660618/9

Glass apothecary bottle used
to store benzoic acid.
SM, A660618/11

Glass apothecary bottle used
to store iron filings.
SM, A660618/12

Glass apothecary bottle used
to store ammonium compound.
SM, A660618/15

Glass apothecary bottle used
to store scurvy-grass water.
SM, A660618/22

Glass apothecary bottle used
to store sambucus water.
SM, A660618/23

Glass apothecary bottle used to
store tilia water. SM, A660618/24

Glass apothecary bottle used
to store an unidentified remedy.
SM, A660618/25

Glass apothecary bottle used
to store cinnamon water.
SM, A660618/28

Glass apothecary bottle used
to store an unidentified remedy.
SM, A660618/37

Glass apothecary bottle used
to store an unidentified remedy.
SM, A660618/48

Glass apothecary bottle used
to store an unidentified remedy.
SM, A660618/49

Glass apothecary bottle used
to store an unidentified remedy.
SM, A660618/50

Glass apothecary bottle used
to store tincture of myrrh.
SM, A660618/51

Green glass medicine bottle.
1880–1960. SM, A657655

Blue glass medicine bottle.
SM, A660665

Blue glass medicine bottle.
SM, A660664

Opaque blue glass medicine
bottle. Probably British.
SM, A660075

Green glass medicine bottle.
SM, A660191/1

Brown glass poison bottle.
SM, A660262

Green glass poison bottle.
SM, A660188/1

Green glass poison bottle.
SM, A660188/2

Green glass poison bottle.
SM, A660188/3

Blue glass measuring cylinder.
English, 1851–1900.
SM, A638729

Blue glass measuring cylinder.
English, 1851–1900.
SM, A638729

Blue glass measuring cylinder.
English, 1851–1900. SM, A63872

Blue glass measuring cylinder.
English, 1851–1900.
SM, A638729

Green glass medicine bottle.
Possibly English, 1801–50.
SM, A140996

Green glass medicine bottle.
Possibly English, 1801–50.
SM, A634217

Green glass medicine bottle.
Possibly English, 1801–50.
SM, A634216

Green glass medicine bottle.
Possibly English, 1801–50.
SM, A634090

Green glass medicine bottle.
Possibly English, 1801–50.
SM, A634171

Blue glass medicine bottle.
English, 1890–1930.
SM, A633534

Blue glass medicine bottle.
English, 1898. SM, A633533

Brown glass poison bottle.
English. SM, A660267

Glass apothecary bottle used to
store antipyrine powder. English,
1860–1920. SM, A638014

Glass apothecary bottle used
to store sulphuric acid. English,
1801–50. SM, A638015

Glass apothecary bottle used to
store potassium iodide. English,
1860–1920. SM, A638011

Glass apothecary bottle used to
store ammonium bromide. English,
1850–1920. SM, A638009

Glass apothecary bottle used
to store paraldehyde. English,
1850–1920. SM, A638010

Glass apothecary bottle
used to store oxymel. English,
1860–1900. SM, A633350

Glass apothecary bottle used
to store an unidentified syrup.
English, 1850–1900.
SM, A190922

Glass apothecary bottle
used to store syrup of saffron.
English.1851–1900.
SM, A190921

Glass apothecary bottle used
to store syrup of orange. English,
1851–1900. SM, A191259

Glass apothecary bottle
used to store syrup of white
horehound. English, 1851–1900.
SM, A660051

Glass apothecary jar used to store
an unidentified remedy. Spanish,
1601–1800. SM, A61740

Glass apothecary jar used to store
iron oxide. Spanish, 1601–1800.
SM, A61736

Glass apothecary jar used to store
powdered caster seed. Spanish,
1601–1800. SM, A61727

Glass apothecary jar used to
store ivory shavings. Spanish,
1601–1800. SM, A61739

Glass apothecary jar used to store
haematite. Spanish, 1601–1800.
SM, A61730

Glass apothecary jar used to
store powdered soot. Spanish,
1601–1800. SM, A61679

Glass apothecary jar used to
store a bull's penis. Spanish,
1601–1800. SM, A61692

Glass apothecary jar used to store
an unidentified powder. Spanish,
1601–1800. SM, A61683

Glass apothecary jar used to
store sedatine salt. Spanish,
1601–1800. SM, A61700

Glass apothecary jar used to store
iron oxide. Spanish, 1601–1800.
SM, A61697

Glass apothecary jar used to
store dragon's blood. Spanish,
1601–1800. SM, A61759

Glass apothecary jar used to store
blue vitriol. Spanish, 1601–1800.
SM, A61761

Glass apothecary jar used to store
scammony or ipomoea. Spanish,
1601–1800. SM, A61791

Glass apothecary jar used to
store a crab's eye. Spanish,
1601–1800. SM, A61772

Glass apothecary jar used to
store western hyacinth. Spanish,
1601–1800. SM, A61769

Glass apothecary jar used to
store emerald fragments. Spanish,
1601–1800. SM, A61774

Glass bottle decorated with
a painted saint, for holy water.
SM, A660494

Glass bottle decorated with
a painted saint, possibly
Saint Peter, for holy water. Italian.
SM, A77271

Glass bottle decorated with a
painted saint, possibly Saint
Nicholas of Myrna, for holy water.
Possibly Spanish, nineteenth
century. SM, A660480

Glass bottle decorated with painted saint, for holy water. SM, A660491

Glass bottle decorated with a painted saint, for holy water. SM, A660489

Glass bottle decorated with a painted saint, for holy water. Nineteenth century. SM, A660490

Glass bottle decorated with a painted saint, possibly Saint Nicholas of Myrna, for holy water. Possibly Spanish, eighteenth–nineteenth centuries. SM, A660481

Glass bottle decorated with a depiction of Saint Nicholas of Bari, for holy water. Italian. SM, A660614

Glass bottle decorated with painted saints, for holy water. SM, A660476/2

Purple glass medicine jar. SM, A660662/1

Purple glass medicine jar. SM, A660662/4

Purple glass medicine jar. SM, A660662

Pink glass tincture bottle. Bohemian. SM, A659176 pt

Pink glass tincture bottle. Bohemian. SM, A659176 pt

Pink glass tincture bottle. Bohemian. SM, A659176 pt

Green glass medicine bottle used to store peppermint water. English, 1780–1850. SM, A181110

Green glass medicine bottle used to store syrup of camphor. English, 1780–1850. SM, A181111

Glass wine flask. SM, A660555

Glass wine flask. SM, A660533

Glass wine flask. SM, A660532

Glass flask. 1551–1650. SM, A660732

Glass flask. SM, A660734

Glass display bottle used to store naval bouquet. English, 1801–1900. SM, A602252

Glass jar bearing the alchemical sign for mercury. English, 1851–1900. SM, A633505

Glass jar bearing the alchemical sign for sulphur. SM, A660693

Glass flask. SM, A660640

Glass flask. SM, A660651

Metal

Finger amputation saw with ivory handle. Nineteenth century. SM, A241782

Finger amputation saw. English, 1901–50. SM, A614941

Small amputation saw. English, 1780–1880. SM, A600870

Metacarpal bow-frame amputation saw. 1751–1850. SM, A106337

Bow-frame amputation saw. 1781–1880. SM, A600807

Bow-frame amputation saw. c. 1580. SM, A121435

Bow-frame amputation saw. Probably Spanish, 1551–1700. SM, A85259

Bow-frame amputation saw, c. 1750. SM, A121434

Bow-frame amputation saw with wooden carved eagle head handle. c. 1680. SM, A85252

Adjustable bow-frame amputation saw. English, c. 1880. SM, A600826

Adjustable bow-frame amputation saw. English, c. 1850. SM, A600830

Metacarpal bow-frame amputation saw. English c. 1750. SM, A600822

Bow-frame amputation saw. c. 1680. SM, A155568

Bow-frame amputation saw. French, 1630. SM, A600810

Amputation saw. English, nineteenth century. SM, A600563

Bow-frame amputation saw. c. 1780. SM, A600813

Post-mortem amputation saw. c. 1830. SM, A600864

Amputation saw. c. 1880. SM, A600871

Bow-frame amputation saw. c. 1840. SM, A600878

Bow-frame amputation saw. English, nineteenth century. SM, A647716

Bow-frame amputation saw. c. 1730. SM, A121432

Bow-frame amputation saw with eagle head handle. c. 1650. SM, A121431

Amputation knife with ebony handle. French, eighteenth century. SM, A622732

Amputation knife with bone handle. c. 1550. SM, A648001

Amputation saw. English, 1831–70. SM, A500502 pt 1

Amputation knife. English, 1831–70. SM, A500502 pt 2

Amputation knife. English, 1831–70. SM, A500502 pt 3

Amputation knife. English, 1831–70. SM, A500502 pt 4

Finger saw. English, 1831–70. SM, A500502 pt 5

Finger knife. English, 1831–70. SM, A5600502 pt 6

Amputation scalpel. English, 1831–70. SM, A500502 pt 7

Amputation scalpel. English, 1822–69. SM, A500502 pt 8

Artery forceps. English, 1822–69. SM, A500502 pt 9

Bone obstetrical forceps. English, 1831–70. SM, A500502 pt 12

Tenaculum. English, 1831–70. SM, A500502 pt 10

Hinged obstetrical forceps. English, 1810–50. SM, A615726

Obstetrical forceps. English, 1851–1900. SM, A500242

Obstetrical forceps. English, 1851–1900. SM, A500210

Obstetrical forceps. *c.* 1750. SM, A615833

Obstetrical forceps. Probably British, 1731–70. SM, A500434

Obstetrical forceps. Scottish, 1871–1900. SM, A615789

Obstetrical forceps. 1831–70. SM, A500213

Obstetrical forceps. English, *c.* 1860. SM, A500382

Obstetrical forceps. 1831–70. SM, A615774

Obstetrical forceps. English, 1783–1843. SM, A615636

Obstetrical forceps. 1750–1850. SM, A500393

Obstetrical forceps with chain. English, 1866–1900. SM, A615231

Obstetrical forceps. 1851–1900. SM, A615784

Obstetrical forceps. English, *c.* 1850. SM, A615792

Obstetrical forceps. 1851–1900. SM, A615821

Obstetrical forceps. English, 1870–1901. SM, A500407

Obstetrical forceps. French, 1850–1930. SM, A615831

Obstetrical forceps. Scottish, 1865–1900. SM, A633695

Obstetrical forceps. 1680–1750. SM, A615836

Obstetrical forceps. 1680–1750. SM, A615857

Obstetrical forceps. Scottish, *c.* 1870. SM, A500373

Obstetrical forceps with traction

rods. Scottish, 1860–80. SM, A615645

Obstetrical forceps. English, 1871–1900. SM, A615728

Obstetrical forceps. French, 1750–1850. SM, A615620

Obstetrical forceps. Norwegian, nineteenth century. SM, A79425

Obstetrical forceps. SM, A500424

Obstetrical forceps. Norwegian, nineteenth century. SM, A79426

Obstetrical forceps. SM, A95923

Votive offerings

Votive female head. Roman, 200 BC–AD 200. SM, A635639

Votive female head. Roman, 200 BC–AD 200. SM, A636864

Votive male head. Probably Etruscan, 400–100 BC. SM, A637016

Votive female head. Probably Roman, 200 BC–AD 200. SM, A636890

Votive male head. Probably Etruscan, 200 BC–AD 200. SM, A636193

Votive face. Probably Roman, 200 BC–AD 100. SM, A634930

Votive face. Etrusco-Roman, 200 BC–AD 200. SM, A636843

Votive face. Etrusco-Roman, 200 BC–AD 200. SM, A636848

Votive hair. Probably Roman, 200 BC–AD 200. SM, A114891

Votive hair. Possibly Roman, 100 BC–AD 300. SM, A634932

Votive mouth and teeth. Probably Roman, 200 BC–AD 200. SM, A636148

Votive tongue. Probably Roman, 400 BC–AD 200. SM, A634928

Votive trachea. Roman, 200 BC–AD 200. SM, A636200

Votive right eye. Probably Roman, 300 BC–AD 200. SM, A166869

Votive right eye. Probably Roman, 200 BC–AD 200. SM, A114897

Votive eye. Probably Roman, 200 BC–AD 200. SM, A636131

Votive eye. Probably Roman, 400 BC–AD 100. SM, A636134

Votive eye. Probably Roman, 200 BC–AD 100. SM, A635569

Votive right ear. Probably Roman, 200 BC–AD 200. SM, A59910

Votive left ear. Probably Roman, 400 BC–AD 100. SM, A636127

Votive right ear. Probably Roman, 200 BC–AD 200. SM, A637008

Votive left ear. Probably Roman, 200 BC–AD 200. SM, A637009

Votive right ear. Probably Roman, 200 BC–AD 200. SM, A636879

Votive left ear. Etrusco-Roman, 200 BC–AD 200. SM, A59913

Votive right leg. Probably Roman, 200 BC–AD 200. SM, A637034

Votive left leg. Roman, 200 BC–AD 200. SM, A129321

Votive right leg. Probably Roman, 200 BC–AD 200. SM, A85622

Votive left leg. Probably Roman, 200 BC–AD 200. SM, A85620

Votive left leg. Roman, 200 BC–AD 200. SM, A69406

Votive right foot. Probably Roman, 200 BC–AD 200. SM, A69290

Votive left foot. Probably Roman, 200 BC–AD 200. SM, A635666

Votive right foot. Probably Roman, 200 BC–AD 200. SM, A635615

Votive right foot. Probably Roman, 200 BC–AD 200. SM, A635609

Votive right foot. Probably Roman, 200 BC–AD 200. SM, A635668

Votive right foot. Probably Roman, 200 BC–AD 200. SM, A655537

Votive left foot. Probably Roman,
200 BC–AD 200. SM, A38705

Votive right foot. Probably Roman,
200 BC–AD 200. SM, A73009

Votive right arm. Roman,
200 BC–AD 200. SM, A636830

Votive left arm. Roman,
200 BC–AD 200. SM, A636831

Votive right arm. Probably Roman,
200 BC–AD 200. SM, A637102

Votive left hand. Roman,
200 BC–AD 200. SM, A637100

Votive right hand. Probably Roman,
400 BC–AD 200. SM, A636172

Votive right hand. Probably Roman,
200 BC–AD 200. SM, A636174

Votive right hand. Probably Roman,
200 BC–AD 200. SM, A95397

Votive left thumb. Probably Roman,
100 BC–AD 300. SM, A634922

Votive female viscera.
Probably Roman, 200 BC–AD 200.
SM, A634939

Votive viscera. Probably Roman,
200 BC–AD 200. SM, A636802

Votive viscera. Probably Roman,
200 BC–AD 200. SM, A635755

Votive viscera. Probably Roman,
200 BC–AD 200. SM, A636803

Votive torso and viscera.
Probably Roman, 200 BC–AD 200.
SM, A634998

Votive bladder. Etrusco-Roman,
200 BC–AD 200. SM, A636057

Votive bladder. Etrusco-Roman,
200 BC–AD 200. SM, A636049

Votive intestine. Probably Roman,
200 BC–AD 200. SM, A73042

Votive intestine. Probably Roman,
200 BC–AD 200. SM, A73043

Votive kidney. Probably Roman,
200 BC–AD 200. SM, A636807

Votive stomach. Probably Roman,
200 BC–AD 200. SM, A659672

Votive organ. Probably Roman,
200 BC–AD 200. SM, A659668

Votive organ. Probably Roman,
200 BC–AD 200. SM, A659677

Votive bone. Probably Roman,
200 BC–AD 200. SM, A659701

Votive figurine of a woman
and child. Believed to be from a
Greek colony in Italy, 350–50 BC.
SM, A655612

Votive infant. Probably Roman,
200 BC–AD 200. SM, A636026

Votive breast. Probably Roman,
200 BC–AD 200. SM, A634927

Votive breast. Probably Roman,
200 BC–AD 200. SM, A635572

Votive breast. Proabably Roman,
200 BC–AD 100. SM, A635551

Votive breast. Probably Roman,
200 BC–AD 100. SM, A635554

Votive uterus. Probably Roman,
200 BC–AD 200. SM, A636076

Votive uterus. Probably Roman,
200 BC–AD 200. SM, A636107

Votive uterus. Probably Roman,
200 BC–AD 200. SM, A636165

Votive vulva. Probably Roman,
200 BC–AD 200. SM, A636058

Votive vulva. Probably Roman,
200 BC–AD 200. SM, A636106

Votive placenta. Probably Roman,
200 BC–AD 200. SM, A635557

Votive male genitalia. Probably
Roman, 200 BC–AD 200.
SM, A636071

Votive male genitalia. Probably
Roman, 200 BC–AD 200.
SM, A635600

Votive male genitalia. Probably
Roman, 200 BC–AD 200.
SM, A635592

Votive male genitalia. Probably
Roman, 200 BC–AD 200.
SM, A636861

Votive male genitalia. Probably
Roman, 200 BC–AD 200.
SM, A69348

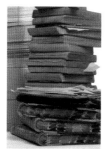

Page 1

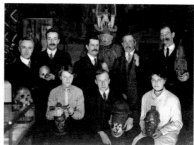

Pages 2/3

Page 1
Part of the archive
documenting the
Wellcome Historical
Medical Museum.

Pages 2/3
Staff in the Wellcome
Historical Medical
Museum, c. 1915.

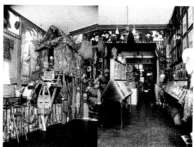

Pages 4/5

Page 4
A head-hunter's hut,
south-east New Guinea,
in the Hall of Primitive
Medicine, Wellcome
Historical Medical
Museum, c. 1914.

Page 5
Hall of Primitive Medicine
in the Wellcome Historical
Medical Museum, c. 1914.

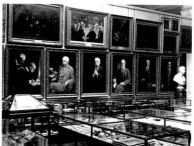

Pages 6/7

Pages 6/7
East wall of the Portrait
Gallery in the Wellcome
Historical Medical
Museum, c. 1914.

Pages 8/9
The galleried Hall of
Statuary in the Wellcome
Historical Medical
Museum, c. 1914.

Pages 10/11
Reconstruction of a seventeenth-century English
apothecary's shop in the Wellcome Historical
Medical Museum, c. 1914.

Pages 12/13
The Anatomy Room in the Wellcome Historical
Medical Museum, c. 1914.

Page 14 top
An exhibition of materia medica in the Wellcome
Historical Medical Museum, 1913.

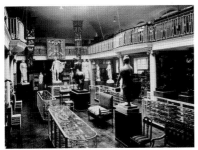

Pages 8/9

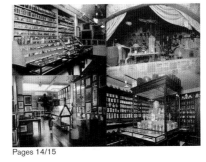

Pages 14/15

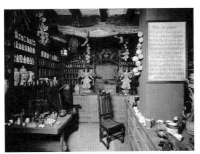

Pages 10/11

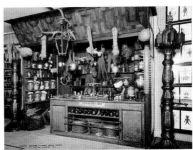

Pages 16/17

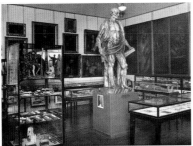

Pages 12/13

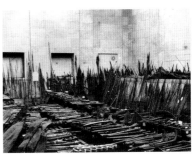

Pages 18/19

Page 14 *bottom*
Chemistry section of the first floor galleries in the
Wellcome Historical Medical Museum, 1926.

Page 15 *top*
Reconstruction of a sixteenth-century alchemist's
laboratory in the Wellcome Historical Medical
Museum, *c.* 1914.

Page 15 *bottom*
A display of pharmacy jars in the Wellcome
Historical Medical Museum, *c.* 1914.

Pages 16/17
Reconstruction of a seventeenth-century
Turkish drug shop in the Wellcome Historical
Medical Museum, *c.* 1914.

Pages 18/19
Weapons originally belonging to the
Wellcome Historical Medical Museum laid
out in the Duveen Gallery at the British
Museum, 1955. The photograph shows one
section of the gallery only. Probably about
one twelfth of the whole.

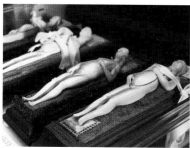

Pages 398/399

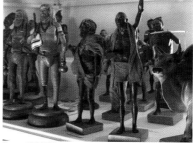

Pages 404/405

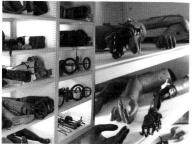

Pages 400/401

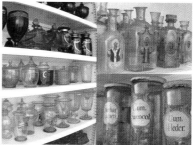

Pages 406/407

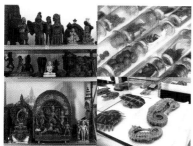

Pages 402/403

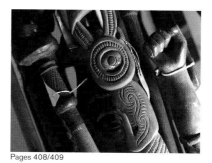

Pages 408/409

Pages 398/399
Ivory anatomical models from the Wellcome collection, now in the Science Museum's Anatomy storeroom.

Page 400
Leg and foot prostheses from the Wellcome collection, now in the Science Museum's Orthopaedics storeroom.

Page 401
Arm and hand prostheses from the Wellcome collection, now in the Science Museum's Orthopaedics storeroom.

Page 402
Objects from the Wellcome collection, now in one of the Science Museum's Oriental storerooms.

Page 403 *top*
Seeds and roots from the Wellcome collection, now in the Science Museum's Materia Medica storeroom.

Page 403 *bottom*
Seahorses and turtle shells from the Wellcome collection, now in the Science Museum's Materia Medica storeroom.

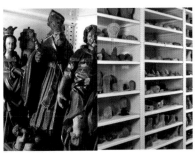

Pages 410/411

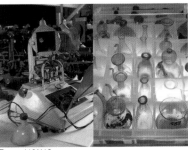

Pages 412/413

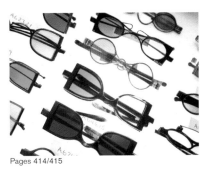

Pages 414/415

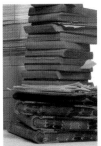

Page 416

Page 410
Medical saints from the Wellcome
collection, now in the Science Museum's
Classical and Medieval Medicine
storeroom.

Page 411
Graeco-Roman terracotta votive offerings
from the Wellcome collection, now in the
Science Museum's Classical and
Medieval Medicine storeroom.

Page 412
Ophthalmological equipment from the
Wellcome collection, now in the Science
Museum's Ophthalmology storeroom.

Page 413
Bottles and jars from the Wellcome
collection, now in the Science Museum's
Medical Glassware storeroom.

Page 404/405
Indian figures from the Wellcome collection,
now in one of the Science Museum's Oriental
storerooms.

Page 406/407
Bottles and jars from the Wellcome collection,
now in the Science Museum's Medical
Glassware storeroom.

Pages 408/409
Detail of staff and spears from the Wellcome
collection, now in one of the Science Museum's
Ethnography storerooms.

Pages 414/415
Spectacles from the Wellcome collection,
now in the Science Museum's
Ophthalmology storeroom.

Page 416
Part of the archive documenting the
Wellcome Historical Medical Museum.

Further Reading

Engineer, A. 2000. 'Illustrations from the Wellcome Library: Wellcome and "The Great Past"' in *Medical History* 44, pp. 389–404.

Hall, A.R. and Bembridge, B.A. 1986. *Physic and Philanthropy, a history of the Wellcome Trust 1936–1986*. Cambridge: Cambridge University Press.

James, R.R. 1994. *Henry Wellcome*. London: Hodder & Stoughton.

Macdonald, G. 1980. *In Pursuit of Excellence*. London: Wellcome Foundation Ltd.

Russell, G. 1986. 'The Wellcome Historical Medical Museum's disposal of non-medical material, 1936–1983' in *Museums Journal* 86, supplement.

Skinner, G.M. 1986. 'Sir Henry Wellcome's Museum for the Science of History' in *Medical History* 30, pp. 383–418.

Symons, J. 1993. *Wellcome Institute for the History of Medicine: A Short History*. London: The Wellcome Trust.

Symons, J. 1998. '"These crafty dealers". Sir Henry Wellcome as a Book Collector' in Myers, R. and Harris, M. (eds), *Medicine, Mortality and the Book Trade*. Kent: St Paul's Bibliographies/Oak Knoll Press.

Turner, H. 1980. *Henry Wellcome: the man, his collection and his legacy*. London: The Wellcome Trust and Heinemann.

UCLA Museum and Laboratories of the Ethnic Arts. 1965. *Masterpieces from the Sir Henry Wellcome Collection at UCLA*. Los Angeles.

Index

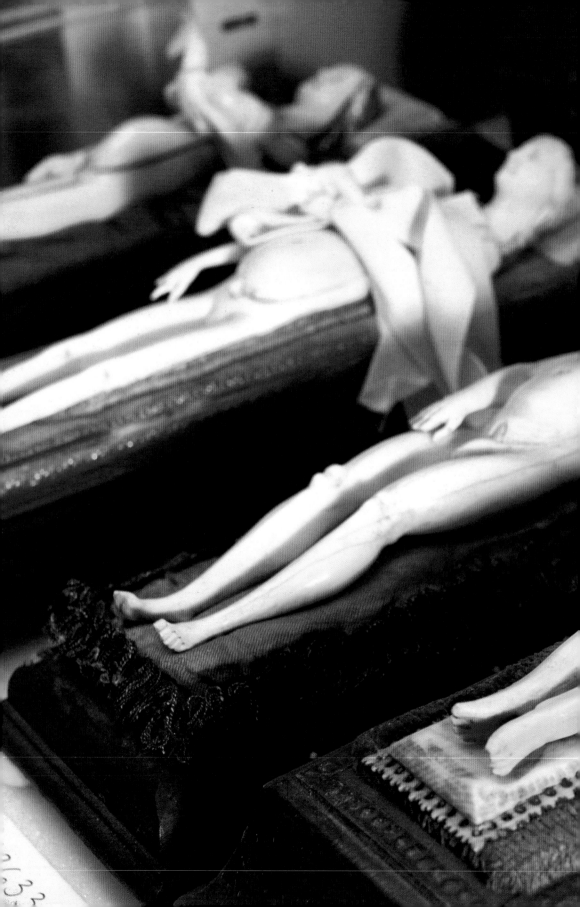

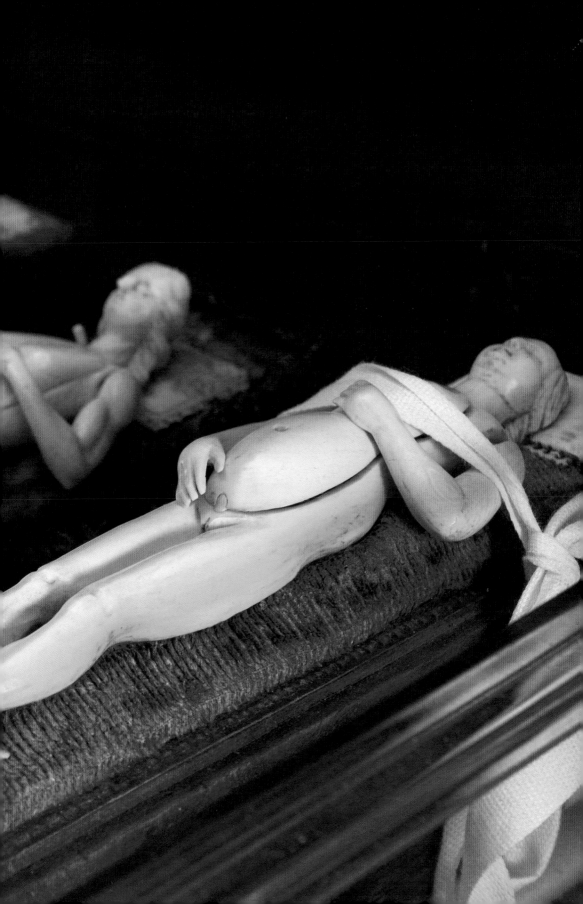

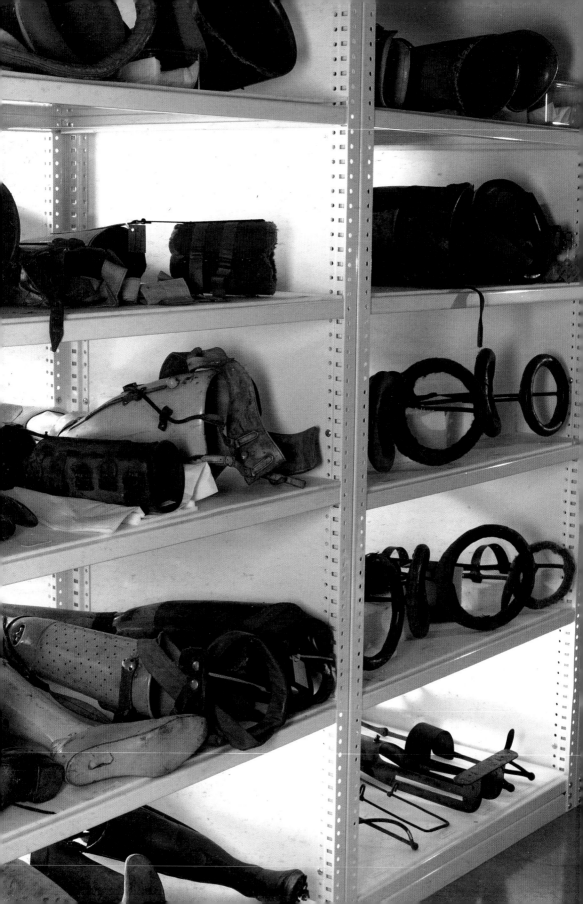

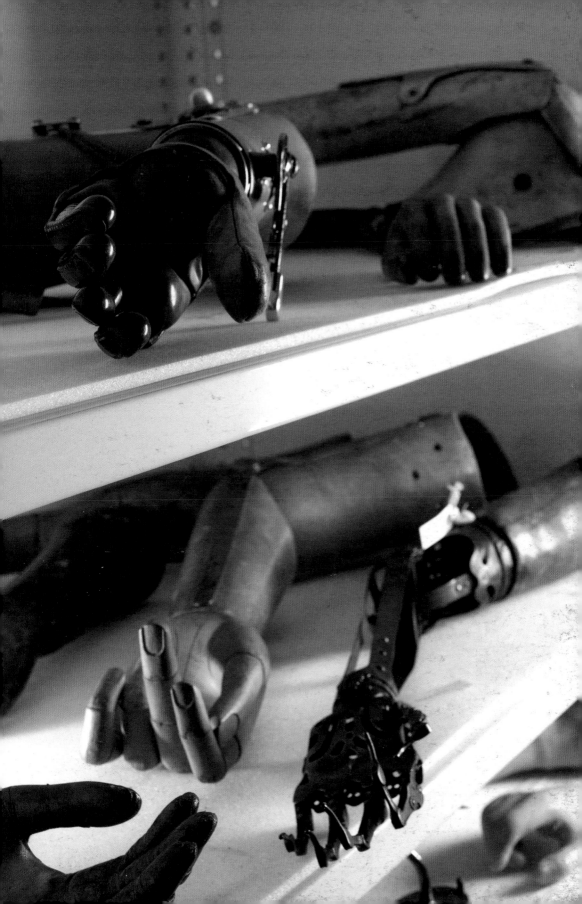

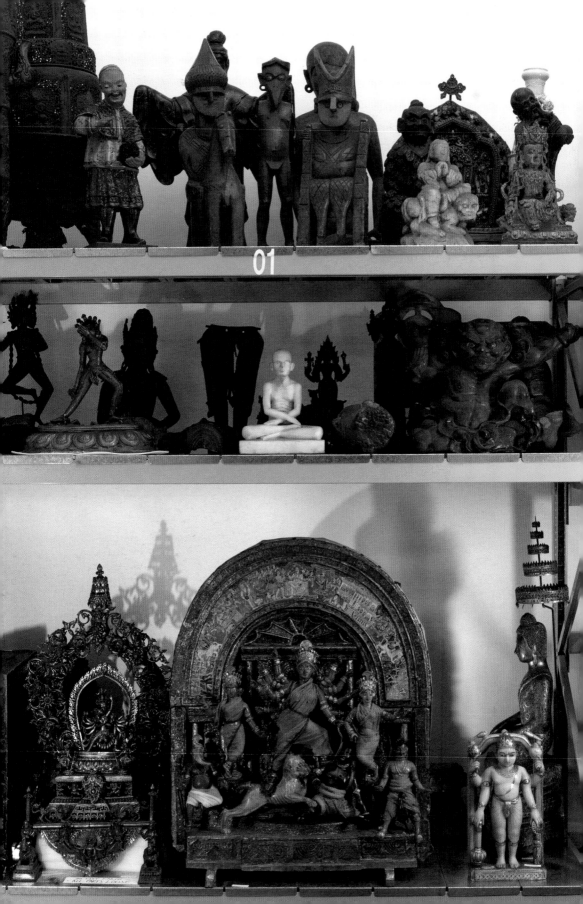

01

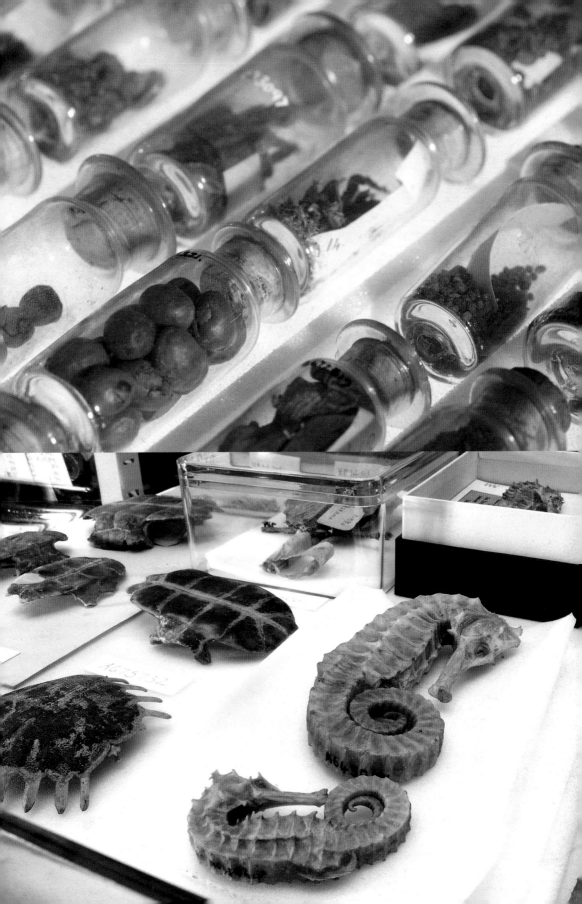

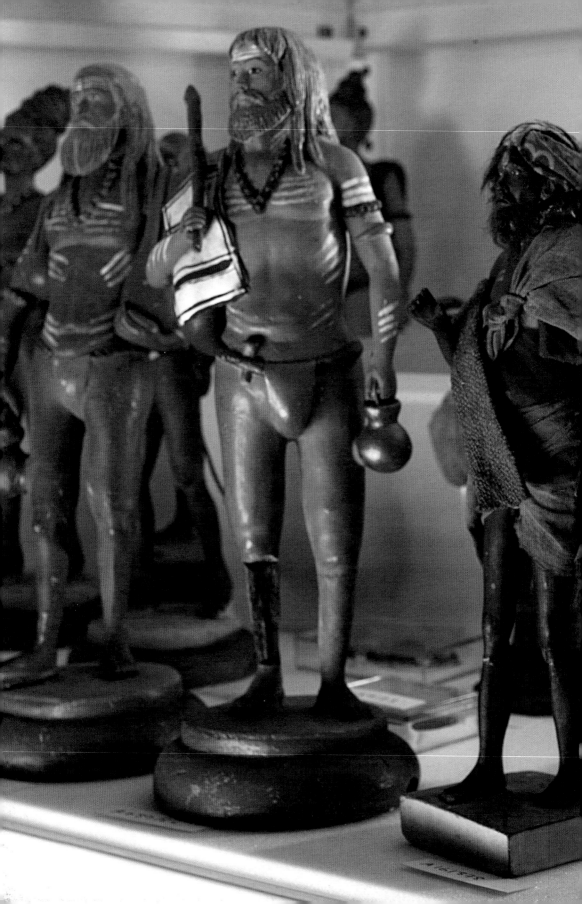

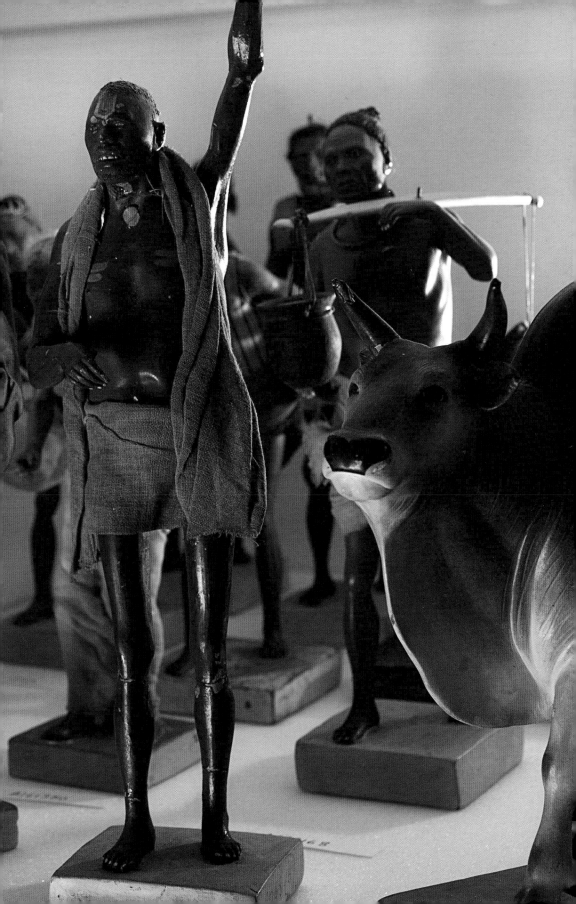

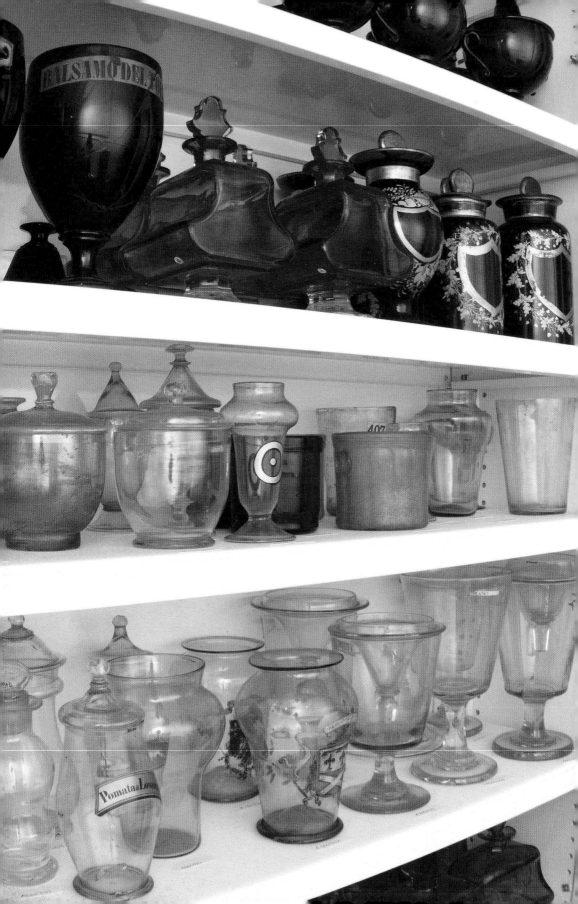

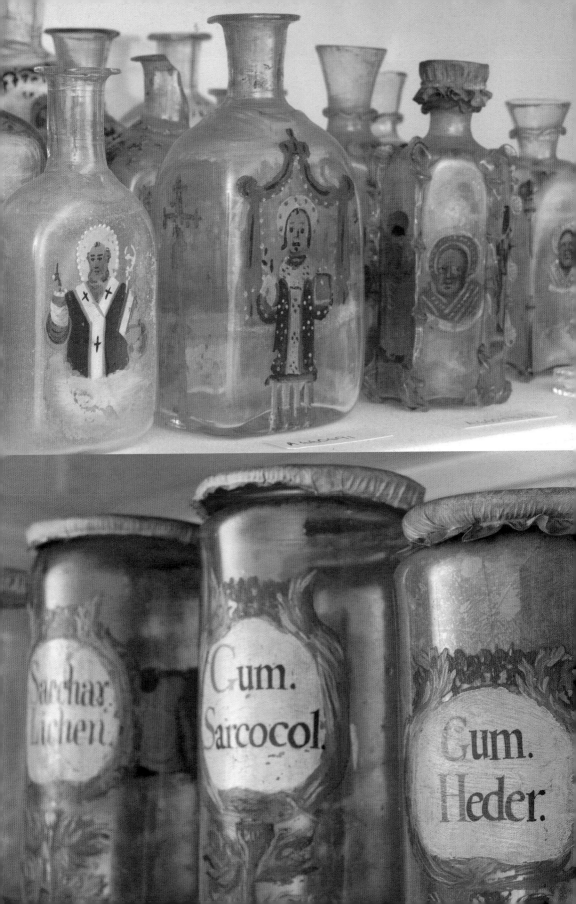

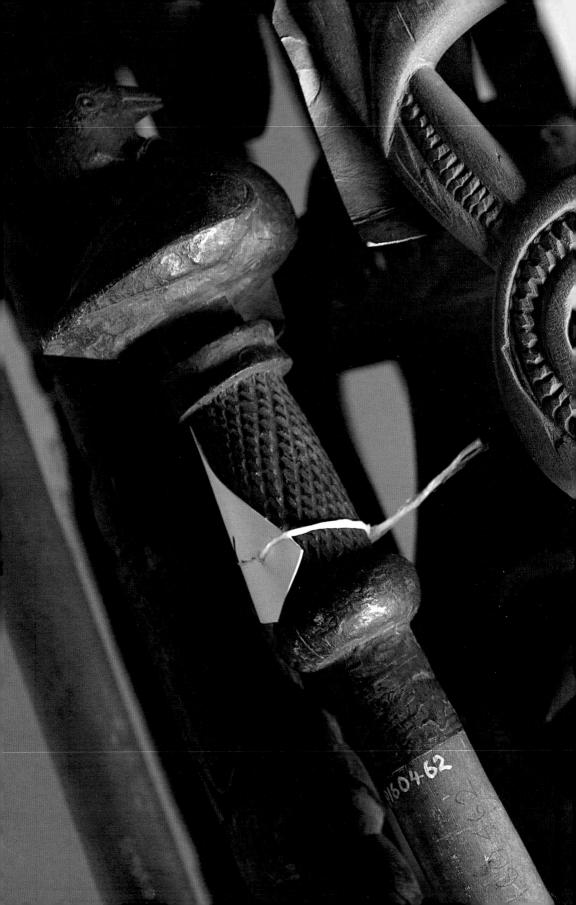

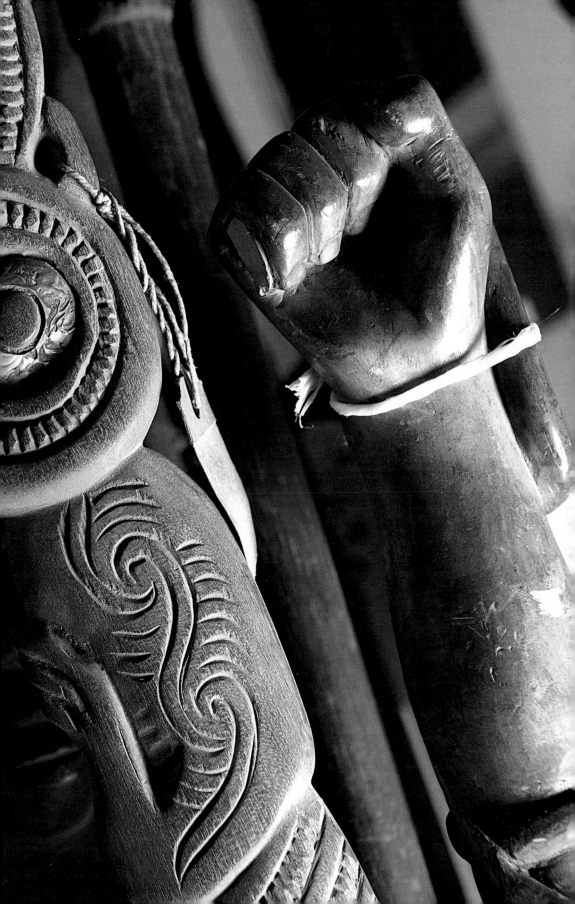

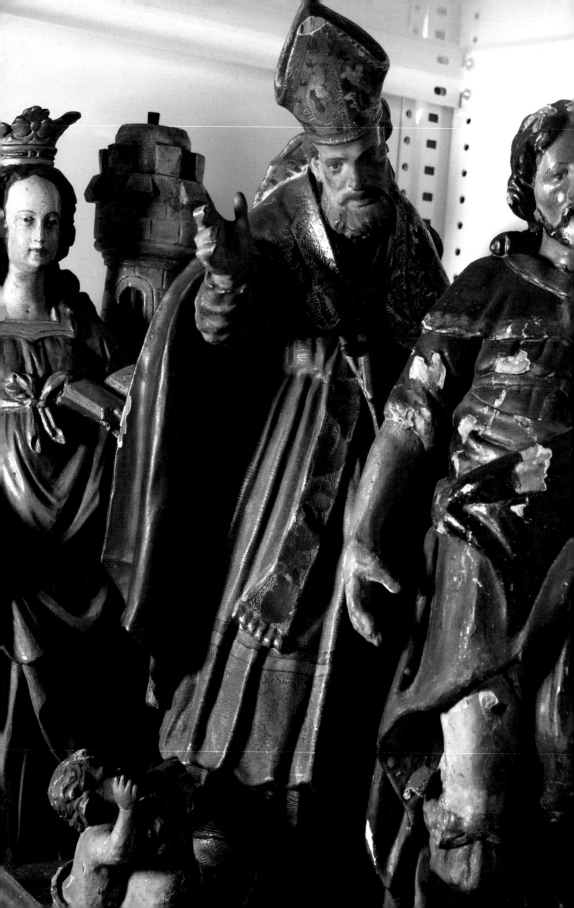

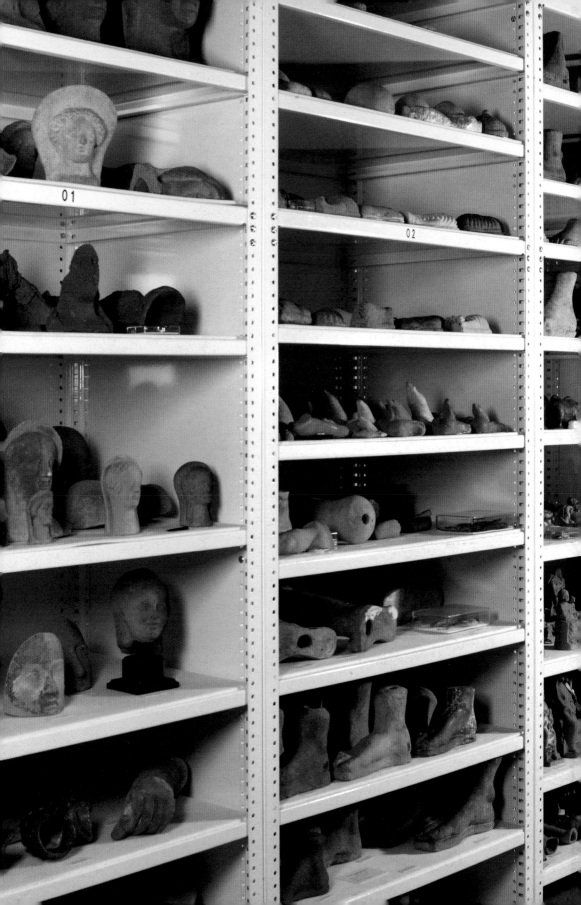

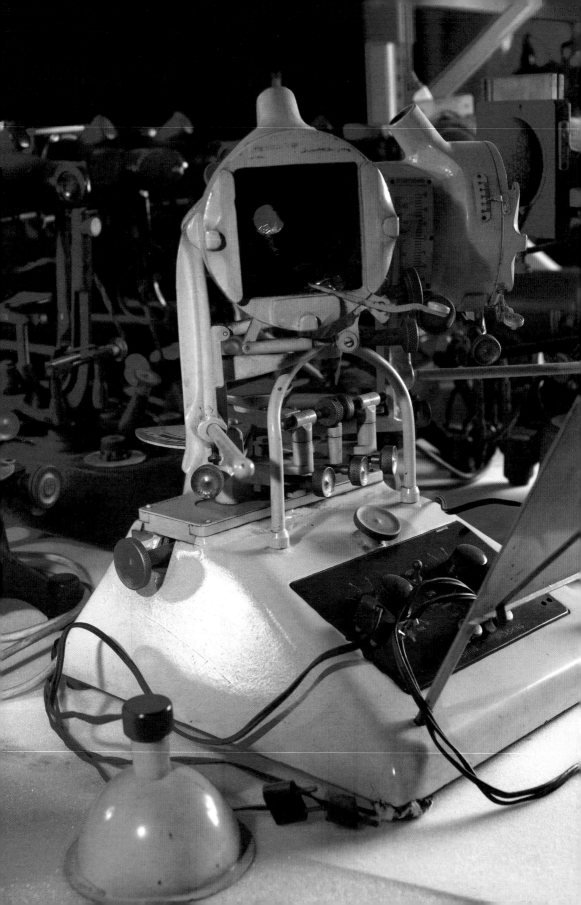

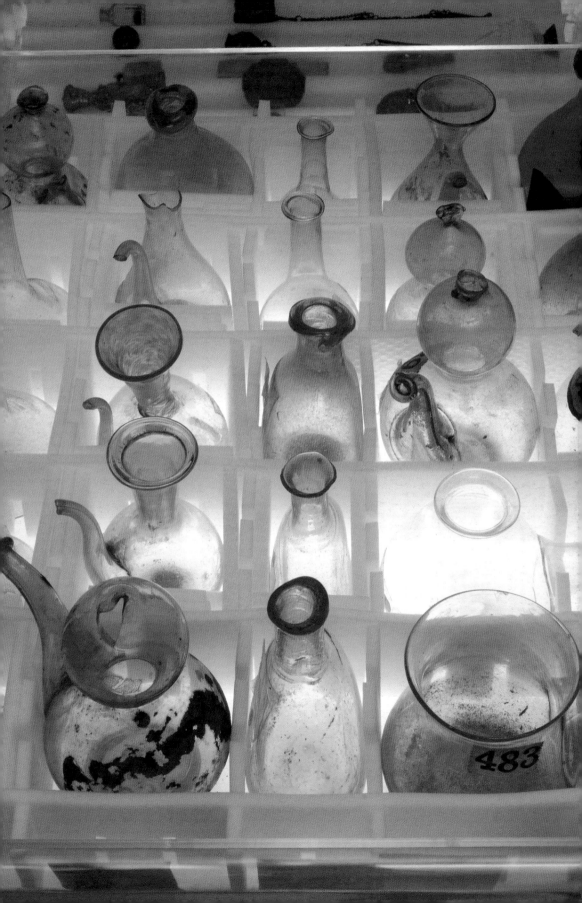

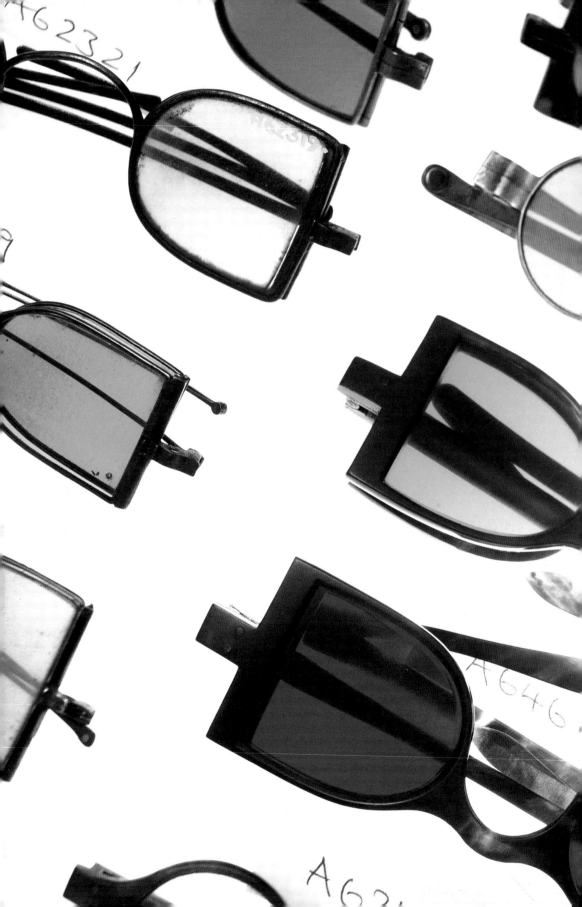

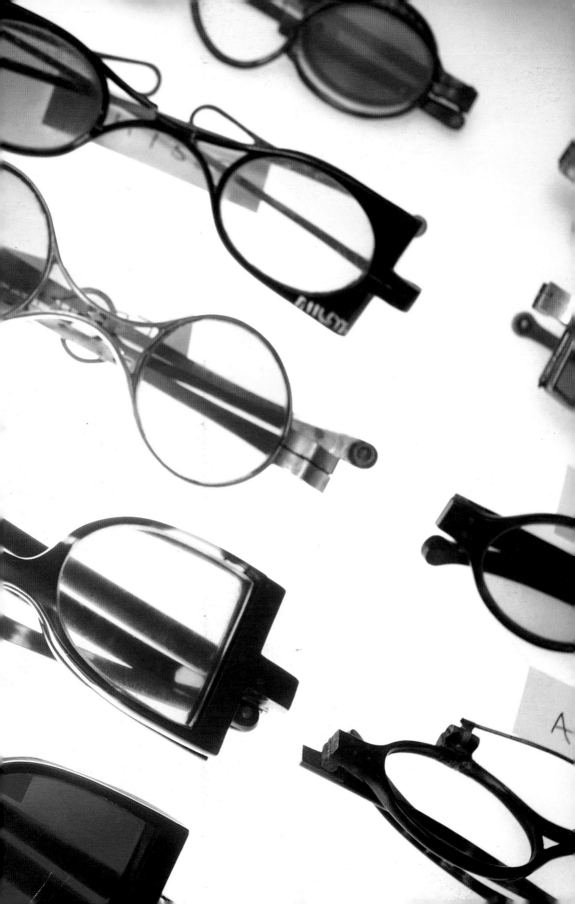

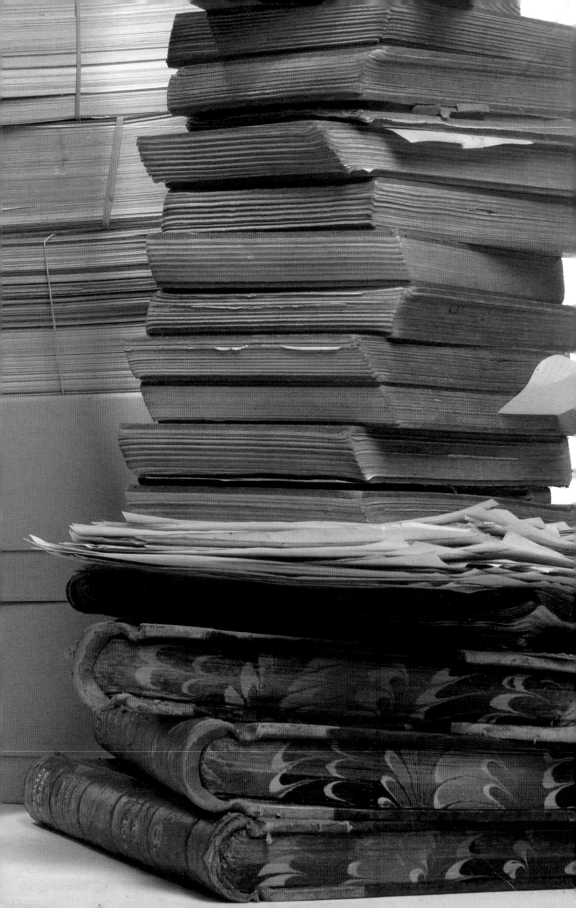